Examination Medicine
A guide to physician training

Fifth edition

Examination Medicine
A guide to physician training

Fifth edition

Nicholas J Talley
MD, PhD, FRACP, FRCP (London),
FRCP (Edin), FAFPHM, FACP, FACG
Professor of Medicine,
Mayo Clinic Rochester, Minnesota;
Consultant Physician

Simon O'Connor
FRACP, DDU, FCSANZ
Cardiologist, The Canberra Hospital;
Clinical Senior Lecturer,
Australian National University
Medical School, Canberra, ACT

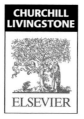

Sydney Edinburgh London New York Philadelphia St Louis Toronto

ELSEVIER

Churchill Livingstone
is an imprint of Elsevier

Elsevier Australia
(a division of Reed International Books Australia Pty Ltd)
30–52 Smidmore Street, Marrickville, NSW 2204
ACN 001 002 357

This edition © 2006 Elsevier Australia. Reprinted 2006

First edition © 1986. Reprinted 1986, 1988 (updated), 1990
Second edition © 1991. Reprinted 1992, 1994
Third edition © 1996. Reprinted 1997 (updated), 1999
Fourth edition © 2001. Reprinted 2002, 2003, 2004

National Library of Australia Cataloguing-in-Publication Data

Talley, Nicholas Joseph
Examination medicine: a guide to physician training

5th ed.
Bibliography
Includes index

ISBN-13: 978-0-7295-3773-5
ISBN-10: 0-7295-3773-0

1. Physical diagnosis. 2. Medical history taking.
3. Internal medicine. I. O'Connor, Simon. II. Title.

616.0754

Publishing Director: Vaughn Curtis
Publishing Editor: Mary Maakaroun
Publishing Services Manager: Helena Klijn
Edited by Carolyn Pike
Proofread by Kerry Brown
Cover and internal design by Tania Edwards
Typeset by Midland Typesetters, Australia
Index by Russell Brooks
Printed in Australia by Southwood Press

Contents

Foreword

There are no two words that strike more fear to the hearts of potential or actual physician trainees than the words 'the examination' and, to an extent, the fear is well-deserved. The training to become a physician is long, intense, rigorous and demanding and not everyone who starts down the path reaches the final destination—the award of FRACP.

However, back in the 'bad old days', the examination was there as the only barrier. There was no curriculum, there was no accreditation of sites, and there were no supervisors or Directors of Physician Training. After a period of self-determined training, one presented oneself for the examination, modelled on the UK examination with Part One (written) and Part Two (clinical) components. After completion of the clinical examination, all those who had participated waited in the College lobby to receive an envelope containing a piece of paper inviting them either to take a sherry in the Council Room with the Chair of the Board of Censors or to go away and to study harder for next year! Success at the examinations resulted in membership of the Royal Australasian College of Physicians (RACP). Advanced training was at one's whim, usually undertaken overseas, and when the individual returned to the Antipodes, he or she commenced practice.

Times have changed and even more changes are afoot, but more about that later.

What Talley and O'Connor have done very successfully, over a number of years, is to demystify the process, with each edition updated to reflect the relevant changes. They provide candidates with the best advice about how to prepare for and be successful at the written and clinical examinations. Most trainees will receive solicited and unsolicited advice from a range of sources—most sensibly and most up-to-date from their Director of Physician Training—but also from other trainees, both basic and advanced, and from clinicians with whom they come into contact on a daily basis. However, the period of basic training is a journey over a minimum of 3 years. The training is intermingled with clinical service delivery and with trying to have a life outside medicine, so unless someone is so obsessive as to have a palm pilot and write down everything relevant when they hear it, they will have no one single source to refer to that relates purely to what they see as their 'mission impossible'—to complete basic training and the examinations, and enter advanced training.

Using a range of sources and written in a user-orientated and friendly fashion, and appropriately light-hearted at times, this book should be on the desk or bedside table of every basic trainee. It covers all the important topics, from the administrative to the theoretical knowledge to the clinical skills and behaviours. Have no doubt, there is both science and art to the practice of medicine, and this is no more evident than in the examinations.

Having been previous Director of Physician Training and Chair of the Board of Censors of Adult Medicine and currently Chair of the Curriculum and Assessment Working Group for the College's education strategy, I have been well placed to observe and participate in some of the changes that have occurred to the RACP training program over the last 15 years. There will be major changes to basic training, the examination and advanced training over the next few years. For a combination of reasons, less emphasis will be placed on the examination in its current form, with greater importance placed on in-training assessment and assessment of the other 'physicianly' skills—communication, health advocacy, teamwork, professionalism and scholarship—and proper curricula will be constructed for basic training and advanced training across the range of subspecialties.

However, in spite of that, there will always be a requirement for an assessment of knowledge and clinical practice through written and clinical assessments, and therefore there will be an ongoing need for a book such as this, whatever changes might occur.

I congratulate Talley and O'Connor (Nick and Simon as they are known to their friends) on this publication, and recommend it highly to all potential trainees.

Rick McLean
Professor and Associate Dean, University of Sydney
23 May 2005

Preface

The FRACP examination continues to evolve. Dr Rick McLean has outlined further changes to the examination that are being considered by the College. Although assessment and basic training reports are likely to become more important in the future, the College still considers its written and clinical examinations to be an essential part of its assessment of doctors who want to become physicians.

There is no doubt that preparation for this difficult examination concentrates the minds of candidates but also that the vast amount of work involved in practising for the examination does help to train doctors in their preparation to become specialist physicians. This training leads to the acquisition of skills that have a lifelong effect on a person's approach to patients and their care.

This new edition has been comprehensively updated and revised. We have tried to keep up with the most recent changes to the examination format and marking system.

We are very grateful to Associate Professor Ross O'Neil who wrote the new chapter on imaging. Candidates are now expected to comment on X-rays, computed tomography (CT) scans and magnetic resonance imaging (MRI) scans and common examples of these have been included in Chapter 9 with commentary and explanation.

Our new publishers, Elsevier Australia, have helped us review and update this book. We hope that senior medical students and clinicians preparing for other specialist examinations will continue to find the book useful.

Nicholas Talley
Simon O'Connor
Rochester and Canberra
November 2005

Acknowledgments

The following specialists have been kind enough to review the text. We are very grateful for their advice and comments.

Associate Professor Ross O'Neil FRANZCR, Radiologist, The Canberra Hospital, Australian Capital Territory, who wrote Chapter 9.

Dr Chris Rayner, Senior Lecturer, Department of Medicine, Royal Adelaide Hospital, South Australia, who reviewed the text.

Dr J D'Rozario FRACP, FRCPA, Haematologist, The Canberra Hospital, Australian Capital Territory, who reviewed the haematology section.

Dr M Hurwitz FCP(SA), FRACP, FCCP, Staff Specialist in Thoracic Medicine, The Canberra Hospital, Australian Capital Territory, who reviewed the respiratory section.

Despite all our best efforts, factual errors may still have been included. As with every book or authority, please check and question everything. Write to us if you have any suggestions.

An historical note

The problem is not so much how to test candidates but how to test examinations.

J Parkhouse, Lancet *1971; i: 905–906.*

Internal medicine at the beginning of last century was still in its infancy. It was practised largely on an empirical basis. Therapeutics was very limited. Surgery was a more popular specialty, partly because of its greater efficacy in treating many diseases. There were consultant physicians in Australia, but medicine was mainly practised by the family doctor.

In 1930 some leading physicians formed the Association of Physicians of Australia. It aimed to foster expansion of scientific knowledge of medicine in Australia and New Zealand. It also allowed physicians to meet socially. It was an exclusive organisation— only physicians who held honorary appointments at teaching hospitals were eligible to join.

Non-members began to lobby, however, for the formation of a college. Eventually, after considerable opposition from members of the Association, the Royal Australasian College of Physicians was legally incorporated in 1938 (the title 'Royal' was conferred by King George VI). The inauguration ceremony occurred, with great pageantry, in the Great Hall of the University of Sydney. Sydney was chosen for the headquarters because the Royal Australasian College of Surgeons had previously been established in Melbourne.

Since its beginning, the College has been responsible for the maintenance of the standards of training and practice of medicine and paediatrics. This was originally achieved by conducting an examination known as 'the Membership'. The College set two major prerequisites for this test:

1. The candidate had to be a graduate of 3 years' standing or more from an acceptable medical school.
2. Two Fellows of the College must vouch for the candidate's integrity and character.

No limits were set on age or experience, no attention was given to previous training, no standard was defined for the examination, and few guidelines were laid down. Although this was a rather subjective test, Censors carried out their obligations well, as is obvious from the high standards of internal medicine practised in Australia and New Zealand today. The Membership examination consisted of two papers of essay questions and a clinical and oral examination. Multiple-choice questions were introduced only in 1967.

With the growth of technology and medical knowledge, the College began to coordinate the flourishing specialty associations and societies. By 1968 the need for a change in evaluation of physician trainees became apparent. In 1976 the Membership examination was replaced by the Fellowship. After considerable discussion within the College, it was decided that the emphasis should be on training, rather than examination. To this end the FRACP (Part One) examination was established as an early examination to admit candidates to advanced training. Candidates successful in this Part One examination would then have 3 or 4 years of supervised training in general medicine or a subspecialty, and in most cases no further examination would be required. An advanced trainee would be elected a Fellow after the required time of supervised training in accredited terms, if the supervisors' reports were satisfactory.

In this the College decided on a different course from the Royal Australasian College of Surgeons, which requires candidates to sit for an examination at the end of advanced training before election to Fellowship. The actual training emphasis of the Colleges still remains different.

Internal medicine today is an extremely popular specialty. The College of Physicians has helped promote ethical and professional standards, as well as the study of medicine. Influence has been extended to South-East Asia. In 1963, teams lectured in advanced medicine to postgraduates in Singapore with the University of Singapore. In 1966 the Asian-Pacific Committee was set up to ensure active participation in the maintenance of standards of medical education in the region. In 1976 the South-East Asian Regional Committee was set up to be responsible for meetings of College members in the region. As well, teachers have been sent to Kuala Lumpur, and lecturers have been provided for the University of Papua New Guinea.

The FRACP examination, with which this book deals, is now held at centres in Australia and New Zealand.

The examination system has its critics. The pass rate for the FRACP is low; on average, in the past only 40% of candidates passed both the written and their first attempt at the clinical examination. Changes to the format of the clinical examination have increased this somewhat in recent years. In the United Kingdom, the MRCP (UK) also has a low pass rate. In an editorial in *Lancet*, it was suggested there are only two possible reasons for a low pass rate in the MRCP: either the training or the examination is of poor quality, and the College is directly or indirectly responsible for each (*Lancet* 1990; i:443–445). The Royal Australasian College of Physicians has tried to tackle some of these issues in recent years, but vigorous debate on the method of examination continues.

There is no doubt, however, that physician training remains very popular. Over 400 candidates presented themselves for the clinical examination in 2005. This is almost three times the number attempting the clinical examination in the mid 1990s.

The objectives of the College remain the same as they were at its inception. Essentially the College strives to promote the study of the art and science of medicine, and to encourage research and dissemination of knowledge, as well as *to promote and ensure the fitness of persons desirous of qualifying for membership of the College*. This book deals with strategies to enable one to satisfy the strict examination requirements of the College.

Basic training requirements

I would live to study, and not study to live.

Francis Bacon (1561–1626)

The requirements for basic training, which after fulfilling the candidate may sit the Royal Australasian College of Physicians' (RACP) written and clinical examinations, are set out in the RACP handbook, *Requirements for Physician Training*. This is published annually. The most current information, however, is available on the RACP website <www.racp.edu.au>. Most registration forms are available from <www.racp.edu.au/members/training/forms.htm>.

The College now requires 3 years of basic training after the intern year in Australia or New Zealand. It insists on at least 36 months of supervised training across the breadth of internal medicine in both general medicine and the other medical subspecialties ('core' training), which must involve the continuing care of medical patients in approved hospitals. Approved hospitals are listed on the website. There are four categories of training hospitals: level 3 hospitals—previously called university teaching hospitals (UTHs); level 2 hospitals—previously called general teaching hospitals (GTHs); level 1 hospitals—generally regional hospitals; and secondment hospitals. At least 12 months must be spent in a level 3 hospital. At least 3 months must be spent in a general medicine term. Only 6 months may be spent in a single subspecialty. Up to 3 months of this time may be undertaken in each of coronary care, relieving, emergency medicine, nuclear medicine, psychiatry, dermatology or an approved secondment post, but the total time spent in these combined cannot exceed 6 months. Approval of the Director of Physician Training (DPT) is required for most of these terms.

Accreditation of terms that are suitable for basic training are now looked at more critically to ensure adequate levels of supervision and support for trainees, and some hospitals have lost accreditation. This applies especially to hospitals that receive resident medical officers on secondment. Up to 3 months of core training may be carried out in a single approved secondment post. It is important to check with the RACP Department of Education if there is any doubt that terms are acceptable. Basic training requirements are now so strict that careful negotiation with the hospital for suitable training terms from the beginning of basic training is the only way to ensure that it is possible to sit the examination in the minimum time.

A DPT is appointed in each hospital with an accredited training scheme. He or she is responsible for supervising basic training.

The College has published the sequence of steps involved in entry to the Fellowship (FRACP).

- Register as a basic trainee (post graduation year 2 [voluntary] or 3 [compulsory]).
- Apply for FRACP examinations (written A$1263 [NZ$1125], clinical A$2433 [NZ$2531.25]).
- Apply for approval of advanced training program (A$1124 [NZ$1181] per year).
- Accreditation of advanced training.
- Apply for admission to Fellowship (A$749 [NZ$506.25]).

The annual registration fee for basic trainees (voluntary in the first year of basic training [or the second postgraduate year] and free but compulsory after that) is A$246 (NZ$225). The forms for registration as a basic trainee should be downloaded from the website. Applications for approval of basic training must be made by early in the year of training and signed by the DPT. Late applications for training and to sit examinations are sometimes accepted (subject to an extra fee) but not always. The exact dates by which all applications are required are set out in the website and must be taken very seriously.

In exchange for the annual payment of this 'small fee', trainees receive regular information from the College. At the moment this includes the College journal *Fellowship Affairs* but not the *Internal Medicine Journal*. The registration fee is paid annually during basic training and is the start of a physician's long financial association with the College.

Interrupted and part-time training are possible. Research may be accepted for part of non-core basic training. Candidates who have a higher degree (MD or PhD) may apply to have accredited 1 year of basic training or 1 year of advanced training. Such acceptance requires negotiation.

All candidates are notified by post when their applications are received and again when approval to sit the examination is granted. This second letter gives the times, date and place of the examination. The application to sit the examination is required in November of the year before.

Success at the written and clinical examinations is *not* recognised as a specialist qualification. To be admitted to Fellowship of the College requires completion of basic and advanced training and success in both examinations. Once a trainee has completed 3 years of basic training, he or she can undertake a conditional year of advanced training. During the year the examinations must be successfully completed for the year to be accredited. If the trainee does not pass the examinations, the year cannot count towards advanced training. All advanced training in general medicine or a subspecialty must be approved by the appropriate Specialist Advisory Committee (SAC) and by the Committee for Physician Training (CPT). There is no longer any exit examination.

In some cases, exemption from the written examination may be granted. This usually applies to people with postgraduate physician training and overseas qualifications—for example, the MRCP, the Diploma of the American Board of Internal Medicine, the FRCP (Canada) or the Master of Medicine (Singapore). The appropriate application form for exemption can be obtained from the College. Approval is not automatic but is at the discretion of the CPT. Exemption from the clinical examination will occasionally be given to highly qualified senior people who trained overseas.

Each year of advanced training is assessed by a supervisor, who is usually one of the consultants that the trainee works for during the year. The supervisor submits a report on the candidate's performance during the year and a recommendation about accreditation of part or all of the year's training. Unsatisfactory reports are rare. An advanced trainee who receives an unsatisfactory report is offered an interview with a member of the CPT and a representative of the appropriate SAC. This committee will also interview the trainee's supervisor. A report is then issued by the Independent Review of Training Committee (IRC). This has replaced the old verification interview. The report and recommendation are considered by the CPT, which makes a final decision. The emphasis, for advanced trainees and their supervisors, is very much on addressing problems with performance during the year, with regular meetings. Supervisors are encouraged to discuss any problems they perceive with a trainee before the end of the year and to suggest ways of improving performance.

Advanced training requirements are very different for the various subspecialties and details can be obtained from the College.

Determination to pass both sections of the examination at the first attempt is an important part of preparation. The first section is a written examination, which is held only once every year, in March, in each of the Australian capital cities and in four main centres in New Zealand. The second part is a clinical viva-voce (live-voice) or 'viva' test. The clinical examination can be attempted only by candidates who have been successful in the written part. Failure in the written examination means waiting a year to sit again. There is now no limit to the number of times one may sit the entire examination. Some persistent individuals have sat many times (the record, we believe, is 11—and the candidate passed).

In December 2004 the College announced that a pass in the written examination now entitles a candidate to sit the clinical examination within 5 years. A candidate who is successful in the written examination in 2005 has until 2009 to pass the clinical examination. It may be possible to defer sitting the clinical examination for a year, under certain circumstances, but a pass must still be obtained within 5 years. These changes to the rules are retrospective and apply even to candidates who have passed the written examination but then failed the clinical examination and failed the written at the second attempt.

Over 85% of those people who continue to sit do eventually get through, if they have the stamina. The pass rates for the last few years are published by the College and given in Table 1.1.

A list of successful candidates is published at each hospital in which the written examination is held. Those who have failed the written examination are sent a feedback sheet indicating their performance in the various subspecialty areas. The DPT of each hospital is sent a list of the average marks for the candidates from that hospital in each subspecialty.

The viva is now held only once each year, in July or August, in a number of cities in rotation. This rotation forms the basis for the unofficial 'FRACP See Australia Travel Plan'. Experienced candidates know this tour well. In Australia, clinical examinations are now held in both major centres (Sydney, Melbourne, Brisbane or Adelaide) and 'less major' centres (Hobart, Canberra, Newcastle, Perth and others). In 1989, for the

Table 1.1 Past examination pass results		
Sat	Passed	Percentage
2004 written examination 500	346	69.2
2003 written examination 475	320	67.4
2003 viva 446	287	64.3
2002 viva 425	259	60.9

first time in living memory, the viva was postponed in Australia for 2 months because of a pilots' strike. Such events cannot be relied on to give more time for preparation. A pass in the viva counts as a pass in the year that the examination was sat. A supplementary examination (SE), or 'post', is offered to fewer than 5% of the candidates who encountered some major disaster, such as sickness on the day of the examination or a patient who was too sick to allow proper examination or had a heart attack during it; it is held about 3 weeks later.

The current fees for the written examination are listed on page 2. The fees rise by about 10% per year. The cost of travel and accommodation must be added to the examination fees. Claiming these expenses as a tax deduction usually seems to be allowed.

An exemption from the written examination entitles the candidate to sit the viva.

The practice of putting up viva results in one location on the day of the examination has now been reintroduced. The story goes that the practice was abandoned in the 1970s because, it is rumoured, a few candidates tied knots in the chains of the grandfather clock and did other damage, necessitating the repainting of the lobby of the Royal College of Surgeons, where the results were to be posted! Currently results are posted at 5 p.m. at a location to be advised; it is usually at the site of the examiners' meeting. A list of successful candidates in the viva examination is also published in the national press within a week. Notification by post occurs a little later.

Unsuccessful candidates receive an offer to arrange an interview with a College examiner to discuss the reasons for failure. The case notes, which are made by the teams of examiners during the 10-minute period provided for discussion of a candidate's performance, will be available to the member of the Committee for Examinations that is providing the advice. Candidates who have been given a 'post' can obtain this information very soon after the examination; for the others it will be available somewhat later. The College no longer sends a detailed critique of the candidate's performance from the notes.

Successful candidates receive a letter of congratulation. The *Handbook of Physician Training* is also sent.

For further information, write to one of the following:

Department of Education
The Royal Australasian College of Physicians
145 Macquarie Street
Sydney NSW 2000 Australia

Department of Education, New Zealand Committee
The Royal Australasian College of Physicians
Kevin Chambers, 16 The Terrace
Wellington 1 New Zealand

The College website (see p 1) contains increasing amounts of information about the training requirements and the examinations. Application forms can be downloaded and the important dates for applications and of examinations are detailed. Past examination papers are also available. It is an essential reference point for candidates and advanced trainees.

The future

There has been much discussion within the College and between the College and the Australian Medical Council (AMC) over the last few years about physician training. As a result of this, a more formal syllabus will probably be introduced within the next few years. This may be followed by changes to basic training that include *formative* and *summative* assessments. Although the clinical examination is often regarded as too subjective to be fair, it still has much support and is very unlikely to be abandoned in favour of a purely written examination, as is used in the United States.

2
CHAPTER

The written examination

No man's opinions are better than his information.

Paul Getty (1960)

The examination format

The written examination is a screening examination to select candidates for further testing. In 1994 the format was changed from three papers to two, which are held on the same day. The aim of the changes was to make both papers more relevant to clinical practice. The written examination is an objective multiple-choice examination, with five choices in each question.

The first paper (Paper A) is set with an emphasis on medical sciences and relevant basic science. It lasts 2 hours and consists of 60 questions. These are all 'A-type' questions—that is, of the five alternatives, only one is correct. Marks are not deducted for wrong answers and therefore it is no longer possible to score a negative mark for the total question. An incorrect or omitted answer will score zero. This is meant to encourage candidates to attempt to answer all questions.

The second paper (called, not unexpectedly, Paper B) contains 100 questions of the 'A type'. There are five alternatives and only one is the correct answer. Again, each correct answer gains a mark and an incorrect one scores zero. The candidate has 3 hours to sit this paper. There is evidence that 'A-type' questions discriminate better between candidates than other formats.

Although most candidates report that 2 hours is plenty of time for the completion of Paper A, this is not the case for Paper B, which is considerably more rushed. Some people have reported difficulty completing Paper B in the time allowed. The questions in Paper B are clinical scenarios and often contain long preambles, which may include a clinical history and the results of numerous investigations. They can be spread over several paragraphs. The clinical application questions are now designed to include tests that a practising clinician must be able to interpret. Various X-ray films (including chest radiographs, computed tomography [CT] and magnetic resonance imaging [MRI] scans), blood films (actual photographs or reports or both), photographs of urinary sediments and histopathology slides (e.g. renal biopsies) may be included. Photographs (both black-and-white and colour) are usually of high quality. Interpretation of biochemistry results (e.g. liver function tests) is also examined. Normal values are always supplied.

A pencil is provided at the test, as well as a well-used eraser. It is advisable, however, to bring a pencil sharpener, a spare soft B pencil, and a good eraser, particularly if you are indecisive.

The marking system is complex. All questions are approved by a test committee. About one-third of the questions on each paper come from previous papers. These are questions that have been found to be particularly discriminating.

There is, unfortunately, no predetermined pass mark. All candidates' papers are first scored. Any question that most candidates get wrong is examined carefully for degree of difficulty and ambiguity and may be eliminated. The best questions discriminate between 'good' and 'bad' candidates and each question is analysed statistically to determine whether it meets this standard. Then various statistical methods are employed to separate candidates into two groups. The exact pass mark is set at approximately 2.5 standard deviations below the mean mark for Australasia, in such a way that the cut-off falls in a gap between clusters of candidates. Approximately 60–70% of candidates are in the 'good' group, and these people pass. This means that one must aim to be better than at least 35% of the other candidates to be successful. The pass mark is not set according to the number of places that are available in the clinicals. It is expected that about two-thirds of candidates will continue to pass the written examination each year.

The examination used to be held in winter, when experienced candidates could be spotted in the centre of Sydney equipped with coats, scarves and thick woollen socks (for some reason the examination room at the University of Sydney was not heated). This problem has been solved by changing the date of the examination to March.

Approaching multiple-choice questions

By the time they sit this examination, most candidates will have had considerable experience with multiple-choice questions. However, it is worth stating a few relevant points.

Ensure that you estimate in advance the amount of time you have for each question. The questions are complicated and each question tests several items of knowledge. The correct answer may be a number of steps removed from the initial statement. This means that it is important to read each question with great care; noting or underlining the salient points may be helpful, and do look especially for negatives and double negatives. Most people find that their first carefully considered answer is more reliable than a change of mind on later review of the paper.

It is worth remembering that the words 'always' and 'never' do not often apply in medicine. The word 'recognised' means that an association has been described, whereas 'characteristic' implies that the given factor is important to the condition and essential to the diagnosis.

It is always better to guess at answers when the question is obscure rather than to leave a question out entirely. To avoid coming to the end of the paper and finding an unexpected unfilled space on the answer sheet, you should keep a constant check that question and answer numbers match.

Preparation for the written examination

The College does not provide a curriculum for the written examination but recommends the use of any major textbook and some journals (see Further Reading). We recommend concentrating on the latest edition of a standard textbook (e.g. the most recent edition of *Harrison's Principles of Internal Medicine* or the *Oxford Textbook of Medicine*); it is a most satisfactory method of preparation. The *Medical Knowledge Self Assessment Program (MKSAP)* of the American College of Physicians is also available and is very useful. It contains brief up-to-date accounts of most areas of internal medicine. It clearly indicates the currently fashionable topics on which questions are likely to be set. It also has a comprehensive series of multiple-choice questions (and excellent critiques) based on the text. Only some of these questions are of a similar standard to the written examination questions.

The College now produces its own self-assessment questions—the *Australian Self Assessment Programme* (ASAP). These ASAP questions are produced regularly and can be recommended. None of these questions is ever likely to appear in the examination paper as the ASAP is primarily educational and therefore tends to have a bias towards positive responses, unlike the written examination.

There is great value in practising multiple-choice questions. Sample questions from past papers are available from the College. These are taken from papers that have been used in recent years. Currently the Committee for Examinations also releases, every second year on the College website, complete copies of written examination papers that were set 3 years previously. Old released questions do not usually appear in the current examination paper. The College has a large bank of questions that are adjusted annually. The Written Examination Committee adds new questions and updates and improves old questions.

Many hospitals conduct their own trial examination, with questions written by the staff. Also available on the market are books of multiple-choice questions, which are based on such other postgraduate examinations as the MRCP but are of less value. Many candidates find that practising multiple-choice questions in a study group of three or four to discuss the various options is very helpful.

The College recommends a number of general medicine journals that candidates should read regularly. These currently include (roughly in order of usefulness):

- *Lancet*
- *New England Journal of Medicine*
- *Annals of Internal Medicine*
- *British Medical Journal*
- *Internal Medicine Journal*
- *American Journal of Medicine.*

We recommend concentrating on editorials and review articles. Study of specialist journals is not required.

Each year, postgraduate institutions hold courses on various topics, which some candidates do find helpful. A course of lectures lasting 34 weeks (one night a week for 17 weeks a year over 2 years) is available for the candidates in Sydney. Short but comprehensive courses are also available in Australia (e.g. Royal Prince Alfred Hospital, Sydney) or New Zealand (e.g. in Dunedin) and can be particularly useful for revision.

As of this year, the comprehensive lecture series given by the Victorian State Committee of the RACP, running over 40 weeks of the year and held once a week in the evening for 3 hours, is being videoconferenced widely across Australia. It covers the entirety of the syllabus in 1 year. This is particularly useful for trainees in regional centres. Details can be obtained from the Department of Education.

A number of cassette tape programs are available on medical topics. The Audio Digest Internal Medicine tapes are available in many libraries and provide updates of topics, but are mostly from a North American perspective and of somewhat patchy quality.

In summary, we have listed a number of conventional but important suggestions for the written examination:

1. Be well rested and avoid travelling long distances on the eve of the examination. Make sure you know where the examination centre is situated.
2. Be familiar with the format of the paper and know how much time to allow for each question.
3. Work through the paper at a leisurely, deliberate pace and return to troublesome questions at the end. Inspiration may well come from other questions.
4. Rely on first careful impressions and do not change an answer if in doubt.
5. Check every tenth question or so to be sure that answer numbers match the question numbers.
6. Have a short rest after the written examination, but begin work for the 'viva' examination then, as time between the two parts of the examination is limited.

3
CHAPTER

Suggested topics for the written examination

Every physician, almost, hath his favourite disease.

Tom Jones, Henry Fielding *(1707–54)*

Introduction

There is, as yet, no syllabus published by the College for the written examination, however, the College website now publishes past written examination papers. Three years of papers, starting from about 3 years ago, are available, with official answers, from the College website. These are an invaluable guide to the topics, standards and subject matter that the College expects candidates to master. In this section, we have compiled a necessarily *incomplete* list of topics from our own and colleagues' experience of the written examination and information from the website, over the past several years. Although greater breadth and depth of knowledge is required to pass, many have found such a list a very useful method of checking progress, and it may also help those who would not otherwise have realised that certain areas (e.g. psychiatry or basic physiology) are examined in the written test.

The closing date for multiple-choice question submissions is approximately 4 months before the examination sitting date. After detailed evaluation, the actual questions are selected in December or January. Remember that any fashionable topic (e.g. mutated human immunodeficiency viruses [HIV]) that has appeared in the popular press in the year prior to the closing date may crop up.

We strongly believe that seeing many cases for the clinical part is a good way of reinforcing theoretical knowledge. Many physicians base their knowledge on cases seen personally.

Do not concentrate on strong areas or only on topics of great interest. This is a certain way to be unsuccessful. Questions are drawn from all branches of medicine, especially the large subspecialties. Medicine relevant to the South-East Asian region is also sometimes examined.

Some areas appear only rarely in the test (e.g. unusual tropical diseases). Much has been asked about the genetic abnormalities associated with disease in recent years, as there have been rapid and important advances in this area.

Important topics for the written examination

Note: Investigations are now likely to be presented as part of a detailed clinical history in Paper B.

Cardiovascular system

Investigations

- Electrocardiographic (ECG) changes in different conditions, including pericarditis or right ventricular infarction, Wolff-Parkinson-White syndrome.
- Chest X-ray films (e.g. left ventricular [LV] aneurysm, aortic aneurysm, valvular heart disease).
- Echocardiography—indications, sensitivity of transthoracic versus transoesophageal, two-dimensional (2D), Doppler colour flow mapping—and M-mode echocardiogram (e.g. hypertrophic cardiomyopathy, septal motion abnormalities, normal anatomy), LV Doppler inflow patterns (e.g. for mitral stenosis, diastolic dysfunction), colour flow map showing a ventricular septal defect or mitral regurgitation.
- Coronary angiography—the different views and the names of the main vessels and their branches, complications (e.g. false aneurysm, stroke). Exercise stress test interpretation, Bayes' theorem, role of sestamibi and dipyramidole sestamibi testing (e.g. for left bundle branch block). Dobutamine echocardiography.
- Positron emission tomography (PET) scanning and detection of viable myocardium.
- Role of magnetic resonance imaging (MRI) scanning. Coronary calcium scoring.
- Role of electrophysiological studies, appropriate indications for cardioverter-defibrillators. Cardiac markers, including troponin I and troponin T.

Physical examination

- Pulse character, jugular venous pressure waves, abnormal heart sounds, clinical signs of severity of valve lesions.

Anatomy

- Coronary arteries, conducting system and accessory pathways, left and right internal mammary arteries.

Physiology

- Metabolic substrate for heart muscle, red blood cells and skeletal muscle; heart failure, free radicals and myocardial damage, myocardial angiotensin-converting enzyme (ACE) activity, nitric oxide, endothelin.

Chronic coronary heart disease

- Coronary artery spasm, causes of non-atherosclerotic angina, ischaemic cardiomyopathy, coronary artery bypass grafting—indications, effect on prognosis, left and right internal mammary artery grafting, coronary angioplasty and coronary stenting complications, role of drug-eluting stents, contraindications, comparison with atherectomy. Coronary risk factors, cholesterol reduction and plaque stabilisation, calcium score.

Acute coronary syndromes

- Measurement of infarct size, right ventricular infarction (features and prognosis), thrombolysis (agents, indications and contraindications), results of major thrombolysis trials, tissue plasminogen activator versus streptokinase versus primary angioplasty, anaesthetic risks following infarction, early complications of infarction, assessment of risk of acute coronary patients, appropriateness of intervention.

Arrhythmias

- Supraventricular tachycardia and its mechanisms, ventricular tachycardia and its mechanisms, antiarrhythmic drugs, proarrhythmic drugs, cardiac arrhythmia suppression trial (CAST) (flecainide), electrical approaches for treatment of lethal ventricular arrhythmias using automatic implantable cardioverter-defibrillators, pacemakers and anti-tachycardia pacemakers, catheter ablation for accessory pathways and ventricular tachycardia, ablation procedures for atrial fibrillation (atrio-ventricular [AV] nodal ablation, ablation around the pulmonary veins).

Valvular heart disease
• Mitral valve prolapse, prosthetic heart valves, valvular heart disease and pregnancy, indications for valve surgery and place of valve repair, balloon valvuloplasty.

Infective endocarditis
• Organisms, diagnostic features, complications, role of echocardiography—trans-thoracic and transoesophageal.

Cardiomyopathy
• Hypertrophic cardiomyopathy, place of cardiac biopsy, cardiac transplantation—indications and contraindications, complications and monitoring.

Pericardial disease
• Viral causes, Dressler's syndrome (features and complications).

Congenital heart disease
• Atrial septal defect, ventricular septal defect, patent ductus arteriosus, Ebstein's anomaly, Fallot's tetralogy, Eisenmenger's syndrome, bicuspid aortic valve, coarctation of the aorta, adults with 'corrected' heart disease, risks of pregnancy.

Pulmonary heart disease
• Pulmonary hypertension, pulmonary embolism—findings on computed tomography (CT), pulmonary angiography, ventilation–perfusion (V/Q) scan.

Peripheral vascular disease
• Acute aortic dissection and its associations.

Hypertension
• Complications, appropriate investigations, phaeochromocytoma—treatment and perioperative management, target levels (e.g. for diabetics), role of different classes of drugs, non-drug treatment.

Congestive cardiac failure
• Ejection fraction, mechanisms of oedema, role of B-type natriuretic peptide, benefits of drug treatment, cardiac transplantation, cardiac myoplasty, physiology of pulmonary oedema, diastolic failure.

Cardiac catheterisation
• Pressures and saturations—interpretation.

Shock
• The major endogenous mediator in sepsis (cachectin or tumour necrosis factor), multi-organ failure, prognosis.

Preoperative assessment
• Patient with a history of ischaemic heart disease/congestive cardiac failure, bifascicular heart block.

Other
• Genetics of hypertrophic cardiomyopathy (HCM)/sudden cardiac death in athletes.

Respiratory system

Investigations
- Chest X-ray file (e.g. silicosis, bronchiectasis, tuberculosis, pneumonia in the immunosuppressed host).
- Respiratory function tests (e.g. flow volume loops, FEV_1 [forced expiratory volume in 1 second], FVC [forced vital capacity], maximal voluntary ventilation, diffusing capacity).
- Arterial blood gas level interpretation (e.g. significance of alveolar–arterial differences).
- Ventilation–perfusion (V/Q) scan interpretation (e.g. pulmonary embolus).
- Sleep apnoea testing.

Lung mechanics
- Pleural pressures, elastic recoil, cough syncope.

Physiology
- Affinity of haemoglobin for oxygen.

Chronic obstructive pulmonary disease
- Aetiology, elastic properties of the lung in emphysema, poor prognostic features, causes of hypoventilation, effect on the pulmonary circulation, tumour necrosis factors and weight loss in patients with emphysema, pulmonary rehabilitation and lung volume reduction surgery.

Asthma
- Bronchopulmonary aspergillosis and its importance, precipitating factors, desensitisation treatment, late-phase reactions, inhaled steroids, long-acting bronchodilators, leukotriene inhibitors.

Small airways disease

Sleep disorders
- Obstructive sleep apnoea—treatment, mechanisms of action, central apnoea, narcolepsy.

Interstitial lung disease
- Silicosis (diagnosis and features), sarcoidosis, pulmonary fibrosis, bronchiolitis obliterans organising pneumonia (BOOP), drug causes, bronchoalveolar lavage and aspirated cell types, place of high-resolution CT scanning and lung biopsy.

Infectious disease
- Pneumococcal vaccine, non-bacterial pneumonia, *Legionella*, fungal disease, tuberculosis, HIV and the lung.

Occupational lung disease
- Asbestosis (including relationship to the amount of exposure and the different types).

Genetic defects
- Cystic fibrosis (diagnosis, management and prognosis), immotile cilia syndrome, alpha$_1$-antitrypsin deficiency.

Lung neoplasms
- Smoking association, additive risk factors, different cell types and their different presentations and management, mesothelioma.

Pulmonary embolus
- Features, role of pulmonary angiography and thrombolytic treatment, diagnosis and effects.

Rhinitis
- Causes, treatment.

Vasculitis
- Wegener's granulomatosis, Churg-Strauss syndrome, treatment.

Adult respiratory distress syndrome

Pneumothorax
- Spontaneous pneumothorax—incidence, recurrence, associations and treatment, emphysematous bullae.

Pleural disease
- Mesothelioma.

Lung transplantation
- Indications and problems, long-term outcome.

Gastrointestinal system

Investigations
- Endoscopy—role, complications, use in screening.
- Barium swallow (e.g. achalasia, diffuse oesophageal spasm, stricture).
- Barium enema (e.g. inflammatory bowel disease).
- Abdominal CT scans (e.g. normal anatomy, lymphoma, pancreatic cancer).
- Small intestinal biopsy findings (e.g. coeliac disease).
- Malabsorption test interpretation (e.g. bacterial overgrowth).
- Liver tests (e.g. assessment of a jaundiced patient, interpretation of hepatitis serology, clues for alcoholic liver disease [and differential diagnosis], tests for autoimmune liver disease).

Oesophagus
- Achalasia, diffuse oesophageal spasm, gastro-oesophageal reflux, transient lower oesophageal sphincter relaxation, role of combination treatment in reflux disease, drugs that change lower oesophageal sphincter pressures, Barrett's oesophagus (short and long segment), motor activity, pH monitoring.

Stomach
- *Helicobacter pylori* gastritis, acid secretion, side-effects of H_2-receptor antagonists, proton pump inhibitors, triple and quadruple *H. pylori* therapy, antibiotic resistance, gastrointestinal hormones (especially gastrin, cholecystokinin and grhelin), control of acid secretion, gastric carcinoma, haemorrhage and the role of endoscopy.

Small intestine
- Fat absorption mechanisms, diagnostic uses of small bowel biopsy, bacterial overgrowth syndromes, vitamin B_{12} malabsorption, intestinal lactase deficiency, coeliac disease, Crohn's disease, small bowel capsule.

Large intestine
- Antibiotic-associated colitis, inflammatory bowel disease (including infliximab side-effects), solitary ulcer in the colon, reactive arthritis, ischaemic bowel, abdominal X-ray changes, screening for carcinoma of the colon.

Pancreas
- Hyperamylasaemia, chronic pancreatitis.

Liver and biliary tract
- Causes of chronic liver disease, non-alcoholic steatohepatitis, associations of chronic hepatitis, genetics of haemochromatosis, Wilson's disease, hepatitis (A, B, C, D, E and G)—differences and modes of transmission, causes of hepatic granulomas, alpha$_1$-antitrypsin deficiency (genetics and effects), bile secretion (e.g. conjugation, phospholipid content), physiology of ascites, cholangitis, hepatitis B vaccine, liver transplantation.

Diarrhoea
- *Yersinia* enterocolitis, traveller's diarrhoea, *Clostridium difficile*, gay bowel syndrome.

Trace elements
- Zinc deficiency.

Haematological system

Investigations
- Full blood count reports (e.g. features of acute/chronic leukaemias).
- Blood film photographs (e.g. microcytic anaemia, haemolytic anaemia, thrombotic thrombocytopenic purpura [TTP]).
- Iron studies (e.g. interpret serum iron level, total iron-binding capacity and serum ferritin level).
- Protein electrophoresis (e.g. multiple myeloma).
- Haemoglobin electrophoresis (e.g. HbE).
- Coagulation/mixing tests.
- Cold agglutinin disease.

Red cell indices
- Causes of change in mean corpuscular volume (MCV).

Anaemia
- Types, causes, Coombs' test interpretation.

Haemopoietic stem cell disorders
- Preleukaemic syndromes, myeloproliferative diseases (polycythaemia rubra vera—distinguishing primary and secondary types, chronic myeloid leukaemia, essential thrombocythaemia, myelofibrosis).

Erythropoiesis and disorders of red cells
- Causes of hypochromic anaemia, iron metabolism, aplastic anaemia, haemolytic anaemia, causes of iron deficiency, vitamin B$_{12}$ and folate metabolism, thalassaemia (complications, types), hereditary spherocytosis.

Granulopoiesis and disorders of white cells
- Causes of eosinophilia, eosinophil function, eosinophilia–myalgia syndrome.

Multiple myeloma
- Diagnosis, complications.

Lymphopoiesis and disorders of lymphocytes

- Angioimmunoblastic lymphadenopathy, lymphoma (new classifications, e.g. mantle zone, cytogenetics and treatment), myeloma and dysproteinaemias, POEMS syndrome (polyneuropathy, organomegaly, endocrine, M protein, skin), acute lymphoblastic leukaemia, cytological features and prognosis.

Haemostasis defects

- Platelets—congenital defects (Bernard-Soulier's disease, Glanzmann's disease, von Willebrand's disease), haemophilia and prophylaxis before surgery, haemophilia B and its laboratory abnormalities, lupus anticoagulant, protein C and S deficiencies, antithrombin III deficiency, factor V Leiden/prothrombin mutation, homocystein-uria, interpretation of coagulation tests, heparin-induced thrombocytopenia, role of fragmin and heparinoids, the new antiplatelet drugs—adenosine diphosphate (ADP) inhibitors, glycoprotein IIb, IIIa (platelet aggregation) inhibitors.

Splenectomy

- Indications and complications.

Transfusion medicine

- Indications for transfusion of blood products, safety of blood products, risk of trans-mission of infection, indications for filtered blood.

Bone marrow transplantation

- Extended indications, role in treating non-haematological malignances. Different indications for autologous and allogenic transplant.

Nervous system

Investigations

- Carotid angiography and duplex scanning.
- CT and MRI scans of the brain (e.g. normal anatomy), differing applications of these techniques (e.g. temporal lobe sclerosis, syringomyelia).
- Electromyogram (EMG) findings (e.g. distinguishing peripheral neuropathy from myopathy).
- Electroencephalogram (EEG)—interpretation of reports, findings in minor seizures and temporal lobe epilepsy, Jakob-Creutzfeldt disease and how this affects the options for treatment.
- Visual-evoked responses.

Electrodiagnosis

- EMG—fibrillation potentials and disease findings, EEG, caloric responses, brain death diagnosis.

Cerebrospinal fluid

- Immunoglobulin changes with disease.

Anatomy

- Spinal cord pain pathways, diagnostic possibilities regarding brain biopsy (pathology).

Dementia

- Reversible causes, Alzheimer's disease, genetics, pathophysiology, Lewy body disease, risk factors, supportive management.

Encephalopathy, mitochondrial disease
• Mitochondrial encephalopathy lactic acidosis stroke-like episodes (MELAS).

Vision
• Causes of unilateral visual loss, causes of bilateral visual loss, visual-evoked responses, treatment of multiple sclerosis.

Muscle disease
• Myasthenia gravis, dystrophia myotonica, EMG interpretation.

Cerebrovascular disease
• Cerebral haemorrhages—common sites and causes, features of internal carotid artery occlusion, transient ischaemic attack features and causes, aphasia, transient global amnesia, lacunar infarcts, use of thrombolysis.

Organic brain syndromes
• Neurological features of liver failure.

Headache
• Cluster headache, migraine.

Nystagmus
• Causes and types.

Tumours
• Cerebellopontine angle tumour (and caloric findings), pituitary tumour and prolactinaemia.

Extrapyramidal syndromes
• Chorea.

Peripheral nerve injuries
Drugs
• Neurological findings with drug overdose, anti-parkinsonian drugs.

Cerebral abscess
• Causes and features.

Psychiatry
Schizophrenia
• Inheritance, risk to relatives, possible causes of schizophrenic-like illnesses.

Organic psychoses
• Distinguishing hypomania from organic psychoses by clinical features and EEG.

Depression
• Difference from dementia/ageing.

Panic attacks
• Recognition, treatment, risk of benzodiazepine treatment.

Anorexia nervosa and bulimia
• Diagnosis.

Defence mechanisms
* Sublimation.

Drugs—mechanism of action and side-effects
* Major tranquillisers, antidepressants (tricyclic, tetracyclic and monoamine oxidase [MAO] inhibitors, selective serotonin reuptake inhibitors [SSRIs]), lithium.

Rheumatology

Investigations
* Joint radiographs (e.g. hands in gouty arthropathy, fingers in psoriatic arthritis).
* Bone scans in ankylosing spondylitis.
* Synovial fluid analysis. Anti-phospholipid antibodies.
* Modern serology (e.g. antinuclear factor, double-stranded DNA, anti-centromere antibody, anti-smooth muscle, anti-Jo-1, Scl-70, ribonuclear protein [RNP]).

Biology of connective tissue
* Different types of collagen.

Rheumatoid arthritis
* Serology (nature of rheumatoid factor), X-ray findings, complications, other causes of polyarthritis, juvenile rheumatoid arthritis (types, clinical features), drugs (particularly methotrexate, gold, penicillamine, chloroquine, anti-TNF [tumour necrosis factor] alpha, leflunamide).

Raynaud's phenomenon
* Associations.

Sjögren's syndrome
* SS-A and SS-B cytoplasmic antibody associations, association with lymphoma.

Systemic lupus erythematosus
* Nervous system and renal complications, problems with pregnancy, anti-cardiolipin antibodies, features of drug-induced lupus.

Systemic sclerosis
* Differential diagnosis, diffuse versus limited (CREST syndrome) disease.

Seronegative arthropathy
* Behçet's syndrome features, diagnosis of Reiter's syndrome, HLA-B27 association with each disease, intestinal bypass surgery—associations, Whipple's disease.

Osteoarthritis
* Primary osteoarthritis—synovial fluid characteristics, pathogenesis, characteristic risk factors and X-ray changes.

Haemochromatosis arthropathy

Vasculitis
* Giant cell arteritis and association with polymyalgia rheumatica, Wegener's granulomatosis, mixed cryoglobulinaemia, Henoch-Schönlein purpura, diagnostic tests (e.g. antineutrophil cytoplasmic antibodies [ANCA]).

Crystal-induced synovitis
• Crystal characteristics of gout, pseudogout and hydroxyapatite arthropathy.

Infectious arthritis
• Lyme arthritis, gonococcal arthritis.

Non-steroidal anti-inflammatory drugs (NSAIDs)
• Prevention of gastrointestinal damage using misoprostol, proton pump inhibitors and high-dose H_2-receptor antagonists, cyclooxygenase (COX-2) inhibitors.

Infectious diseases

Investigations
• Cerebrospinal fluid findings (e.g. meningitis).
• Syphilis serology interpretation.
• Gallium and indium scans.

Fever
• Mechanisms, types.

Viral diseases
• Epstein-Barr virus (associations with Burkitt's lymphoma and nasopharyngeal carcinoma, complications including cranial nerve palsies, diagnosis), cytomegalovirus (CMV), herpes simplex virus (HSV) (complications including encephalitis, diagnosis, treatment), HSV-8 (Kaposi's sarcoma), measles (complications, diagnosis), arboviruses (e.g. dengue fever), viral gastroenteritis (e.g. rotavirus incubation period and diagnosis), lissavirus, enterovirus (acute haemorrhagic conjunctivitis), influenza, slow prion diseases (e.g. Jakob-Creutzfeldt disease, pathological findings, sterilisation of instruments), teratogenic viruses, HIV/AIDS (seroconversion and clinical disease, risks after needlestick injury, post-exposure prophylaxis, $CD4^+$ count, viral loads, HAART [highly active anti-retroviral therapy] and its side-effects).

Bacterial diseases
• Gram-negative aerobes (e.g. *Campylobacter jejuni*—clinical features and treatment), anaerobes (e.g. *Clostridium difficile* and its toxin, *Bacteroides fragilis*), mycobacterial infection (including atypical mycobacteria), Lyme disease.

Fungi and parasites
• Mycotic disease (e.g. cryptococcosis, aspergillosis), parasitic diseases (e.g. resistant strains of malaria, exoerythrogenic phases and types, transmission, treatment, drugs interfering with thick films), *Pneumocystis carinii* (organism, diagnosis, treatment).

Syphilis serology
• Causes of false-negative results.

Worms
• Appearance of hookworms, roundworms, worms known to migrate, worms that cause eosinophilia.

Antibiotics/resistance
• Methicillin-resistant *Staphylococcus aureus* (MRSA), vancomycin-resistant *Staph. aureus* (VRSA, VRE), streptococcal pneumonia, resistance to penicillin, new quinolones, fourth generation cefalosporins.

Vaccines
- Hepatitis B vaccine, dangers and value.

Diseases in specific populations
- Homosexual men—particularly HIV and gay bowel syndrome, immunocompromised hosts.

Other topics
- Organisms persisting after primary infections (as in varicella, tuberculosis), bacterial endotoxins, exotoxins and superantigens, Kawasaki disease, non-specific urethritis, toxic shock syndrome, blood cultures—diagnostic value in aerobic and anaerobic infections.

Oncology

Tumour induction
- Cigarettes, benzene, Epstein-Barr virus.

Tumour-associated markers
- Alpha-fetoprotein, carcinoembryonic antigen, prostate-specific antigen, beta-human chorionic gonadotrophin (β-HCG), CA-19-9.

Antitumour drugs
- Mode of action and side-effects of each (e.g. tamoxifen). Mechanisms of drug resistance.

Radiotherapy
- Indications, mechanisms of action, complications.

Breast carcinoma
- Oestrogen receptor status importance, role of adjuvant therapy, treatment of disseminated disease.

Prostatic carcinoma
- Prostate-specific antigen.

Colon carcinoma
- Adjuvant therapy, treatment for metastases.

Malignant melanoma
- Poor prognostic features, new chemotherapeutic approaches.

Retinoblastoma
- Inheritance, prognosis.

Testicular tumours
- Common types, investigations, treatment.

Sarcomas
- With Paget's disease, radiosensitivity.

Manifestations of cancer
- Paraneoplastic syndromes, neurological manifestations, superior vena cava syndrome, malignant effusions, infection in the compromised host, common metastatic sites.

Biological response modifiers
- Interferons.

Genetics of cancer
- *BRCA1, BRCA2, p53* genes, genetic abnormalities in carcinoma of the colon (e.g. DNA mismatch repair gene).

Endocrine system

Investigations
- Pituitary function tests.
- Thyroid function tests.
- Diagnosis of Cushing's syndrome.
- Electrolyte changes (e.g. in Addison's disease).
- Insulinoma and hypoglycaemia.
- Interpretation of dual energy X-ray absorptiometry (DEXA) scans (osteopenia/ osteoporosis), prophylaxis for osteoporosis.

Hormonal activity
- Sites of action, receptor sites, changes during pregnancy.

Anterior pituitary lobe
- Diagnostic tests of function, 'empty sella' syndrome, prolactin-secreting tumours, acromegaly.

Posterior pituitary lobe
- Antidiuretic hormone—structure, drugs affecting levels, psychogenic polydipsia.

Ectopic hormone secretion/multiple endocrine neoplasia syndromes

Adrenal cortex
- Cushing's syndrome tests, aldosterone (stimulators and inhibitors of secretion, sites of production, synthesis), Addison's disease and its associations, risk of antibiotics inducing adrenal insufficiency, steroid-responsive aldosteronism (GRA).

Adrenal medulla
- Phaeochromocytoma, adrenal mass.

Thyroid gland
- Thyroxine (T_4), triiodothyronine (T_3), reverse T_3, sensitive thyroid-stimulating hormone (TSH), changes in health and disease (sick euthyroid), drugs affecting conversion of T_4 to T_3, multinodular goitre, eye disorders in Graves' disease, de Quervain's thyroiditis, thyroxine replacement, management of hypothyroid states, congenital hypothyroidism, postpartum thyroiditis.

Reproductive system
- Causes of gynaecomastia, infertility and galactorrhoea, testosterone-binding activity and control of secretion, hormonal control of spermatogenesis, hirsutism, Klinefelter's syndrome, hormone replacement therapy—benefits and risks, indications for use, polycystic ovaries. Causes of galactorrhoea.

Bone and mineral disorders
- Primary hyperparathyroidism, biochemical features in various diseases, vitamin D metabolism, oestrogen therapy, side-effects of bisphosphonates. DEXA scans—indications and interpretation.

Atrial natriuretic factor
- Effects, site of origin.

Diabetes mellitus
- Biochemical control of gluconeogenesis, insulin antibodies, viruses associated with diabetes, reversible abnormalities in diabetes (e.g. red cell deformability, capillary leaks, triglycerides, neuropathy), drugs causing diabetes, pathogenesis of ketoacidosis, hypoglycaemia and its association with immunoreactive insulin, gestational diabetes, glycosylated proteins, treatment of retinopathy, characteristics of amyotrophy, detecting incipient nephropathy, ACE inhibitors, beta-blockers and nephropathy, control of blood sugar and complications, new treatment (e.g. trigliatazone and its side-effects—fluid retention), treatment trials—Diabetes Control and Complications Trial (DCCT)/UK Prospective Diabetes Study (UKPDS).

Anorexia nervosa
- Endocrine changes.

Hormones and growth
- Effects on skeletal maturity, somatomedins (including IGF-1), growth hormone.

Gynaecomastia
- Hormonal drug causes.

HIV and endocrinological complications

Renal system

Investigations
- Intravenous pyelograms (e.g. polycystic kidney disease).
- CT scans (e.g. polycystic kidney disease).
- Bone radiographs (e.g. hips showing renal osteodystrophy).
- Urine sediment photograph (e.g. red and white cell casts).
- Renal biopsy photographs (e.g. crescentic glomerulonephritis, vasculitis).

Electrolyte and water disturbances
- Inappropriate antidiuretic hormone secretion, diabetes insipidus, sodium disorders, potassium disorders, calcium disorders, countercurrent multiplication and exchange.

Acid–base disturbances
- Metabolic acidosis and alkalosis, causes of a high, normal and low anion gap.

Urinary protein excretion
- Nephrotic syndrome.

Urine microscopy

Glomerulonephritis
- Classification, immunoglobulin A (IgA) nephropathy, complement changes, Goodpasture's syndrome, nephritic and nephrotic syndromes.

Systemic diseases
- Vasculitis, diabetes and systemic lupus erythematosus in the kidney.

Tubulointerstitial nephritis
- Causes, clinical course.

Hypertension
- Causes, plasma renin levels in various disorders, natriuretic hormones, therapy.

Drugs and the kidney
- Safe antibiotics to prescribe in renal failure, effects of NSAIDs in renal failure, analgesic nephropathy.

Chronic renal failure
- Reversible causes, manifestations, treatment (e.g. erythropoietin, transplantation, dialysis), polycystic disease.

Acute renal failure
- Contrast nephropathy and its management/prevention.

Renal stones and hypercalciuria

Urinary tract infection
- Urinary incontinence, urinary catheterisation.

Bartter's syndrome

Rhabdomyolysis

Pregnancy (physiology and disease states)

Renal transplant
- Indication, complications and treatment.

Immunology

Basic immunology
- T helper cells (TH-1, TH-2), inhibitory proliferative cytokines and CD28 deficiency. Natural killer (NK) cells, important CD T cell types. Vaccination and immunodeficiency. Immunological response to bacterial infection.

Hypersensitivity reaction
- Types I–IV.

Urticaria, angio-oedema

Complement system
- Physiology, C1 esterase deficiency.

Geriatrics

Normal ageing

Falls/osteoporosis

Dementia/delirium

Constipation/urinary incontinence

Polypharmacy

Clinical pharmacology

Ionisation of drugs and movement across membranes
- Drugs with lipid solubility.

Dose–response curve
- Competitive and non-competitive antagonists, pharmacokinetics versus pharmacodynamics.

Drug receptors
- Alteration with chronic therapy.

Cardiovascular system and drugs
- Alpha and beta effects of catecholamines, diuretics (site of action), digoxin (differences from digitoxin and ouabain, effects of intoxication), antihypertensive drugs (e.g. withdrawal hypertension), antiarrhythmic drugs (classes and effects, arrhythmic effects, contraindications), cholesterol and drugs.

Respiratory system and drugs
- Aminophylline (half-life in different conditions).

Gastrointestinal system and drugs
- Paracetamol toxicity, side-effects of laxatives, toxicity of immunosuppressives, liver P450 enzyme levels, COX-2 inhibitors and gastric bleeding, role of acid suppression in prevention of gastrointestinal complications with NSAIDs.

Haematological system and drugs
- Warfarin (how levels are increased or decreased and the causes of such changes), heparin (antibodies, toxicity), fractionated versus unfractionated heparin, ximelagatran, aspirin versus clopidogrel, folate antagonists.

Nervous system and drugs
- L-dopa (contraindications, side-effects), neurotoxic antibodies, cholinergic and anticholinergic drugs.

Endocrine system and drugs
- Drugs precipitating diabetes mellitus (e.g. diuretics, diazoxide, phenytoin), prednisone (side-effects, half-life compared with other steroid agents), general effects of steroids, vitamin D (metabolism, effects on parathyroid hormone and calcium), drugs affecting bone and calcium metabolism.

Psychiatry and drugs
- Neuroleptic drugs (mechanisms of action, side-effects), lithium (absorption, interactions, indications, routine management).

Antibiotics
- Penicillin G (mode of action, mechanisms of resistance, structure, effect of renal failure), sulfonylureas (side-effects), metronidazole, cefalosporins, imipenem, fluoro-quinolones. Azithromycin versus doxycycline.

Antiviral agents
- Indications, treatment of HIV infection, drug interactions (e.g. prothrombin index), treatment of herpes simplex with antiviral drugs.

Cytotoxic drugs
- Adriamycin (mechanism of action, usefulness, cardiotoxicity, monitoring), methotrexate (indications, mechanism of action, treatment of overdosage, interaction with salicylates, activation, protein binding, excretion, antagonist factors, side-effects including monitoring for liver toxicity), cyclophosphamide (absorption, mechanism of action, prevention of side-effects), azathioprine (interaction with allopurinol, use in pregnancy, half-life), 5-fluorouracil (mode of action, administration, indications, complications), cell-cycle-specific drugs, drug-eluting stents (e.g. paclitaxel).

Other topics
- Heroin withdrawal features, drugs affecting free water clearance (e.g. increased by ethanol and lithium, decreased by nicotine, vincristine and clofibrate), pharmacology of alcohol, tobacco and cocaine. Plasma half-life and drug clearance.

Genetically determined drug reactions
- Malignant hyperpyrexia, succinylcholine apnoea.

Pregnancy
- Physiological changes, effect on chronic disease, drug use in liver disease and pregnancy.

Statistics/epidemiology
- Study designs, odds ratio versus relative risk; sensitivity, specificity and predictive value (and influence of prevalence), *number needed to treat* (NNT) and *intention to treat* (ITT) analysis of trials.

An approach to the clinical examination

This is a very testing part. It is more difficult than the written test.

Talley & O'Connor (1986)

The examination format

The clinical examination consists of two sessions of two parts each and now takes up a whole (rather exhausting) day. There is evidence that lengthening a clinical examination improves its reliability. The College believes that the new format has improved reliability. Candidates are notified of the starting time of the ordeal after their success in the written papers. Be on time: the examination runs to a strict timetable and no allowances can be made for late arrival.

For half of the candidates the day begins with a long case. At the appropriate moment, candidates are escorted to the patient by a 'bulldog'—a term apparently derived from the name of proctors' attendants at the universities of Oxford and Cambridge. The bulldog is usually a resident medical officer working at the examining hospital who has an interest in sitting the clinical examination. If ever candidates have the opportunity to work as a bulldog, they should take it. The bulldog introduces the candidate to the patient and then leaves. There are never any examiners in the room during a long case. The time is limited to 60 minutes with the patient. A 5-minute warning is given after 55 minutes. At the end, candidates are escorted by the bulldog from the patient's room to a chair outside the examiners' room. Ten further minutes are allowed for candidates to pull themselves together and get to the examination room. A glass of water or weak orange juice is usually offered at this stage. If not, do ask for a drink if you need one.

A bell then rings and candidates are taken in separately, seated, and introduced to the examiners. Try to appear self-possessed (even if weak at the knees), but don't give an air of nonchalance (e.g. by slouching in your chair).

As a rule there are two examiners, but there may be three in the room (one an observer only). One is a member of the Committee for Examinations (CFE) or National Examining Panel (NEP) (who previously held the more intimidating title of 'Censor'). The others are experienced examiners who are local physicians, and may include the Director of Physician Training (DPT). Local examiners undergo 'calibration' exercises before they examine. All see the patient before the examinations begin. There may be a bulldog sitting in the room as well.

Immediately before the examination, the examiners interview the long-case patient blind, that is, without reference to the patient's case notes. This is to ensure that the history is up to date and also to gauge any difficulty in terms of the patient's ability to give a history and to check for signs.

The examiners will assess the candidate's ability to take a detailed history and complete examination; they will also assess the candidate's ability to identify the patient's active problems and to recognise priorities for investigation and management. The examiners will also be interested in seeing if the candidate recognises the impact of the patient's disease on the patient and his/her family. The examiners will mark the performance in each of these domains according to set key criteria, which are available to all candidates. It would be wise for candidates to examine these anchor statements carefully—they are available on the Royal Australasian College of Physicians' website (see Ch 1) or from the DPT at each hospital. Concise, standard questions will usually be asked. Only two examiners will ask questions—one 'leads' the discussion and the other follows near the end for 5–7 minutes. For reasons of fairness, it is unusual for specialists to 'lead' the examination of a candidate on a patient with problems in their own field. Twenty-five minutes are spent with the examiners, presenting the case and discussing diagnosis and management. The discussion period is critical to passing (or failing).

At the end of the time a bell will ring and the candidate is taken to begin the short-case examination. There are a few minutes available, however, for drinking weak orange juice. Many candidates ask the bulldog's opinion of their performance. We believe this to be an unwise policy, as the resident medical officer is usually junior to the examinee and so is often incorrect in his or her assessment.

The candidate is then introduced to the short-case examiners. The examiners for the first short case are never the same as the ones who examined for the long case but you may see the long-case examining team for your second short case. Again, one examiner in each team is a member of the CFE. Fifteen minutes are allowed for the first short case. A second short case is then examined without a break. The new examination system does not allow for more than two cases per short-case session. This, and the extension of time from 22 to 30 minutes, means that examination of each patient is a little less rushed. The result of this extra time means that there is a greater opportunity for the examiners to ask questions related to the physical findings. The examiners assess five domains during the short-case examination, including the way the candidate approaches the patient, the thoroughness of the examination technique, the accuracy of detecting physical signs, the ability to offer a diagnosis on the basis of the findings and the ability to use investigations to support the physical findings. Examining centres have also been told to have X-rays, computed tomography (CT) scans, magnetic resonance imaging (MRI) scans and electrocardiographs (ECGs) available for discussion. The key criteria and the skills that are required to achieve a satisfactory standard are available from the College or the DPT.

The other half of the candidates do this routine in the reverse order.

After lunch a second session begins, and this time the order of short and long cases is reversed for each candidate. There is no longer provision for extra short cases for candidates who are thought to be borderline.

In conjunction with these new arrangements comes a new marking system, which was introduced in 1996. The mark required to pass the examination is 40. Each long case is worth 21 marks and each short case is worth 7 marks—so the total mark possible is 70.

The mark awarded for each short case is now out of seven as follows: 1, very poor performance; 2, well short of expected standard; 3, short of expected standard; 4, expected standard; 5, better than expected standard; 6, much better than expected standard; 7, exceptional performance. In 2006 part marks were introduced for the short case as well. It is thought this will help some candidates who are very close to a pass overall. This means that when the marks are added up at the end of the day, 4+ for example will be 4.33 and 5– will be 4.67.

In the long case, the scoring system also incorporates positives and negatives (part marks) between 1 and 7, giving a 19-point scale. For example, if the examiners agree that a candidate's performance was better than a 4 but not deserving of a 5, a 4+ is awarded, while if the performance was much better than 4 but not deserving a 5, the mark will be a 5–. Once a 'raw score' out of 7 is awarded, it is weighted; the long-case scores are multiplied by three.

The examiners try very hard to be fair. Each candidate's performance is discussed at the end of each long- and short-case segment. Each examiner scores independently. If there is disagreement about a mark, this is discussed and a consensus mark is chosen. Examiners record any special considerations that may have caused difficulties for the candidate (and flag the assessment sheet with the infamous 'red dot') so that these can be considered later by the executive, if necessary. The Chief Examiner of the day (always a member of the CFE) is responsible for collecting the marked score sheets and dealing with any red dot issues. The examiners do not know the candidate's marks in other sections, and therefore they do not know the effect of their own mark on the candidate's overall success or failure. The examiners see the same short case four times with four candidates. They give a mark at the end of each session and cannot change this after assessing the other candidates' attempts at the same case.

The written examination mark is not taken into account. However, examiners are not trying to pass candidates, as at undergraduate level—they are trying to evaluate the true standard of the candidate. The examinees must prove to the College that they are 'good enough'—that is, they must demonstrate that they have reached the required standard. The standards are very high, but the College emphasises to the examiners that the standard is that which is required for a person to enter advanced training and not the standard expected of a consultant physician.

Overseas-trained physicians (OTPs) will be examined on one long case in their subspecialty area. The standard expected in this case is higher (i.e. at specialist or consultant physician level rather than end of basic training level).

To achieve uniform standards, the CFE has been constantly working on improve-ments. Senior members of the CFE examine more often with less experienced examiners. The CFE also holds regular formal calibration exercises, in which all the examiners view videotapes and mark a candidate's performance. A general discussion is then held to try to develop a uniformity of approach. There is no doubt that problems continue, as it remains difficult (if not impossible) to judge ability accurately in such a short period; however, the CFE is working towards eliminating obvious mistakes. One innovation in the future may be that an examiner will sit in when a candidate interviews and examines the long-case patient.

The overall pass rate (for the written *and* viva examinations) in any one year in the past has been about 40%. The eventual pass rate after success at the written examination and over four vivas (the old system) approached 85%. Under the new system, the pass rate is about 65% for the clinical year, although the results in 2005 were better than this.

Preparation for the clinical examination

For one mistake made for not knowing, ten mistakes are made for not looking. JA Lindsay

The examination aims to test not only clinical ability but also attitudes and interper-sonal skills. For most candidates the successful approach to the viva depends on seeing a large number of long and short cases. It is usually too late to start seeing practice cases only after having passed the written examination. Preparation should start at least several months before. To practise for the long case, try to set aside a regular time each week. Most physicians, if approached, are only too willing to test-run candidates. Exposure to many different examiners is desirable—this will help iron out mistakes and provide practice in answering different types of questions. Although most teaching hospitals have a training scheme in which long cases are examined by consultants or senior registrars, this is not enough. It is difficult to quote numbers, but we believe

40 formal long cases across all disciplines in which different specialists or senior registrars act as examiners represent the bare minimum requirement for preparation. Remember also that each time a patient is admitted to hospital, practice can be gained in the long-case technique—this turns overtime into useful preparation time. Practising cases is also critical in order to be able to cope with management issues in Paper B of the written examination.

Practice for the short cases is also important. More examinees used to fail these than in the long case, although this has changed now that the long case is receiving more emphasis. It is valuable to have senior colleagues as well as peers take candidates on short cases. Travelling to other hospitals to practise is worthwhile because one has to examine in strange surroundings while being watched by unfamiliar examiners. It also relieves the boredom somewhat. The best practice examiner is the one who frightens candidates a little but does not demolish them when they make an error. Seek out constructive criticism. For example, many candidates also practise in pairs, each person taking turns to be the examiner. Practising being an examiner makes one appreciate the bad habits that annoy the real examiners.

Equipment is always provided at the hospital where the examination is held. However, it is important to bring the following:

1. a familiar stethoscope that has been used for a long time—do not buy a newer, fancier stethoscope the day before the test—it takes time to get used to a new instrument
2. a hand-held eye card—obtainable from OPSM for a moderate charge and essential for cranial nerve or eye examinations (see Ch 8)
3. a red-tipped hat pin—candidates can buy a plain one and paint the top with nail polish; this is invaluable for visual field testing (see Ch 8)
4. paper and pens.

It is debatable whether candidates should bring in their own bags of instruments. Many favour bringing their own ophthalmoscope and pocket torch (with fresh batteries in both). Others also like to have cotton wool, pins (an unused one for each case) and spatulas, as well as tuning forks (256 and 128 Hertz) and a patella hammer, which is too much to carry in the pockets. This has led to a trend for leather briefcases to house all the equipment (see Fig 4.1). However, the occasional difficult examiner has been known to complain about this! There is a story about one candidate's briefcase, which was filled with such elaborate equipment, including an inverted cardigan for testing dressing apraxia, that his examiners spent their time inspecting the contents rather than watching him examine the patient.

During practice sessions, it is always a good idea to place equipment in the same pockets. Candidates do not want to be fumbling at this crucial time—it will only create a poor impression. Consultants, other than cardiologists, carry their stethoscopes or put them in their coat pocket; rarely do they place them around their neck. This seems a sensible policy for aspiring consultants also. A candidate who does carry a briefcase into the test (and many neurologists carry one everywhere) can usually place it on the patient's bedside table and leave it open there, so that its contents are easily accessible.

Some candidates take beta-blockers on the day of the test to remain calm. An interesting story from the *Lancet* highlights this very situation. A Scottish physician refers to a British censor who had the habit of counting the temporal pulse of candidates; if he found that the pulse rate was less than 60 beats/minute, he would take this fact into account when giving his mark (Bamber MG 1980 Dope test for doctors. *Lancet* ii:1308). We are unaware of a similar practice in Australasia. However, it is important for candidates intending to use these drugs to give themselves a dose during a practice session. One doctor learnt only at the actual examination, to his horror, that beta-blockers caused him severe bronchospasm (he failed).

Nervous individuals with a tendency to sweat can have problems. One candidate (now a professor) who was balding and wore glasses, found that, during times of

Figure 4.1   A candidates bag.

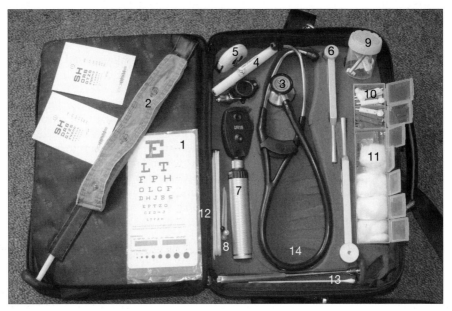

Note:

1. Eye charts and patella hammer
2. Buttons
3. Stethoscope
4. Torch
5. Tape measure
6. Tuning forks
7. Ophthalmoscope and auroscope
8. Hat pins (red and white)
9. Jar with lid (containing key for key grip assessment)
10. Disposable neurology pins
11. Cotton wool
12. Spatula
13. Cotton buds
14. Carefully shaped foam inserts

intense stress, rivers of sweat rolled down from his forehead to fog up his glasses and wash them from his nose. His solution was antiperspirant (unscented of course) applied to the forehead (he passed).

Dress is important. The medical establishment is well known for its conservatism and non-verbal communication should not be forgotten when dressing. Traditionally, men wear a conservative suit and a non-committal tie. Other important considerations are short, tidy hair, a neatly trimmed beard if you cannot bear to shave it off, and a neutral smell. Candidates should dress formally, with care to project an air of quiet efficiency. White coats are never worn. However, being well dressed is no guarantee of success. There is a story of two male candidates, wearing grey suits and with recently cut hair, who were viewing with satisfaction a third examinee whose long hair was tied neatly in a bun—they felt their own success seemed assured with such competition. However, it turned out that they were unsuccessful and that their colleague passed.

Preparation is the key to success. Like an Olympic athlete, obtain plenty of sleep in the week before the ordeal; take no alcohol or tranquillisers in the 48 hours before it, and do not study during the final 24 hours. Make sure that you eat something on the day of the examination and avoid a long trip to the examination city on the morning of or the night before the test.

The long case

The man who confesses his ignorance shows it once; he who tries to conceal it shows it many times.

Japanese proverb

When the examiners discuss a long case with a candidate, they are expecting to find out how the candidate would manage the patient and his or her problems. They want to know if the candidate has a practical grasp of what is required in consultant practice. Candidates are expected to have a mature and sensible approach to the patient and his or her problems. It may help to picture yourself as the physician taking over the care of a new patient. Practising long cases trains candidates to be better clinicians.

Careful allocation of time with the patient is vital. The exact proportions will depend on the case itself but, as a rough guide, spend 25 minutes on the history, 20 minutes on the examination, and the rest of the time preparing discussion and reviewing vital facts with the patient. Nothing is more important than ensuring you leave enough time to put your thoughts in order.

People favour many different systems for recording long case details (as an aid to memory). There are two we recommend. One is to use a small pad that can be held comfortably in the hand and the pages turned unobtrusively. The other is a small card system. One side is used for the history and the other for the examination findings; a second card (if necessary) is used for relevant investigations, management and short lists of facts the candidate may wish to mention. Obviously, numbering each side is important so as not to mix up the order of presentation. These cards are now usually provided to candidates who want them at the examination site. Mixing up the cards can be a disaster. One candidate was sitting, preparing to enter the examination room, when the side door opened and a puff of wind blew the cards out of her hands. She was then ushered straight into the examination room with the cards in random order. She began the long case badly and failed.

Candidates who do not want to rewrite the whole long-case presentation before facing the examiners (time is often a problem) may find it helpful to number the paragraphs with a red pen in the order in which they wish to present the story.

Once you have said 'How do you do?' to the patient at the beginning of the long case, we suggest initially following the steps outlined below. These may help you ascertain rapidly the patient's major problems so that you can direct further questioning more easily.

1. Explain to the patient that this is a very important examination. Gain his or her interest and support. This is a test of bedside manner.
2. Ask the patient what is wrong. If he or she says 'Am I allowed to tell you?', look confident and firm and say 'Yes, of course'. Candidates are entitled to all the information the patient can offer.

3. Ask why the patient is in hospital this time (i.e. is he or she an inpatient or an outpatient?) and, if relevant, the presenting symptoms when he or she was admitted. A number of patients are brought in specifically for the examination and will have no acute medical problems.
4. Ask early what medications the patient is taking. This will give valuable information about both current and past problems.
5. Ask about any recent tests, again to obtain clues about the current problem.

In the majority of long cases, the patient has a chronic illness about which he or she may be very well informed. It is sensible to make use of this knowledge, but remember the trap that patients may be biased in their opinions and give (inadvertently) false information. Having established the main diagnosis early, confirm this with specific questioning. On finding symptoms not fitting the diagnosis, decide the likely possibilities and follow them up with further questions. Never blindly believe the patient.

Inquire about other problems next. Most long-case patients are chosen because they have multiple medical problems. An example might be an elderly woman with pulmonary fibrosis as her major presenting illness who also has significant ischaemic heart disease and moderate renal impairment, and peptic ulceration secondary to aspirin use. It is a terrible experience to discover another major illness only minutes before the end of the time. List all the important diseases chronologically. Obtain full details about each. Organise to present the most important (i.e. often the current) problem first, followed by the others in order of importance. Some healthy scepticism about the patient's opinion of the diagnosis is usually warranted. A history of exotic previous illnesses without a history of appropriate investigations or treatment for such conditions should prompt a careful retaking of the history.

It is important to appreciate the great amount of detail the examiners will expect about the patient's past history. A lot of time needs to be spent on this. Failure to uncover a medical problem from long ago that the examiners found, when they saw the patient, counts against the candidate. Remember that the patient's history is often well rehearsed after the examiners and perhaps another candidate have taken it.

Don't forget the social history. This is especially important, as the examiners (and society) are keen to have caring specialists who are fully aware of the complete social environment of their patients. The examiners will expect great detail here as well. Always ask about:

- *occupation*—now and in the past
- *adequacy of income*—particularly if the patient is on a pension
- *current housing arrangements*—e.g. renting, mortgage
- *ability to cope* at home and the quality of life if this is a chronic disease problem— the activities of daily living (ADLs) should be assessed
- *mobility*—particularly the number of steps that need to be climbed at home and at work, and on which floor the patient lives
- *hobbies*—e.g. contact with animals or chemicals or dusts
- *marital status* and number of children
- *sexual problems*—particularly ask about erectile dysfunction in men (e.g. diabetic patients)
- *place of birth*
- *overseas travel* in relationship to the illness.

A family history must also be taken. This sort of information is easy to obtain, and fills in discussion time neatly, but disaster can threaten if it is not known. The most important aspects should be outlined in the initial presentation and the rest kept in reserve to be unleashed if the examiners show an interest.

As one examines the patient, one should always ask when the examiners came, what parts were examined, and whether any comments were made about the signs.

One candidate was told by his patient that, during a fundoscopic examination, the examiner had said: 'What an interesting Roth's spot!'. However, this is no substitute for a thorough examination.

Even though you should spend most time on the relevant systems, remember that sometimes unexpected signs will crop up, such as a large breast mass, gross papilloedema or an abdominal mass. The examiners always have in front of them a list of the signs and have always gone to the trouble of checking that, in fact, these signs are present. The candidate will be expected to have found all the important signs, so be thorough. Any very equivocal findings should probably be ignored. Ask the bulldog for the results of the urinalysis and the rectal examination. The candidate is not expected to perform these personally. Also, don't forget to take the blood pressure at some stage and check for a postural change, if at all relevant (e.g. diabetes mellitus, p 189).

At the end of the history-taking and the physical examination, always ask: 'Is there anything else you think I should know?'. Amazingly important information is often volunteered at this point. Then ask yourself, 'Could this be anything else?' and 'Can I tie all the multisystem problems into one disease?'.

During the 20 minutes or so remaining, decide what type of case it is—that is, is this a *management* problem, or a *diagnostic* problem, or both? Sort out the active from the inactive problems. Draft the introductory statement (e.g. 'I saw Mrs J Smith, a 50-year-old woman, who presents with the management problem of active rheumatoid arthritis, and also the diagnostic and management problem of chronic liver disease').

Next, mentally rehearse presenting the history and examination concisely and clearly. The concluding statement should reiterate the problems (in order of importance). It is usual to end the presentation by requests for relevant investigations. Always formulate a differential diagnosis, even if the history and examination lead to a positive diagnosis. Create a list of the findings on history and examination that support (or refute) the diagnoses considered. If a positive diagnosis cannot confidently be made, you should try to decide on the most likely diagnosis.

The whole presentation to the examiners should take 8–10 minutes. Leave out any irrelevant detail—padding the presentation never impresses. Also, remember never to use abbreviations when presenting (e.g. don't use JVP for jugular venous pressure, or MCP joint for metacarpophalangeal joint). The examiners are only human too: sometimes they are hungry, tired or just bored after previous presentations (particularly if yours is the last long case of the afternoon). Show interest and enthusiasm while speaking. Don't read notes in a monotone. The notes are meant to be a memory aid. Ideally, the long case should be a discussion between consultants, with the candidate being a respectful junior colleague. The examiners only occasionally interrupt during the presentation. At the end they may try to clarify a particular point. Sometimes they direct the candidate to a particular line of discussion.

The discovery of a major problem with a particular long case (e.g. the patient with obvious dementia) shouldn't lead to panic. By recognising the problem, fully examining the patient, and having a plan of management (finding reversible causes, eliciting from relatives the social set-up etc.), you will pass. One candidate who was faced with a demented patient in the long-case examination became angry and complained bitterly to his examiners. He failed.

Occasionally there are other difficulties, such as language problems (usually the candidate is supplied with an interpreter, often a relative), or the patient becomes ill during the time (cardiac arrests have occurred). Be sure to inform the bulldog of any difficulties—everyone goes out of his or her way to be fair in such circumstances. The examiners will usually make a note of any such problems on their scoresheet, so that this can be taken into account by the executive later on.

It is likely that the examiners will want to discuss the patient's active problems. These should be the areas of management that the candidate is best prepared for. It is very unsatisfactory for an examiner to feel that he or she has not been told all of the major problems, and what the management plan for each problem is, by the end of the discussion. At the end of the candidate's presentation and before discussion of management, the examiners may ask some questions to clarify aspects of the history or examination findings. This should be no cause for alarm. After this the candidate is usually given the opportunity to outline a plan of management, or the examiners may ask specific questions. Examining styles differ, but the candidate should strive to direct the discussion tactfully. Being allowed to do this is usually a good sign, but not being allowed to control the discussion is not necessarily a bad sign.

When appropriate, ask for one or two important investigations relevant to the problems, rather than for a string of routine tests. *A reason should be given for ordering every test.* For a diagnostic problem it may be useful to ask for the results of previous investigations. Any mentioned test may have to be discussed in detail with the examiners. We suggest that you write down the results you are told (it is embarrassing to have to ask for the figures to be repeated). Don't ignore any information that is given: for example, if the haemoglobin value is normal, comment on this and explain how it helps. Remember not to touch X-ray films or criticise the quality of the material shown. Pathological specimens are not shown in the clinical examinations.

Always prepare answers to the obvious lines of question and try to think like a consultant physician who is in charge of the patient's care (and hypothesise that the patient is a close relative of the examiner!). If there is a diagnostic dilemma, consider the tests you want and how positive and negative results will support or refute your proposed diagnoses. In a management case, prepare an outline of the suggested treatment and be able to justify it. Always set management goals for all key therapeutic interventions. The examiners may ask about theoretical aspects of the condition. Most often, they will concentrate the testing of factual knowledge in areas that are necessary for the formulation of adequate management decisions or interpretation of test results. You should think about these areas beforehand. Always consider whether the patient's current treatment is justified and whether the diagnosis previously made is consistent with the history and examination; it may not be. Do not be afraid to contradict the current management if there is clear justification.

The examiners will not usually ask hypothetical questions unrelated to the patient being discussed. If the candidate is answering well, the line of questioning may change, or the depth may become overwhelming. Do *not* be frightened to say, in the latter situation, 'Sir (or Madam), I don't know', when asked a very difficult question. Obvious wild guesses will be detrimental. If the examiner persists in asking a question, it usually means he or she is trying to establish a basic fact. Talk sensibly around the topic—often a supplementary question will result in recall of the appropriate information. With an especially difficult issue it is reasonable to say you would consult the literature or an appropriate subspecialist for advice. Remember that examiners are instructed to avoid making snap judgments or failing candidates because of one small mistake.

You must be able to discuss sensibly anything that you mention in a viva, so don't casually allude to rare diseases that you know nothing about (e.g. kala-azar as a cause of massive splenomegaly).

6

Common long cases

In what manner are the examiners elected? Are they elected by the profession or any part of the profession whose interests are equal to those of the whole, and are they responsible to the profession at large for their conduct? Neither the one nor the other.

Lancet *1824; i:20*

The long case is a test of history-taking, physical examination, interpretation of findings, construction of a diagnosis (and differential diagnosis) and of the candidate's approach to management (investigation and treatment). Important and common long cases are presented in some detail in this section. The list (Table 6.1) is not exhaustive but gives an idea of the range of possible cases. Most (but not all) are discussed here—some other relevant aspects are dealt with in Chapter 8.

The cases are written as a guide to dealing with the long-case examination but are not meant to replace textbook descriptions. To pass you must really know and understand your general medicine. Remember that usually several problems occur in the one case. A patient with an unusual diagnosis will often have one or more common problems as well.

The examiners will often ask if the candidate would like the results of appropriate investigations. Be prepared to interpret any results you have asked for. Electrocardiograms (ECGs), chest X-rays, and computed tomography (CT) and magnetic resonance imaging (MRI) scans may be shown to a candidate. Echocardiogram tapes are not usually shown to candidates but they are expected to be able to interpret echocardiography reports. Some common examples are included here and in Chapter 8. At the end of each report is a comment that gives an idea of the sort of interpretation expected from the candidate.

Cardiovascular system

Ischaemic heart disease

Patients with unstable angina or recent myocardial infarction are always available for long cases if required. Many patients with more exotic medical problems will also have ischaemic heart disease. The whims of the long-case examiners may lead to concentrated questioning about the ischaemic heart disease of a patient in hospital for the management of, for example, renal transplant rejection. These patients are more likely to present management rather than diagnostic problems once they reach the status of long-case patients.

Table 6.1   Common long cases

Cardiovascular system
1. Ischaemic heart disease (p 33)
2. Infective endocarditis (p 41)
3. Congestive cardiac failure (p 46)
4. Hyperlipidaemia (p 56)
5. Hypertension (p 58)
6. Cardiac arrhythmias and atrial fibrillation (p 67)
7. Heart transplantation (p 62)
8. Valvular heart disease (p 232)
9. Revascularisation (p 38)
10. Pacemaker or implantable cardioverter-defibrillators (ICD) (p 72)

Respiratory system
1. Bronchiectasis (p 77)
2. Lung carcinoma (p 79)
3. Chronic obstructive pulmonary disease (chronic airflow limitation (p 83))
4. Tuberculosis (p 103)
5. Pulmonary fibrosis (p 88)
6. Pulmonary hypertension (p 91)
7. Sarcoidosis (p 97)
8. Cystic fibrosis (p 100)
9. Sleep apnoea (p 86)
10. Lung transplant (p 106)

Gastrointestinal system
1. Peptic ulcer (p 108)
2. Malabsorption (p 110)
3. Inflammatory bowel disease (p 115)
4. Carcinoma of the colon (p 119)
5. Chronic liver disease (p 122)
6. Hepatitis B (p 127)
7. Hepatitis C (p 128)
8. Liver transplantation (p 130)

Haematological system
1. Haemolytic anaemia (p 132)
2. Myeloproliferative diseases, e.g. polycythaemia rubra vera (p 141), idiopathic myelofibrosis (p 145) and essential thrombocythaemia (p 145)
3. Lymphomas (p 146)
4. Leukaemia (p 146)
5. Multiple myeloma (p 152)
6. Thrombophilia (p 138)
7. Bone marrow transplant (p 155)

Central nervous system
1. Multiple sclerosis (p 205)
2. Myasthenia gravis (p 208)
3. Guillain-Barré syndrome (p 210)
4. Transient ischaemic attacks and funny turns (p 212)

Rheumatology
1. Rheumatoid arthritis (p 159)
2. Ankylosing spondylitis (p 283)
3. Systemic lupus erythematosus (p 164)
4. Antiphospholipid syndrome (p 173)
5. Scleroderma (p 174)
6. Systemic vasculitis (p 170)

Endocrine system
1. Thyrotoxicosis (p 266)
2. Hypothyroidism (p 267)
3. Panhypopituitarism (p 267)
4. Cushing's syndrome (p 269)
5. Acromegaly (p 272)
6. Addison's disease (p 273)
7. Phaeochromocytoma (p 247)
8. Paget's disease of the bone (p 184)
9. Diabetes mellitus (p 189)
10. Hypercalcaemia (p 182)
11. Osteoporosis (and osteomalacia) (p 177)

Renal system
1. Chronic renal failure (p 196)
2. Renal transplantation (p 204)
3. Nephrotic syndrome (see Table 6.71)

Infectious disease
1. Pyrexia of unknown origin (PUO) (p 215)
2. Human immunodeficiency virus (HIV) infection (p 218)

There have been important changes in the classification of patients with episodes of acute coronary ischaemia. These are based on electrocardiogram (ECG) changes and on the detection of new markers of myocardial damage (troponins), which have prognostic as well as diagnostic usefulness for patients with chest pain. Patients with chest pain and raised troponin levels have had a myocardial infarction even if the creatine kinase level is not elevated. Those who present with chest pain and ECG changes of ST elevation have an ST elevation infarction (STEMI). Those without ST elevation but with abnormal cardiac markers have a non-ST elevation myocardial infarction (non-STEMI). Patients with ST elevation benefit from urgent action to reopen the blocked coronary artery (angioplasty or thrombolytic treatment). Those with non-STEMI are usually treated medically in the first instance. The presence of abnormal cardiac markers indicates an adverse prognosis (increased risk of further infarction or death) and these patients benefit from early but not immediate intervention (angioplasty or coronary surgery) and from immediate aggressive antiplatelet treatment. Non-STEMI patients who have ST depression on the ECG have a worse prognosis than those with T wave inversion or flattening.

The history

1. Find out whether the patient has been or is in hospital because of a recent myocardial infarction or an acute coronary syndrome (unstable angina) or for some other cardiac

or non-cardiac reason. Unstable angina may reasonably be diagnosed in a patient who has experienced the recent onset of angina, a change (for the worse) in the pattern of existing angina or episodes of angina at rest. The most unstable patients are those with chest pain and ECG changes at rest. Clearly, these may represent different pathophysiological states, varying from occlusion of a coronary artery and inadequate collateral flow to rupture of a lipid-rich plaque with thrombus formation. There may be obvious precipitating factors, such as a gastrointestinal bleed or the onset of an arrhythmia. The patient may well know about these events. Questions need to be asked about the character of the chest pain and what precipitated the admission.

Remember that the diagnosis of angina can be suspected from the history but needs to be established by investigations—an abnormal ECG or exercise test at least. One should be suspicious of the diagnosis unless it has been confirmed by investigations. The most common differential diagnosis is gastro-oesophageal reflux disease (GORD). This can be difficult to prove with endoscopy but response to a trial of proton pump inhibitors (PPIs) is very suggestive.

2. The patient's current treatment must be detailed. Oral medications will probably include aspirin, a beta-blocker or calcium antagonist, and nitrates (intravenous, oral or topical). Unstable angina is traditionally managed with heparin and aspirin but additional benefit may be obtained with glycoprotein IIb/IIIa (platelet aggregation) inhibitors in certain subsets of patients (those with resting ECG changes, especially ST depression and those with increased troponin levels). Thrombolytic treatment is probably not effective for unstable angina. This is possibly because unstable angina is not a single pathological entity and also because a state of increased thrombogenesis may follow initial thrombolysis with these drugs.

3. If the patient has had an infarct during this or previous admissions, find out about the management, which may have included primary angioplasty or thrombolysis and treatment of complications such as arrhythmias, cardiac failure, further angina and embolic events.

4. In many hospitals a comprehensive cardiac rehabilitation program will have been offered to the patient. Ask whether this has been helpful, and ask about explanations from hospital staff to the patient about his or her condition and prognosis. Other questions about the effect of this illness on the patient's life and work must be asked.

   Next come standard questions about risk factors in addition to age and male sex:

   - previous ischaemic heart disease
   - hyperlipidaemia
   - diabetes mellitus (the increased risk in these patients is as high as that in non-diabetics who have already had an ischaemic event)
   - hypertension
   - family history (in particular, first-degree relatives with ischaemic heart disease before the age of 60; 92-year-old great-uncles with heart trouble do not count)
   - smoking
   - oral contraceptives or premature menopause
   - obesity and physical inactivity
   - high serum homocysteine levels, which may have been measured if the patient has premature coronary disease and few other risk factors; levels in the top population quintile increase coronary risk twofold; trials of treatment (mostly with folate) are underway
   - the long-term use, in high doses, of the cyclo-oxygenase 2 (COX-2) inhibitors.

   Remember that the presence of multiple risk factors is more than additive.

5. Then find out whether risk factor control has been reasonable. Remember the important results of recent secondary prevention trials. Aggressive cholesterol lowering to below a level of 4 mmol/L of total cholesterol is now considered

appropriate for patients with established coronary disease. There is some evidence that statins have beneficial effects beyond their effect on cholesterol levels (pleomorphic effects).

6. Find out what investigations the patient can remember. An echocardiogram may have been performed to assess ventricular function and possible complications of infarction, such as a pericardial collection, a left ventricular thrombus, mitral regurgitation or a ventricular septal defect (VSD). A gated blood pool scan is sometimes performed to measure left and right ventricular ejection fractions. An exercise test or a sestamibi or thallium scan or a stress echocardiogram may have been performed to assess ischaemia or myocardial viability. Cardiac catheterisation is perhaps the most memorable of the investigations for ischaemic heart disease. The patient may know how many coronaries are abnormal. Complications such as acute mitral regurgitation or an infarct-related VSD are usually treated surgically but have a relatively poor prognosis. All complications are less common if early coronary patency has been achieved.

The examination

Examine the cardiovascular system (p 226). Note the presence of intravenous treatment. This might include heparin, platelet aggregation inhibitors (abciximab or tirofiban), nitrates, inotropes, vasopressors or antiarrhythmic drugs. Record the blood pressure. Look for signs of valvular heart disease, cardiac failure, rhythm disturbances (e.g. atrial fibrillation, frequent ectopic beats) and murmurs suggesting mitral regurgitation or a VSD caused by an infarct. There may be spectacular bruises at venipuncture or femoral puncture sites if the patient has had thrombolytic treatment. Abdominal wall bruising suggests subcutaneous low-molecular-weight heparin therapy, and a bruise (sometimes very large) over one of the femoral arteries suggests cardiac catheterisation or angioplasty. More general complications include a stroke owing to embolism from the heart.

Management

It is best to concentrate on discussing the management of the presenting problem. If the patient has only recently been admitted with an infarct, this means a discussion of thrombolysis and primary angioplasty. Candidates should have some knowledge of the major thrombolysis and angioplasty trials. These have shown that early treatment has improved mortality. Treatment up to 6 hours after the onset of an infarct is worthwhile. Treatment up to 12 hours may be beneficial, especially by angioplasty. The indications and contraindications to the use of these techniques need to be well understood. The major differences between streptokinase and tissue plasminogen activator (tPA or alteplase) are important. Streptokinase is much cheaper than alteplase. Alteplase has been shown to produce a small survival advantage, probably because it is more effective in opening occluded vessels, but it has a slightly increased risk of causing a stroke. Alteplase is the drug of choice for patients who have had a previous dose of streptokinase more than a few days before. This is because antibodies to streptokinase develop within a few days and may cause an allergic reaction to a second dose, thus reducing its effectiveness. This effect lasts at least a year and may persist indefinitely. Reteplase, another thrombolytic drug which is a recombinant plasminogen activator, is given as a double bolus injection with a 30-minute interval.

Urgent coronary angioplasty, if available, is now of proven benefit and has been shown to reduce mortality compared with treatment with thrombolytic drugs. This treatment is being used increasingly in centres equipped to perform it. The advantages, theoretical and real, include definite reopening of the infarct-related artery in over 90% of patients (compared with <60% of patients given thrombolytics), normal flow in the infarct-related artery in most cases, dilatation and stenting of the offending (culprit) lesion as well as removal of clot, very low risk of stroke and shortening of hospital stay, often to only 3 days. Patients are often treated with potent antiplatelet drugs, clopidogrel and one of the platelet aggregation inhibitors. There is now trial evidence that transport of patients to a hospital where this procedure can be performed is preferable to treatment with thrombolytic drugs, if transport times are less than 2–3 hours.

If the history has suggested complications resulting from the infarct, these will have to be discussed. Common complications include:

1. ventricular arrhythmias
2. bradyarrhythmias (especially following an inferior infarct)
3. cardiac failure
4. further ischaemia or reinfarction.

It is important to have planned an approach to the management of these problems.

Investigations

These are aimed at assessment of the infarct size, complications and presence of further ischaemia:

1. left ventricular function—echocardiogram, left ventriculogram, gated blood pool scan
2. complications—echocardiogram for valvular regurgitation, left ventricular thrombus, infarct-related VSD
3. further ischaemia—exercise test, sestamibi stress test, cardiac catheterisation.

Long-term treatment

Early revascularisation is of proven benefit for high-risk patients with acute coronary syndromes (ST elevation, troponin elevation). Prognosis is also improved with aspirin, beta-blockers and, for large infarcts (ejection fraction <40%), angiotensin-converting enzyme (ACE) inhibitors. Carvedilol has been shown to improve prognosis for patients with large infarcts and is probably the beta-blocker of choice for them. Patients with three-vessel disease and significant left ventricular damage or with left main coronary artery stenosis benefit from coronary artery bypass surgery even if their symptoms have settled on medical treatment. Those with tight proximal (before the first diagonal branch) left anterior descending lesions probably also benefit from surgery or angioplasty.

Secondary prevention

Control of cardiac risk factors is even more important once the presence of coronary artery disease has been established. It should be a routine part of the management of these patients. Dietary advice for weight and lipid reduction may be indicated. Lipid-lowering drug treatment should be introduced for patients with a total cholesterol level of 4.0 mmol/L or more. Patients should be encouraged to take part in a cardiac rehabilitation program if this is available. Here, advice about safe exercise, weight reduction and changes to dietary and smoking habits can be encouraged.

Revascularisation

For some long-case patients with ischaemic heart disease the emphasis will be on revascularisation (coronary surgery or angioplasty). These procedures are so common that many patients with other presenting problems will have had them.

The history

Similar information to that outlined in the ischaemic heart disease long case is required.

1. Careful questioning about risk factor control, both before and after surgery or angioplasty, is very important. The patient should know whether he or she has ever had an infarct, and may know whether there was significant left ventricular damage.
2. Find out what procedure (or procedures) the patient has had and whether there has been complete relief of symptoms.
3. If coronary artery surgery was performed, ask how many grafts were inserted and whether internal mammary or other arterial (e.g. radial artery) conduits were used. It may be possible from the history to work out whether surgery was performed to improve symptoms or prognosis, or both.
4. The patient will probably know how many vessels were dilated if angioplasty was performed, and whether stents were inserted. Ask whether the angioplasty was performed in the setting of a myocardial infarction.

The examination

Examine the patient as for the ischaemic heart disease long case. Note the presence of a median-sternotomy scar. Patients who have had a left internal mammary artery graft often have a numb patch to the left of the sternum. This may be permanent. Look at the sternal wound for signs of infection; osteomyelitis of the sternum is a rare but disastrous complication of surgery. Look and feel for sternal instability. Sternal wires are often palpable. Examine the arms for the very large scar that results from radial artery harvesting. Examine the legs for saphenous vein harvesting wounds. Infection and breakdown of these wounds is more common than in the sternal wound.

Management

Surgery

Use of the left internal mammary artery (LIMA) to graft the left anterior descending (LAD) coronary artery has been routine for 15 years. Other arterial conduits are less often used, but 'all arterial revascularisation' is performed routinely in some centres or where saphenous vein grafts (SVGs) are not possible (previous coronary artery bypass graft [CABG] or varicose veins in both legs and thighs). In these cases the right internal mammary artery (RIMA) may be used, usually to graft the right coronary, or the radial artery is used as a free arterial graft. The RIMA may also be used as a free graft attached to the aorta if that is necessary to make it reach.

There is excellent evidence that LIMA grafts have a higher long-term patency rate (>90% at 10 years) than SVGs (50% at 10 years). There is less information about other arterial conduits.

In response to the increasing numbers of angioplasty procedures surgeons, have begun to perform less invasive bypass procedures. The most widely used is the 'off-pump' LIMA graft to the LAD coronary artery. A median sternotomy incision is still used but the LIMA is attached to the LAD coronary artery on the beating heart. This avoids the need for cardiopulmonary bypass, speeds recovery and possibly reduces the risk of intraoperative cerebral events. Minimally invasive bypasses are carried out in some centres. Here a series of lateral chest incisions are used as ports for surgery using thoracoscopic equipment. The technique is not easy and the chest wound, although small, is not necessarily less painful than a median sternotomy.

Angina may recur at any time after CABG. Very early angina suggests a technical problem, such as mammary artery spasm, thrombosis of an SVG or grafting of the wrong vessel, or grafting of the correct vessel but proximal to the area of stenosis. Sometimes revascularisation may be 'incomplete' because one or more vessels were unsuitable for grafting—usually because of distal disease in the target vessel.

Recurrence of angina is more common if risk factors have not been aggressively controlled. Low-dose aspirin has also been shown to prolong graft survival. When angina recurs the patient usually describes symptoms similar in character to the old ones. Recurrent chest pain that is different from the old angina is less likely to be ischaemic.

Angioplasty

Angioplasty is now performed more often than surgery in many centres. Unequivocal evidence that it improves the prognosis for patients with stable angina is not available. A number of studies have shown a similar outcome to surgery in patients with three-vessel disease but at the expense of a higher number of repeat procedures. Diabetics were a subgroup with a worse outcome from angioplasty than from surgery. Many angioplasties are performed to provide symptom relief for patients with one- or two-vessel disease. Increasingly, however, patients with acute coronary syndromes and especially those with raised troponin levels are treated with early angioplasty. There is now good evidence that this group of patients has an improved prognosis (fewer deaths and fewer large infarcts) and a shortened hospital stay when treated aggressively with angioplasty.

The majority (>80%) of dilated vessels are now stented. This has made a considerable difference to the risk of acute closure of the artery or the need for urgent surgery (now a rare event). It has also reduced the clinical restenosis rate (i.e. recurrence of symptoms and angiographic evidence of >50% loss of luminal diameter) from almost 40% to 10%.

Aggressive anticoagulation regimens with heparin then warfarin, previously used after stenting, have been replaced with antiplatelet treatment with aspirin and clopidogrel. These drugs have made subacute stent thrombosis a rare event (<1%). The drug is ideally given for 48 hours before angioplasty and for at least 4 weeks afterwards.

When a dilated vessel seems threatened with closure because of a dissection that cannot be stented or because of the presence of a large amount of thrombus, the potent platelet aggregation inhibitor abciximab (a receptor antibody) may be used as a bolus, followed by infusion for some hours. This drug is very effective in preventing closure of the vessel but is also expensive. Abciximab and tirofiban (which is a small molecule platelet aggregation inhibitor) are very valuable drugs for the management of acute coronary syndromes with angioplasty. Tirofiban has a shorter half-life than abciximab but should be used for at least 24–48 hours before intervention unless started in the catheter laboratory with a double bolus dose.

Primary angioplasty of the infarct-related artery is increasingly used in the treatment of STEMI as an alternative to treatment with thrombolytic drugs, and results in a lower mortality and shortened hospital stay when performed in experienced centres.

The 'open artery hypothesis' suggests that having a patent artery after an infarct is an advantage (possibly because of its effects on remodelling). For this reason occluded arteries may be opened and dilated even late after an infarct, especially if the patient has evidence of persisting ischaemia. Occluded arteries become very difficult to reopen after a few months.

Restenosis remains a problem after angioplasty. It is very unusual after 6 months. It is more common in diabetics, in calcified and complex and long lesions, and in dilated vein grafts. A combination of these factors can result in a restenosis rate of over 60%. Treatment until recently has involved redilatation, which is not very successful, or intra-coronary irradiation.

Drug-eluting stents are now available and appear to have reduced dramatically the incidence of restenosis. The currently available stents have either paclitaxel or sirolimus bound via a polymer to the metal surface of the stent. These antineoplastic drugs are eluted for about a month and prevent the migration of smooth muscle cells into the lumen of the vessel that is the cause of restenosis. Very low restenosis rates of a few per cent have been obtained in trials, even when diabetics are included. They also seem to be effective in preventing further restenosis when used in a restenosed 'bare metal' stent. These stents are very expensive—five to six times the cost of a bare metal stent.

The delayed healing caused by these drugs has been associated with late stent thrombosis. As a result, antiplatelet treatment with aspirin and clopidogrel should be continued for at least 6 months.

Infective endocarditis

As patients with infective endocarditis stay in hospital for weeks, they are often available for long cases. The disease presents diagnostic, plus short-term and long-term management problems. Cases combine cardiological, microbiological and immunological problems. The diagnosis is usually known to the patient. An intravenous infusion containing antibiotics is a valuable clue.

The history

Ask about:

1. details of presenting symptoms (e.g. malaise, fever, symptoms of anaemia)
2. symptoms suggesting embolic phenomena to large vessels (e.g. brain, viscera) or small vessels (e.g. kidney, with haematuria or loin pain)
3. recent dental or operative procedures—a precipitating event is only identified in about 5% of cases; the time between procedure and diagnosis may be up to 3 months
4. use of antibiotics for prophylaxis, either before an invasive procedure or for rheumatic fever, or both
5. a past history of rheumatic fever
6. a history of other heart disease or heart operations, especially of valve replacement
7. a history of intravenous drug abuse, particularly for its association with tricuspid and pulmonary valve infection
8. antibiotic allergies
9. how the diagnosis was made—including the number of blood cultures, and the use of transthoracic or transoesophageal echocardiography
10. management since admission to hospital, including the names of the antibiotics used, the duration of treatment, and whether the possibility of valve replacement has been discussed
11. a history of other major diseases, particularly those associated with immune suppression, such as renal transplantation, or steroid use.

The examination

Start by examining for the peripheral stigmata of endocarditis.

1. Hands:
   (a) clubbing (a late sign)
   (b) splinter haemorrhages
   (c) Osler's nodes on the finger pulp (probably an embolic phenomenon—these are rare)
   (d) Janeway lesions (non-tender erythematous maculopapular lesions containing bacteria, on the palms or pulps—very rare).
2. Eyes: Roth's spots in the fundus, conjunctival petechiae.
3. Abdomen: splenomegaly (a late sign).
4. Urine analysis for haematuria and proteinuria.
5. Neurological signs of embolic disease.
6. Joints (occasionally resembles rheumatic fever pattern).

Next examine the heart. Assess for predisposing cardiac lesions. These are, in order:

1. Acquired:
   (a) prosthetic valve (mechanical)
   (b) mitral regurgitation, mitral stenosis

(c)   aortic stenosis
(d)   aortic regurgitation
(e)   prosthetic valve (tissue)
(f)   repaired mitral valve
(g)   mitral valve prolapse with mitral regurgitation.
2. Congenital:
(a)   bicuspid aortic valve
(b)   patent ductus arteriosus
(c)   ventricular septal defect
(d)   coarctation of the aorta.

Note: Remember, an atrial septal defect of the secundum type is almost never affected. Twenty per cent of endocarditis patients have no recognised underlying cardiac abnormality. Coronary stents and pacemaker leads do not appear to involve any risk of endocarditis.

Examine for the signs of cardiac failure. Look for signs of a prosthetic valve (see Table 8.4) and for scars that may be present from previous valvotomy or repair operations. Look for a source of infection and take the patient's temperature.

Investigations

1. Three to six blood cultures (at least) over 24 hours (98% of culture-positive cases will give positive results in the first three bottles).
2. Full blood count and erythrocyte sedimentation rate (ESR). Look for anaemia (normochromic, normocytic), neutrophilia, an elevated ESR, which may be >100 mm/h, and a raised C-reactive protein (CRP). The ESR tends to remain elevated for months, even when treatment has been successful, but the CRP level falls quite quickly and may be useful for assessing the effectiveness of treatment.
3. Renal function. A freshly spun urine sample will often show red cell casts.
4. Chest X-ray film. Look for left or right ventricular hypertrophy, increased pulmonary artery markings, Kerley's B lines, frank cardiac failure and valve calcification (lateral film).
5. ECG. Atrial fibrillation in the elderly (particularly common) and conduction defects may occur but are not specific.
6. Echocardiography (Fig 6.1) (2D and Doppler). Vegetations must be larger than 2 mm to be detected. This procedure cannot distinguish active from inactive lesions. Vegetations are seen in approximately 40% of cases. They tend to occur downstream of the abnormal jet (e.g. on the aortic surface of the aortic valve in cases of aortic stenosis and endocarditis). Colour Doppler examination is a very sensitive means of detecting new valvular regurgitation, which may be an important sign of endocarditis. Transoesophageal echocardiography (TOE) allows better definition of valvular involvement. It is more likely to detect vegetations. Perhaps more importantly, it is much more likely to detect such complications as valve abscesses. It is now in routine use for the assessment of endocarditis.
7. Serological tests. These include tests for immune complexes, and classical pathway activation of complement causing low C3, C4 and CH50 levels. The test for rheumatoid factor gives positive results in 50% of cases and that for antinuclear antibody in 20% of cases.

Notes

Organisms
Streptococci account for approximately half of these infections.

1. *Streptococcus viridans* (non-haemolytic)—usually presents subacutely. The names of the viridans streptococci are subject to frequent revision but current important types for endocarditis include: *Strep. sanguinis*, *Strep. gordonii* and *Strep. mitis*.

Figure 6.1 Echocardiography report in a patient with possible infective endocarditis.

Echocardiography Report

Reason for study
AR ?; endocarditis

Study quality: Good   Satisfactory   Poor

RV	18	(mm) (N 10–26)
Sept.	10	(mm) (N 7–11)
LVEDD	68	(mm) (N 36–56)
LVESD	42	(mm) (N 20–40)
LVPW	10	(mm) (N 7–11)
Aorta	34	(mm) (N 20–35)
LA	36	(mm) (N 24–40)
FS	38	% (N 27–40)
EF	67	% (N 55–70)

Valves

Mitral	Mild MR
Tricus.	Mild TR
Aortic	Thickened, bicuspid
Pulm.	Appears normal

Doppler—2D
The left ventricle is dilated. The fractional shortening is in the normal range. The aortic valve is thickened and probably bicuspid. A mobile mass 2 mm in diameter is visible on the LV side of the valve and represents a probable vegetation.

Doppler—colour flow mapping
There is no aortic gradient. A large jet of aortic regurgitation is present, extending three-quarters of the way into the LV cavity. Mild-to-moderate MR is present. Mild TR. RV pressure = 28 mmHg.

Conclusions
Severe AR, probable vegetation, bicuspid valve.

Comment
The diagnosis of endocarditis cannot really be made on the basis of echocardiography alone. Even what appears to be a vegetation may be sterile. Nevertheless, a mobile mass attached to a valve in a patient with positive blood cultures makes the diagnosis of endocarditis almost certain.

An abnormal echocardiogram adds weight to the diagnosis. It also enables detection of left ventricular enlargement, which suggests haemodynamic compromise. Serial echocardiograms allow assessment of the treatment of endocarditis and help with the decision about the timing of possible surgery.

The underlying valve abnormality may be obvious. Here the aortic valve is congenitally bicuspid.

More detailed analysis of the heart is possible with transoesophageal echocardiography, which is now routine in cases of endocarditis. It enables smaller vegetations to be identified, as well as complications such as valve ring abscesses.

(cont.)

Figure 6.1 Echocardiography report for a patient with possible infective endocarditis (cont.).

Key

AR = aortic regurgitation; EF = ejection fraction; FS = fractional shortening; LA = left atrium; LVEDD = left ventricular end-diastolic dimension; LVESD = left ventricular end-systolic dimension; LVPW = left ventricular posterior wall; MR = mitral regurgitation; Pulm. = pulmonary; RV = right ventricle; Sept. = septal thickness; TR = tricuspid regurgitation; Tricus. = tricuspid.

---

2. *Streptococcus faecalis*—traditionally more common in older men with prostatism and younger women with urinary tract infections but now in intravenous drug users.
3. *Streptococcus bovis*—associated with bowel polyps and carcinoma.
4. *Staphylococcus aureus*—particularly in drug addicts; usually presents acutely. Note, though, that only a small minority of *Staph. aureus* bacteraemias are associated with endocarditis.
5. *Staphylococcus epidermidis*—more common in patients with recent valve replacement but can also be a contaminant in blood cultures.
6. Gram-negative coccobacilli—rarely a cause; more common with prosthetic valves. The responsible organisms are called the HACEK group: *Haemophilus, Actinobacillus, Cariobacterium hominis, Eikonella* spp. and *Kingella kingae.*
7. Fungi (e.g. *Candida, Aspergillus*)—particularly in drug addicts and immunosuppressed patients.

Causes of culture-negative endocarditis

Note: This diagnosis should be made with caution. It condemns a patient to prolonged treatment with intravenous antibiotics.

1. Previous use of antibiotics.
2. Exotic organisms (e.g. *Haemophilus parainfluenzae*, histoplasmosis, *Brucella, Candida,* Q fever).
3. Right-sided endocarditis (rarely).

Post-valve surgery endocarditis

Early infection is acquired at operation; late infection occurs from another source. This condition has a worse prognosis than native valve endocarditis.

Diagnosis

The diagnosis is usually a clinical one. The Duke criteria are often used to assist. Two major criteria, one major and three minor, or five minor criteria secure the diagnosis.

Major criteria

1. Typical organisms in two separate blood cultures.
2. Evidence of endocardial involvement: echocardiogram showing a mobile intracardiac mass on a valve or in the path of a regurgitant jet, or an abscess or new valvular regurgitation.

Minor criteria

1. Predisposing cardiac condition or intravenous drug use
2. Fever
3. Vascular phenomena or stigmata
4. Serological or acute phase abnormalities
5. Echocardiogram abnormal but not meeting above criteria

Treatment

Early involvement in the management by a cardiac surgeon in a cardiac surgical unit is usually indicated, particularly for staphylococcal infection.

1. Intravenous administration of a bactericidal antibiotic. If the organism is a sensitive *Strep. viridans*, give benzylpenicillin, 6–12 g daily for 4–6 weeks. If it is an enterococcus, at least 4 weeks of intravenous treatment are necessary, and the choice of antibiotic depends on the organism's sensitivity. For prosthetic valves, 6–8 weeks of intravenous treatment is necessary.
2. Follow the progress by looking at the temperature chart, serological results and haemoglobin values.
3. The decision to go on to valve replacement is a difficult one; it is best made with the assistance of a cardiac surgeon who has been involved from the start. Indications for surgery include:
   (a) resistant organisms (e.g. fungi)
   (b) valvular dysfunction causing moderate-to-severe cardiac failure (e.g. acute severe aortic regurgitation)
   (c) persistently positive blood cultures in spite of treatment
   (d) invasive paravalvular infection causing conduction disturbances, or a paravalvular abscess or fistula (detected by echocardiography)
   (e) recurrent major embolic phenomena, although this is controversial (an isolated vegetation is not in itself an indication for surgery).

Factors suggesting a poorer prognosis

1. Shock
2. Congestive cardiac failure
3. Extreme age
4. Aortic valve or multiple valve involvement
5. Multiple organisms
6. Culture-negative endocarditis
7. Delay in starting treatment
8. Prosthetic valve involvement
9. Staphylococcal, Gram-negative and fungal infections

Differential diagnosis

1. Atrial myxoma
2. Occult malignant neoplasm
3. Systemic lupus erythematosus
4. Polyarteritis nodosa
5. Post-streptococcal glomerulonephritis
6. Pyrexia of unknown origin
7. Cardiac thrombus

Prognosis

Prior to antibiotic use, this was an invariably fatal disease. Over 70% of patients with endogenous infection now survive, as do 50% of those with a prosthetic valve infection. Intravenous drug users have a good prognosis.

Prophylaxis

Confusion about rheumatic fever and endocarditis prophylaxis is rife. Rheumatic fever prophylaxis consists of long-term, low-dose antibiotic administration. Prophylaxis against endocarditis requires high-dose, short-term treatment in any patient with a prosthetic heart valve, congenital heart malformation (except for uncomplicated atrial septal defect), acquired valve disease, surgically constructed pulmonary shunt, hypertrophic cardiomyopathy, or a past history of endocarditis.

Prophylaxis regimens are as follows (recommendations from *Therapeutic Guidelines— Antibiotic*):

1. *Dental procedures* (e.g. gum cleaning) or oral surgery—amoxycillin 2 g 1 hour before the procedure. For patients unable to take oral antibiotics, ampicillin IV or IM just before the procedure. If the risk is high (e.g. a prosthetic valve), give ampicillin and gentamicin as described below. For those allergic to penicillin, clindamycin 600 mg, given orally 1 hour before the procedure is adequate.
2. *Enterococcal risk* (e.g. cystoscopy)—ampicillin 2 g plus gentamicin 2 mg/kg IM or IV half an hour before the procedure, and amoxycillin 0.5 g orally 6 hours later. For those allergic to penicillin, vancomycin 1 g IV plus gentamicin is adequate.

Remember that the effectiveness of antibiotic prophylaxis has not been proven. Patients also need to be reminded of the need for good dental hygiene and regular dental review.

Congestive cardiac failure

This is a common therapeutic problem. It may be a diagnostic problem. It is uncommonly the only major problem in a long case in the examination.

The history

1. It is important first to find out what may have precipitated episodes of cardiac failure. Precipitating problems include:
   (a) arrhythmias (especially atrial fibrillation)
   (b) discontinuation of medications (particularly important)
   (c) myocardial infarction
   (d) anaemia
   (e) infection and fever
   (f) the introduction of negatively inotropic drugs (e.g. beta-blockers—this may even include beta-blocker eye drops used for glaucoma)
   (g) thyrotoxicosis
   (h) anaesthesia and surgery
   (i) pulmonary embolism
   (j) high salt intake, drugs that cause salt and water retention (e.g. traditional non-steroidal anti-inflammatory drugs [NSAIDs], COX-2 inhibitors), or excessive physical exertion
   (k) pregnancy.
   Note: Chronic lung disease can be a cause of, or a precipitating factor for, right and left ventricular failure.
2. Then ask about the symptoms of left ventricular failure (e.g. dyspnoea, orthopnoea, paroxysmal nocturnal dyspnoea) and right ventricular failure (e.g. oedema, ascites, anorexia and nausea). Ask about symptoms of ischaemic heart disease (e.g. angina). These may help distinguish dyspnoea caused by lung disease from that caused by cardiac failure.
3. History of previous heart disease:
   (a) hypertension
   (b) ischaemic heart disease—infarcts, angina
   (c) rheumatic or other valve disease
   (d) congenital heart disease
   (e) cardiomyopathy

  (f) previous cardiac surgery (e.g. coronary artery bypass grafting, valve replacement or resection of an aneurysm)

  (g) cardiac transplantation.

4. Coronary risk factors, in addition to age and male sex, including:

  (a) hyperlipidaemia

  (b) hypertension

  (c) smoking

  (d) diabetes mellitus

  (e) family history of early coronary heart disease

  (f) oral contraceptives or premature menopause

  (g) obesity

  (h) physical inactivity.

5. Risk factors for dilated cardiomyopathy:

  (a) excessive alcohol intake

  (b) family history of cardiomyopathy

  (c) haemochromatosis.

6. Medications currently taken.

7. Investigations undertaken—particularly echocardiography, stress ECG testing, nuclear studies and cardiac catheterisation.

8. How the disease affects the patient's life and ability to cope at home (e.g. climbing stairs, sexual difficulties etc.). Remember to classify the patient according to the New York Heart Association (NYHA) guidelines:

  I Patients have disease but are asymptomatic

  II angina/dyspnoea on moderate activity

  III angina/dyspnoea on mild activity

  IV angina/dyspnoea at rest.

The examination

Perform a detailed cardiovascular system examination. Note wasting as a result of cardiac cachexia. Look particularly for signs of cardiac failure, the underlying causes of the problem, and any precipitating factors. Take the blood pressure lying and standing. Treatment with ACE inhibitors and beta-blockers often results in mild hypotension.

Investigations

1. Chest X-ray film. Look for cardiomegaly and chamber size (e.g. left atrium), cardiac aneurysm, valve calcification, sternal wires suggesting previous cardiac surgery, signs of lung disease and pulmonary congestion.

2. ECG. Look for arrhythmias, signs of ischaemia or recent or old infarction (see Fig 6.2), left ventricular hypertrophy and persisting ST elevation (aneurysm). Left bundle branch block is a common ECG finding in these patients (see Fig 6.3).

3. Electrolytes and creatinine levels to exclude hypokalaemia (as a cause of arrhythmia), hyponatraemia (which may indicate severe longstanding cardiac failure, a poor prognostic sign) and renal failure. Measure B-type natriuretic peptide (BNP, previously called brain natriuretic peptide). Although there is doubt about the reference range, a definitely elevated level may help distinguish cardiac from non-cardiac dyspnoea. Since BNP falls when heart failure is treated, trials of monitoring BNP are underway as a means of assessing the adequacy of cardiac treatment.

4. Haemoglobin value. Exclude anaemia as a precipitating cause.

5. If the diagnosis is not already obvious, consider dilated cardiomyopathy. Investigations for this include the following:

Figure 6.2 Sinus rhythm. There are Q waves from V1 to V5. This is diagnostic of an extensive old anterior infarct, which is likely to be the cause of this patient's heart failure.

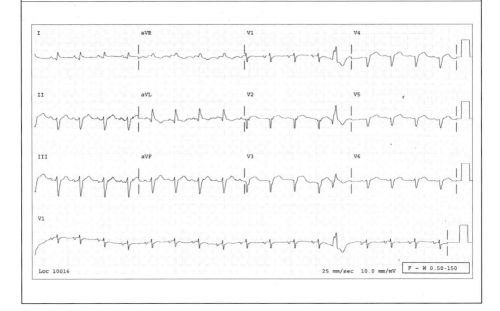

Figure 6.3 Sinus rhythm. Left bundle branch block (LBBB). The QRS complexes may widen further as heart failure progresses. LBBB is a common finding in heart failure but is not diagnostic.

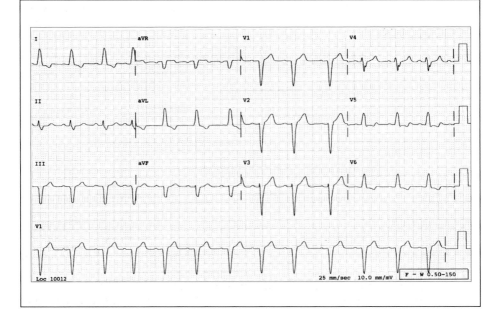

(a) Echocardiography (Fig 6.4). This will show generalised or segmental wall motion abnormalities and reduced fractional shortening. An estimate of left ventricular ejection fraction can be made. Segmental hypokinesia suggests that ischaemia is the cause of the cardiac failure. Doppler echocardiography will usually show at least some mitral and tricuspid regurgitation in these patients. The presence of more severe valvular disease suggests a different aetiology for the cardiac failure. Serial echocardiograph measurements of left and right ventricular dimensions can be useful for following the patient's progress.

(b) A gated blood pool scan for the ejection fraction. The right ventricular ejection fraction is normally >45% and the left ventricular ejection fraction is >50%. The scan will also show whether hypokinesis is global or segmental, and to what extent the right ventricle is affected.

(c) Coronary angiography. This is often necessary to exclude coronary artery disease.

(d) Right ventricular biopsy. This may help determine the aetiology in selected patients.

Treatment

1. Remove precipitating causes. Atrial fibrillation and other incessant tachycardias can be a cause of cardiac failure—tachycardia-induced cardiomyopathy. The prognosis is good if normal heart rates can be restored.

2. Correct underlying causes if possible (e.g. thrombolysis for an acute infarct, or coronary artery bypass grafting or angioplasty for ischaemia) (Table 6.2).

3. Control the failure.

(a) Decrease physical activity (e.g. avoid exertion to the point of breathlessness, bed rest).

(b) Control fluid retention (e.g. by diuretics, low-salt diet, fluid restriction [1000–1500 mL for severe failure]).

(c) Reduce preload and afterload. ACE inhibitors are considered to be the drug class of choice for cardiac failure as they prolong life; symptomatic hypotension is the major side-effect in cardiac failure. ACE inhibitors are indicated for all classes of heart failure, even for asymptomatic patients with left ventricular dysfunction. There is some controversy about the appropriate doses of these drugs. The doses used in clinical trials (e.g. 50 mg tds of captopril) are higher than those achieved in usual clinical practice. Every effort should be made to titrate the dose up to the maximum tolerated. The usual limitation is symptomatic hypotension.

Long-acting nitrates are useful venodilators. The combination of nitrates and hydralazine also improves the prognosis and should be considered in patients unable to take ACE inhibitors.

The most common reasons for the cessation of ACE inhibitors are cough and deterioration in renal function (usually in patients with renovascular disease). Renal function may improve again if the ACE inhibitor and diuretic doses are reduced and hypovolaemia is corrected. There is little therapeutic difference between the various ACE inhibitors.

The angiotensin-receptor (AR) blocking drugs are a newer class of anti-hypertensives. Their usefulness in heart failure has now been demonstrated in a number of clinical trials. They should be second-line treatment for patients intolerant of ACE inhibitors because of cough. They are associated with a very low incidence of cough but are as likely to cause renal impairment as the ACE inhibitors. Trials have also demonstrated some additional benefit when ACE inhibitors and AR blockers are combined. The treatment of cardiac failure involves polypharmacy. It is probably only the minority of patients who will be prepared to take an AR blocker as well as all the other

Figure 6.4 Echocardiography report in a patient with cardiac failure caused by anterior myocardial infarction.

Echocardiography Report

Reason for study

Assess left ventricular function, cardiac failure

Study quality: Good   Satisfactory   Poor

RV   13   (mm) (N 10–26)

Sept.   8   (mm) (N 7–11)

LVEDD   66   (mm) (N 36–56)

LVESD   49   (mm) (N 20–40)

LVPW   10   (mm) (N 7–11)

Aorta   22   (mm) (N 20–35)

LA   36   (mm) (N 24–40)

FS   26   % (N 27–40)

EF   50   % (N 55–70)

Valves

    Mitral   Mild-to-moderate MR

    Tricus. Mild TR

    Aortic   Thickened, not stenosed

    Pulm.   Appears normal

Doppler—2D

The left ventricle is dilated. There is extensive antero-apical hypokinesis.

    The aortic valve is slightly thickened and there is mitral annular calcification. The mitral valve is not stenosed and there is no mitral valve prolapse.

Doppler—colour flow mapping

There is no aortic gradient, mild-to-moderate MR is present. MR jet to two-thirds of LA. Mild TR. RV pressure = 38 mmHg.

Conclusions

Severe segmental LV dysfunction, moderate MR.

Comments

This echocardiography report demonstrates the typical findings when a patient has cardiac failure caused by previous anterior myocardial infarction. The left ventricular dysfunction is not global (typical of cardiomyopathy) but involves the infarcted area. There is overall LV dilatation with an increase of the LVEDD. The FS is the percentage change in LV size from diastole to systole measured at the base of the heart. It can be in the normal range despite the presence of LV dysfunction, if the base of the heart is not involved.

    The ejection fraction can be estimated from the LVEDD and LVESD measurements. There are a number of formulas, which are applied automatically by the calculation software of the echocardiograph machine. It is difficult to obtain an accurate ejection fraction, which is a volume change measurement on the basis of two 2D image measurements. These calculated ejection fractions tend to have a higher reference range than those obtained by nuclear heart pool scanning. MR is almost always detected when moderate LV dysfunction is present.

Mitral annular calcification is a common finding in elderly patients; it can be associated with MR but not with mitral stenosis. The presence of left atrial enlargement suggests that the mitral regurgitation is not acute but can also be associated with hypertension.

TR is commonly found in patients with heart failure but may also be present in normal people. Interrogation of the regurgitant jet with continuous wave (CW) Doppler allows measurement of its velocity. This can be used to calculate the pressure difference across the valve. Since the pressure in the right atrium is usually close to 5 mmHg, the pressure in the RV can be calculated by adding 5 to the pressure difference. In this case the pressure difference across the valve is about 33 mmHg.

Key

EF = ejection fraction; FS = fractional shortening; LA = left atrium; LVEDD = left ventricular end-diastolic dimension; LVESD = left ventricular end-systolic dimension; LVPW = left ventricular posterior wall; MR = mitral regurgitation; Pulm. = pulmonary; RV = right ventricle; Sept. = septal thickness; TR = tricuspid regurgitation; Tricus. = tricuspid.

drugs usually prescribed. Questions to the patient about the difficulties of compliance with a complicated drug regimen may be useful at this point.

(d) Increase myocardial contractility (e.g. with digoxin).

  Note: The use of digoxin in cardiac failure is no longer controversial. Recent trials have suggested an increase in symptoms if cardiac failure patients who are in sinus rhythm and on treatment with digoxin, diuretics and ACE inhibitors have their digoxin withdrawn. Digoxin mortality trials have shown no difference in mortality but definite improvement in symptoms (when used in combination with a diuretic and ACE inhibitor). Patients most likely to benefit have more severe heart failure, an S3 gallop, impressive cardiomegaly and an ejection fraction <20%.

(e) Give beta-blockers. Trials with carvedilol, a non–cardioselective beta-blocker and vasodilator, have shown improvements in symptoms and mortality for this drug used in patients with classes II–IV heart failure. The drug is usually surprisingly well tolerated but must be introduced at a low dose (e.g. 3.125 or 6.25 mg bd) and titrated upwards as tolerated to 25 mg bd. Patients may initially feel worse as catecholamine support to the heart is blocked. More recent trials with metoprolol (Carvedilol or Metoprolol European Trial [COMET]) suggest slight superiority for carvedilol over metoprolol. Bisoprolol is a cardioselective beta-blocker. It is also of proven benefit for cardiac failure and available in a once daily preparation.

(f) Spironolactone in a small dose of 12.5 mg a day has been shown to be an additional effective drug in the treatment of chronic heart failure.

(g) Intravenous inotropes (e.g. dopamine or dobutamine) may have a place in the short-term treatment of severe cardiac failure. Patients may be admitted for a 'dobutamine holiday' and have improved symptoms for some months. Levosimendan is a promising new intravenous drug that works as a calcium channel activator. A 24-hour course may improve symptoms and possibly prognosis. No effective oral inotrope is yet available. Trials of previous drugs have been associated with an increased mortality.

Table 6.2   Causes of ventricular failure

Left ventricular failure
1. Volume overload
    (a) Aortic regurgitation
    (b) Mitral regurgitation
    (c) Patent ductus arteriosus
2. Pressure overload
    (a) Systemic hypertension
    (b) Aortic stenosis
3. Myocardial disease
    (a) Ischaemic heart disease
    (b) Dilated cardiomyopathy—causes include:
        (i)   Idiopathic (most common)
        (ii)   Alcohol
        (iii) Myocarditis
        (iv)   Familial (autosomal dominant)
        (v)   Peripartum
        (vi)   Neuromuscular disease (e.g. dystrophia myotonica)
        (vii) Connective tissue disease (e.g. scleroderma)
        (viii) Haemochromatosis
        (ix)   Sarcoidosis
        (x)   Drugs (e.g. doxorubicin)
        (xi)   Radiation
        (xii) Diabetes mellitus

Note: Restrictive cardiomyopathy and hypertrophic cardiomyopathy can be causes of heart failure also.

Right ventricular failure
1. Volume overload
    (a) Atrial septal defect
    (b) Tricuspid regurgitation
2. Pressure overload
    (a) Pulmonary stenosis
    (b) Pulmonary hypertension
3. Myocardial disease
    (a) Cardiomyopathy secondary to left ventricular failure
    (b) Right ventricular infarction (rare)

(h) Rhythm control. Remember, cardiac failure has a poor prognosis. About 50% of these patients die suddenly of a ventricular arrhythmia. There may be an improvement in survival in at least selected patients with the use of amio-darone. The detection of high-grade ventricular arrhythmias is an indication for an implanted defibrillator. This is associated with a proven improvement in prognosis. Routine use of these devices in patients with a low ejection fraction has been shown to improve survival even when ventricular arrhythmias have not been recorded.

(i) Cardiac transplantation may now be offered to certain patients. The reduced availability of donor hearts and the improvement of many patients who would otherwise be suitable for transplant with beta-blockers has reduced the frequency of this procedure.

(j)   Ventricular assist devices are sometimes used as a bridge to transplant in very ill patients. Survival for weeks or months is possible with these devices. Trials of entirely artificial hearts continue in small numbers of patients.

(k)   Biventricular pacing or cardiac resynchronisation may be helpful for heart failure patients with very wide QRS complexes. The LV pacing wire is placed via the coronary sinus into one of the left ventricular veins. This complicated procedure enables both ventricles to be paced and asynchronous contraction of the ventricles associated with a very wide QRS to be corrected.

Diastolic heart failure

Most breathless patients with heart failure have abnormal left ventricular systolic function, which is characterised by dilatation and hypokinesis. Some cardiac failure, however, may be caused by diastolic dysfunction. In such cases, the myocardium is stiff, often because it is hypertrophied, and does not relax normally. The condition seems to be more common in elderly patients. Hypertension is a common cause. The diagnosis is difficult but an echocardiogram will show preserved or increased systolic contraction without dilatation and there may be left ventricular hypertrophy. Doppler echocardiography may show abnormalities of left ventricular filling caused by the stiffness of the ventricle. However, this is not easy to quantify and is very dependent on variations in preload and afterload.

The condition has probably a better prognosis than systolic heart failure. Treatment is similar but verapamil and beta-blockers are used early and only small doses of diuretics should be required. At least in theory, digoxin should be avoided if the patient is in sinus rhythm. Every effort should be made to control hypertension.

Hyperlipidaemia

Hyperlipidaemia may be present in patients under investigation for vascular disease, pancreatitis, hypothyroidism or diabetes mellitus. It often presents both diagnostic and management problems.

The history

1.   The patient should be able to indicate whether the main problem is vascular or not. If the problem is one of premature coronary artery disease, hypercholesterolaemia is the likely lipid problem. The most important inherited cause is *familial hypercholesterolaemia*, which is caused by a defective or absent low-density lipoprotein (LDL) receptor. The heterozygous form occurs in about one person in 500. As the transmission is autosomal dominant, the patient may know of first-degree relatives who have been affected. There may even be family members with the homozygous form. These people usually present with a tenfold elevation in serum cholesterol levels as a result of an increase in plasma LDL levels, and have a myocardial infarction before the age of 20 years. People with the heterozygous form typically have myocardial infarctions in their 30s and 40s and have a twofold to threefold elevation in cholesterol level. Over 80% of affected men and nearly 60% of affected women have had myocardial infarcts by the age of 60 years. Find out whether the patient has already had a myocardial infarct and which of his or her relatives has been affected.

Familial combined hyperlipidaemia is associated with obesity or glucose intolerance and may be expressed as type IIa, IIb or IV hyperlipidaemia (Table 6.3). This is also an autosomal dominant trait. Patients develop hypercholesterolaemia and often hypertriglyceridaemia in puberty. Once again, there usually is a strong family history of premature coronary artery disease. There is no doubt that an elevated triglyceride level adds to the risk of hypercholesterolaemia.

Table 6.3 Hyperlipoproteinaemias

Type	Lipoprotein elevated	Electrophoretic mobility	Mechanism	Secondary causes	Clinical features	Associations
I	Chylomicrons	Origin	Deficiency Extrahepatic lipoprotein lipase or apo C-II deficiency	Rarely SLE	Eruptive xanthomata; lipaemia retinalis	Pancreatitis
IIa	LDL	β	Receptor defect	Cushing's; hypothyroidism	Xanthelasma; corneal arcus	CAD, PVD
IIb	LDL & VLDL	β & pre-β		Cholestasis; nephrotic syndrome	Tendon xanthomata	
III	IDL	Broad β	Oversynthesis and/or abnormal apo E	Renal and liver disease	Palmar crease and tuboeruptive xanthomata; xanthelasma	CAD, PVD
IV	VLDL	Pre-β	Oversynthesis and/or under catabolism of VLDL	Diabetes mellitus; alcoholism; chronic renal failure	Usually no xanthomata	
V	VLDL & chylomicrons	Origin and pre-β	Saturation lipoprotein lipase by VLDL	As for IV	As for I	As for I

Notes:
- Apo A-1 deficiency is associated with the absence of plasma HDL and severe premature CAD.
- Apo B deficiency is the defect in abetalipoproteinaemia (autosomal recessive), which is characterised by haemolytic anaemia (acanthocytosis), fat malabsorption and neurological defects (proprioceptive loss, retinitis pigmentosa).
- LCAT deficiency results in decreased HDL, cloudy corneas and progressive renal disease.

apo = apolipoprotein; CAD = coronary artery disease; HDL = high-density lipoprotein; IDL = intermediate-density lipoprotein; LCAT = lecithin cholesterol acyltransferase; LDL = low-density lipoprotein; PVD = peripheral vascular disease; SLE = systemic lupus erythematosus; VLDL = very-low-density lipoprotein.

Familial dysbetalipoproteinaemia is also associated with coronary artery disease. These patients have elevated cholesterol and triglyceride levels and are usually found to have obesity, hypothyroidism or diabetes mellitus. Find out whether there is any history of these and whether there has been atheromatous disease or vascular disease involving the internal carotid arteries and the abdominal aorta or its branches. Ask about claudication, which occurs in about one-third of patients.

2. The patient may be able to tell you his or her cholesterol and triglyceride levels and what they have been in the past. Some even know the LDL and high-density lipoprotein (HDL) levels.

3. If there is no history of coronary artery disease and the patient either knows the triglyceride level to have been very high or has a history of pancreatitis, the likely diagnosis is *familial hypertriglyceridaemia*. This is also a common autosomal dominant disorder and is associated with obesity, hyperglycaemia, hyperinsulinaemia, hypertension and hyperuricaemia. Although there is a slightly increased incidence of atherosclerosis, this is probably related to diabetes, obesity and hypertension rather than to the hypertriglyceridaemia itself.

   Ask about the patient's alcohol consumption or any history of hypothyroidism or the ingestion of oestrogen-containing oral contraceptives. Any of these can precipitate a rapid rise in the triglyceride level, which may precipitate pancreatitis or the characteristic eruptive xanthomas. Between attacks, patients have moderate elevations of the plasma triglyceride level.

4. Next, find out about treatment. In familial hypercholesterolaemia, this will have been aimed at the cholesterol level itself and at any cardiovascular complications that have occurred. The patient should be well informed about a low saturated fat diet and may be aware of side-effects from medication usage.

5. The need for drug treatment of hyperlipidaemia depends on the lipid levels and on the patient's other vascular risk factors. Ask about a family history of premature coronary disease (first-degree relatives under the age of 60), previous vascular disease (coronary, cerebral or peripheral), smoking, diabetes and elevated homocysteine levels.

6. A history of cutaneous xanthoma. These may have resolved with treatment or been surgically removed.

The examination

Examine the cardiovascular system, where there may be evidence of cardiac failure from previous myocardial infarcts or a sternotomy scar from previous coronary surgery. Occasionally one sees the scandalous situation of a patient with untreated hyperlipidaemia presenting with more angina after initially successful coronary surgery.

Look specifically for the interesting skin manifestations of these conditions. Patients with the heterozygous or homozygous form of familial hypercholesterolaemia may have *tendon xanthomas*. These are nodular swellings that tend to involve the tendons of the knee, elbow, dorsum of the hand and the Achilles tendon. They consist of massive deposits of cholesterol, probably derived from the deposition of LDL particles. They contain both amorphous extracellular deposits and vacuoles within macrophages. They sometimes become inflamed and cause tendonitis.

Cholesterol deposits in the soft tissue of the eyelid cause *xanthelasma* and those in the cornea produce *arcus cornea* (previously insensitively called *arcus senilis*). Xanthelasma occur in about 1% of the population and arcus senilis in 30% of people over 50. When corneal arcus is seen in younger people it is more often associated with hyperlipidaemia. Surveys of people with xanthelasma indicate a slightly higher than average cholesterol level.

The tendon xanthomas are diagnostic of familial hypercholesterolaemia but the other signs are not so specific. Up to three-quarters of patients with the heterozygous form have these signs.

The majority of patients with the homozygous form have even more interesting signs. Yellow xanthomas may occur at points of trauma and in the webs of the fingers. Cholesterol deposits in the aortic valve may be sufficient to cause aortic stenosis; occasionally mitral stenosis and mitral regurgitation can occur for the same reason. Painful swollen joints may also be present. Obesity is uncommon in these patients.

These skin manifestations may or may not resolve with treatment of the cholesterol level. Surgical treatment is sometimes indicated.

Eruptive xanthomas are a sign of hypertriglyceridaemia (levels often over 20 mmol/L). This is type V hyperlipoproteinaemia. Eruptive xanthomas occur on pressure areas, such as the elbows and buttocks, and resolve rapidly with treatment. The association here is with pancreatitis. The problem is often hereditary but exacerbated with obesity, diabetes and alcohol consumption. It is a less definite risk factor for cardiovascular disease. *Palmar xanthomata* are a sign of dysbetalipoproteinaemia (type III hyperlipoproteinaemia). They also resolve with treatment.

If the history suggests combined hyperlipidaemia or hypertriglyceridaemia, obesity is likely to be present. Look also for signs of the complications of diabetes mellitus, and for signs of hypothyroidism or the nephrotic syndrome (see Table 6.71). In sick patients with hypertriglyceridaemia, there may be signs of acute pancreatitis.

Investigations

A cholesterol level over 8 mmol/L with a normal triglyceride level suggests one of the familial hyperlipidaemias. This diagnosis can be confirmed by an assay of the number of LDL receptors on blood lymphocytes. The diagnosis is more often made from a combination of the lipid pattern, the history and the clinical examination (see Table 6.3). The other necessary investigations are those required for coronary artery disease.

Investigation of hypertriglyceridaemia includes tests to exclude possible underlying causes, such as hypothyroidism, diabetes and excessive alcohol intake. In familial hypertriglyceridaemia the plasma triglyceride level tends to be moderately elevated— 3–6 mmol/L (type IV lipoprotein pattern). The cholesterol level is normal. The triglyceride level may rise to values in excess of 12 mmol/L during exacerbations of the condition.

Familial combined hyperlipidaemia produces one of three different lipoprotein patterns—hypercholesterolaemia (type IIa), hypertriglyceridaemia (type IV), or both hypercholesterolaemia and hypertriglyceridaemia (type V).

Familial dysbetalipoproteinaemia (type III hyperlipoproteinaemia) results in the accumulation of large lipoprotein particles containing triglycerides and cholesterol. These particles resemble the remnants and intermediate-density lipoprotein (IDL) particles normally produced from the catabolism of chylomicrons and very-low-density lipoproteins (VLDL). These patients are homozygous for the apolipoprotein E2 (apo-E2) allele, which is unable to bind to hepatic lipoprotein receptors, thus preventing the rapid hepatic uptake of IDL and chylomicrons. The condition is usually expressed only in patients with hypothyroidism or diabetes mellitus, and tests for these disorders are necessary. Apo-E genotyping may sometimes be useful.

Management

A combination of diet and treatment of the underlying condition is usually required. Underlying diabetes and hypothyroidism must be treated. Some patients with dysbetalipoproteinaemia respond dramatically to the introduction of thyroxine. Effective management of the condition tends to cause disappearance of the skin signs and improves the prognosis as far as vascular disease goes. Effective treatment of familial hyperlipidaemia from early adult life delays the onset of coronary artery disease.

Treatment is almost always begun with hydroxymethylglutaryl coenzyme A (HMG-CoA) reductase inhibitors (statins, e.g. pravastatin, lovastatin, atorvastatin). These work by inhibiting the synthesis of cholesterol in the liver by impeding the activity of the rate-limiting enzyme. Patients need to have their liver function checked after about a month. They are effective drugs; total cholesterol levels may be expected to fall at least 30%.

The Four-S trial in Scandinavia was the first of a number of trials to show a definite survival advantage for patients treated with these drugs for secondary prevention (i.e. those patients who have already had an ischaemic event). Secondary prevention trials for high- and intermediate-risk patients have also been positive. It is now clear that patients with existing coronary artery disease or multiple risk factors benefit most from lipid-lowering treatment. Previous concern about an apparent increase in overall mortality associated with lipid lowering seems to have been allayed.

The current indications for drug treatment of cholesterol allow a statin for patients with established coronary artery disease and a total cholesterol level of >4 mmol/L. The most frequent problem with these drugs is the occurrence of myalgias. These are, however, uncommon. The relatively long experience with the statins suggests they are safe in quite large doses and current starting doses are two to four times those used in the past. Atorvastatin is the most potent of the statins and should be the drug of choice for severe hypercholesterolaemia. It also has more effect on triglycerides than the other statins. All the statins favourably affect the HDL/LDL ratio.

There is controversy about the need to treat levels that are already below 4 mmol/L. There is evidence that there are pleomorphic effects of the statins that reduce coronary risk separately from their effect on cholesterol. This also implies that, for secondary prevention, the use of statins may be beneficial for patients whose total cholesterol is below 4 mmol/L before drug treatment.

Ezetimibe reduces cholesterol absorption from the gut and thus interrupts its enterohepatic circulation. It does not seem to interfere with the absorption of fat-soluble vitamins. Its effect on cholesterol levels is substantial although not as great as that of the statins. It is useful for patients who are intolerant of the statins or, when used in combination with a statin, for patients whose cholesterol level is not controlled on a statin alone.

Gemfibrozil increases the activity of lipoprotein lipase and is useful in hyper-triglyceridaemia as a result of increased VLDL or IDL levels. Its main role is for patients with elevation of both cholesterol and triglyceride levels. Clofibrate is no longer in common use for lipid control.

A few patients may be taking one of the bile-sequestering resins—cholestyramine or colestipol. These are less often used as initial treatment now that the HMG-CoA reductase inhibitors (statins) are generally available. Some patients may use a statin and a resin in combination. Resins bind bile salts in the gut so that cholesterol is withdrawn from the circulation by the liver to make more. They are not absorbed but can cause constipation and flatulence, and can block the absorption of other drugs. The patient may need to take up to two sachets (8 g) three times daily. If the cholesterol cannot be brought down to normal levels with diet and a resin, nicotinic acid (which blocks VLDL synthesis) can be added. This is an effective drug and may help block the compensating increase in hepatic cholesterol synthesis that occurs with bile-sequestering resins. Side-effects include flushing, pruritus, abnormal liver function tests, hyperglycaemia and aggravation of peptic ulcer disease. The patient will probably have been begun on a small dose and had this gradually increased as tolerance improved. In practice it is a very difficult drug to use because of its side-effects.

The indications for treatment of hyperlipidaemia with drugs on the pharmaceutical benefits scheme (PBS) are complicated. Total cholesterol, HDL, LDL and triglyceride levels, as well as the presence of other risk factors, are all part of the formula. Candidates should be familiar with the latest PBS rules.

Patients with homozygous familial hypercholesterolaemia are unlikely to live long enough to be present in clinical examinations, but treatment for these people can sometimes involve repeated plasma exchange and even liver transplantation.

A patient with one of the combined hyperlipidaemias is likely to need to lose weight as well as to control the cholesterol and saturated fat intake, and with dysbetalipoproteinaemia may require treatment for hypothyroidism. All these patients need to avoid alcohol and oral contraceptives. Diet is the mainstay of treatment for reducing triglyceride levels; gemfibrozil or one of the newer fibrates may be used if diet fails.

A patient with familial hypertriglyceridaemia will have been managed in a similar way and may have required treatment for acute pancreatitis.

Hypertension

Many long cases are likely to provide the examiners with an opportunity to ask about the management of hypertension. Although it is an increasingly complicated subject, it is unlikely to be the major problem of the patient. The examiners will want to hear sensible discussion from the candidate about a number of aspects of hypertension, including the diagnosis, appropriate investigations and approaches to treatment.

The history

1. Many patients are well informed and very interested in their blood pressure. Find out when the diagnosis was made and what sorts of blood pressure readings were obtained before and after treatment. It is common for measurements to be made in a number of ways and in different settings. Apart from clinic measurements, the patient may have taken and continue to take his or her own blood pressure at home. There may have been ambulatory blood pressure (ABP) recordings made. It seems clear that hypertensive risk is more closely related to non-clinic and ABP results than to those obtained in the surgery. ABP should, however, be lower than clinic readings to be considered normal. Measurements of <135/85 mmHg during the day and <120/75 mmHg at night are considered normal for ABP recordings. See Table 6.4 for the current classification of clinic blood pressure levels.
2. Ask about current and past antihypertensive treatment and about problems or side-effects caused by treatment. Next find out about possible complications of hypertension. These include stroke, heart failure, peripheral vascular disease and renal failure.
3. Very occasionally there may be symptoms that suggest a primary cause of hypertension: paroxysmal sweating, palpitations and headache (phaeochromocytoma) or daytime sleepiness (sleep apnoea). Rarely the patient may be aware of a diagnosis of renal artery stenosis, coarctation of the aorta or an adrenal tumour.

Table 6.4 **Diagnosis of hypertension***

	Systolic (mmHg)	Diastolic (mmHg)
Normal	<120	<80
High–normal	130–139	80–89
Grade 1 (mild)	140–159	90–99
Grade 2 (moderate)	160–179	100–109
Grade 3 (severe)	≥180	≥110
Isolated systolic hypertension	>140	<90

* Based on National Heart Foundation guidelines 2004 and derived from JNC-7 and European Society of Hypertension.

---

4. Ask about other risk factors for vascular disease, especially type 2 diabetes but also hyperlipidaemia, a family history of premature coronary disease or stroke. The presence of any of these conditions, or of existing heart failure, coronary or cerebrovascular disease is a strong indication for treatment.
5. Although primary causes of hypertension are rare there are often a number of factors that contribute to the problem. These include obesity, excess alcohol consumption, lack of physical exercise and a high salt intake. Other factors, such as cigarette smoking, add to the patient's overall risk. Ask what the patient knows about these factors and what efforts (if any) have been made to correct them. Some racial groups have a high risk of premature vascular disease and will benefit more from early and aggressive treatment. These include Australian Aboriginals and Torres Strait Islanders and Pacific Islanders.

The examination

See page 226.

Investigations

1. Test the urine for protein. Measure the serum electrolyte and creatinine, blood sugar, cholesterol and haemoglobin levels.
2. The presence of hypokalaemia in patients who are not on diuretics should prompt investigations for primary aldosteronism. Measurement of plasma renin activity (PRA) and plasma aldosterone (PA) levels may be indicated. A high PA and low PRA level is consistent with primary hyperaldosteronism. The test must be performed off treatment. Other causes of hypokalaemia and hypertension include renovascular disease, Cushing's syndrome and, in young patients, renin-secreting cancers rarely.
3. A history of snoring and obesity should be investigated with sleep studies for sleep apnoea.
4. Intractable hypertension, especially in a young person, is an indication for renal angiography. This is the most sensitive test for renal artery stenosis.
5. Symptoms consistent with a phaeochromocytoma need investigation with 24-hour urinary catecholamines.
6. Any clinical suspicion of Cushing's syndrome should be investigated.
7. An ECG should be routine to look for evidence of ischaemic heart disease and for voltage changes that suggest left ventricular hypertrophy (LVH) (Fig 6.5). The presence of LVH on the ECG in hypertensives is associated with an adverse prognosis. Occasionally an echocardiogram is indicated if there is doubt about the presence of LVH.

Treatment

The decision to begin drug treatment is an important one since it is likely to be lifelong. The current recommendations are that a blood pressure of >140 mmHg systolic or >90 mmHg diastolic, or both, warrants a 'treatment plan'. It is now very clear that the aggressiveness of intervention depends very much on factors other than the blood pressure level. The whole gamut of cardiovascular risk factors must be taken into account. Tables have been published by many cardiovascular societies, which show the calculated risk of vascular events and the calculated reduction in number of events over time with treatment for patients with different risk factors. The decision to use drug treatment should be based on information of this sort. Typically, calculators of risk take into account age, sex, smoking status, level of blood pressure, cholesterol, race and existing cardiovascular disease.

Except for very severe hypertension, attempts should be made to bring the blood pressure down by modifying the factors that are known to increase it. Many patients,

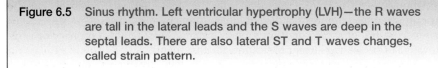

Figure 6.5 Sinus rhythm. Left ventricular hypertrophy (LVH)—the R waves are tall in the lateral leads and the S waves are deep in the septal leads. There are also lateral ST and T waves changes, called strain pattern.

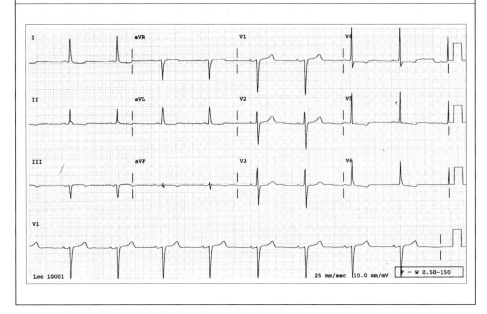

when faced with the threat of lifelong drug treatment, are amenable to suggestions to change the way they live.

Primary hyperaldosteronism can be treated effectively with spironolactone. Renal artery stenosis may be amenable to balloon angioplasty. This usually makes blood pressure control easier but does not cure the condition. Treatment of sleep apnoea with an appropriate continuous positive airways pressure (CPAP) mask (p 88) can also make blood pressure control easier.

Blood pressure reduction without drugs

1. Weight reduction. On average, 1 kg of weight loss will reduce systolic blood pressure by 2 mmHg. The goal should be reduction to a body mass index (BMI) of 25 kg/m^2 and of waist circumference to <94 cm for men and <80 cm for women. Even lower BMIs should be recommended for some racial groups, such as Asians and Australian Aboriginals, whose cardiovascular risk increases at lower BMIs than does Europeans.
2. Exercise. Thirty minutes of moderately intense exercise (e.g. brisk walking) at least 5 days a week can lower blood pressure by about 4/2.5 mmHg.
3. Alcohol. Reductions of 4–5 mmHg can be achieved by alcohol restriction to two standard drinks a day for men and one for women.
4. Salt. Reduction in salt consumption to 90 mmol/day can reduce blood pressure by over 5 mmHg. Warn patients that prepared and snack foods are usually heavily salted.

The cumulative effect of these measures can be considerable but repeated encouragement is likely to be required for patients to achieve them.

Drug treatment

Patients with only a mild risk of cardiovascular problems and blood pressure <150/<95 mmHg should probably continue with these conservative measures. At higher levels of blood pressure than this, drug treatment should be considered. Patients with very high risk (e.g. those with target organ disease or of Aboriginal race) should begin drug treatment if the blood pressure remains above 140/90 mmHg. Otherwise, drug treatment is probably indicated at levels above 150/95 mmHg.

Remember that all classes of drugs (Table 6.5) are fairly similar in their effect on blood pressure. The majority of patients will require more than one drug for effective blood pressure control.

Table 6.5 Classes of antihypertensive drugs
Thiazide diuretics ACE inhibitors Beta-blockers Non-dihydropyridine calcium channel blockers Dihydropyridine calcium channel blockers Angiotensin II receptor antagonists Others: centrally acting (methyldopa), vasodilators (prazosin, hydralazine)

There are many factors to be taken into account when a choice of antihypertensive drug is made (Table 6.6):

1. Previous intolerance to a class of drugs
2. Known contraindications to a class of drugs (e.g. renal artery stenosis and ACE inhibitors)
3. Convenience of drug regimen (e.g. once daily dosage)
4. Interaction with other medications (e.g. concerns about bradycardia with antiarrhythmics and verapamil)
5. Existing medical problems that favour the use of a class of drugs (e.g. cardiac failure and ACE inhibitors)
6. Cost
7. Possible additional protective effects of some antihypertensives (e.g. ACE inhibitors and patients who have had a stroke or have diabetes)

The current National Heart Foundation recommendation is that treatment be begun with a small dose of a single drug. Intolerance suggests the need to try a different class. Failure to achieve control, it recommends, should be managed with the addition of a small dose of another class of drug. The idea is to minimise side-effects. The disadvantage of this approach is that patients will almost all end up on multiple drugs. This can be a problem for compliance and cost. The other approach is to titrate up the dose of one drug to the maximum recommended unless side-effects occur. Then a second drug from another class is added. Some drugs are especially effective in combination:

1. beta-blocker and dihydropyridine calcium channel antagonist
2. ACE inhibitor or AR antagonist and thiazide
3. ACE inhibitor or AR antagonist and calcium antagonist
4. beta-blocker and alpha-blocker
5. beta-blocker and thiazide.

Fixed dose combinations of some of these are available: ACE inhibitor and thiazide, beta-blocker and alpha-blocker (labetalol). These combination drugs should not be

Table 6.6	Factors affecting choice of antihypertensive drug
Condition	**Drug**
Contraindication or relative contraindication	
Asthma or COPD	Beta-blocker
Bradycardia or heart block	Beta-blockers, non-dihydropyridine calcium channel blockers (verapamil, diltiazem)
Cardiac failure	Calcium channel blockers
Diabetes	Thiazides, beta-blockers (relative contraindication)
Gout	Diuretics
Peripheral vascular disease	Beta-blockers
Pregnancy	Most antihypertensives, especially ACE inhibitors; methyldopa is safe
Renal vascular disease	ACE inhibitors, AR antagonists
Possible indication or beneficial effect	
Angina	Beta-blocker, calcium channel blocker
Cardiac failure	ACE inhibitors, AR antagonists, diuretics, some beta-blockers
Myocardial infarction	ACE inhibitors, beta-blockers
Diabetes	ACE inhibitors, AR antagonists

ACE = angiotensin-converting enzyme; AR = angiotensin II receptor; COPD = chronic obstructive pulmonary disease.

used to initiate treatment. Candidates should be familiar with the doses of the common antihypertensive drugs and their important side-effects.

Heart transplantation

Cardiac transplantation is now an accepted form of treatment for intractable cardiac failure. Increasing numbers of patients who have either had a transplant or are on the waiting list for one are available for clinical examinations. Those awaiting transplantation are sick enough to require frequent admissions to hospital and those who have had a transplant are often readmitted for various routine investigations. Patients are usually well informed about their condition and should be able to supply a lot of useful information to the candidate.

Although this fact should not be discussed with our surgical colleagues, heart transplantation is technically not a very difficult operation. Improvements in prognosis have followed medical advances, particularly in the area of the management of rejection. The 5-year survival rate is now slightly over 75% for patients who have received a transplant since 1981, and the 1-year survival rate is currently about 90%.

The examiners will expect a candidate to be familiar with the indications for, and contraindications to, the procedure. It is also important to know what investigations are required before a patient can be accepted for surgery and to understand the management problems that can occur in patients who have had the operation (Table 6.7).

Table 6.7   **Evaluation for heart transplantation**

1. History and examination
2. Body weight
3. Cardiac assessment
   (a) Ejection fraction: estimated by resting gated blood pool scan
   (b) Echocardiogram: with measurement of left ventricular dimensions and assessment of the cardiac valves; examination for left ventricular thrombus
   (c) Coronary angiography in patients with suspected ischaemic heart disease
   (d) 24-hour Holter monitoring to evaluate for ventricular arrhythmias
   (e) Right heart catheterisation to measure pulmonary vascular resistance and its response to vasodilators; fixed pulmonary hypertension is a contraindication to cardiac transplantation
4. HLA tissue typing
5. Chest X-ray and respiratory function tests if indicated
6. Full blood count, ESR and coagulation studies
7. Biochemical profile, including liver function tests, electrolyte levels and estimation of creatinine clearance, serum cholesterol, triglycerides and blood sugar levels
8. Serology for antinuclear antibodies and immunoelectrophoresis
9. Bacteriology: swabs for methicillin-resistant *Staphylococcus aureus* and a Mantoux test if indicated; hepatitis A and B, toxoplasma, CMV, EBV, HIV and herpes simplex serology
10. Psychiatric, renal and dental consultations if required
11. Social work report
    If the cause of the cardiomyopathy is unknown, a myocardial biopsy, viral titres (including coxsackie A virus, echovirus, adenovirus and influenza titres) and iron studies (for haemochromatosis) are required.
    Contraindications for heart transplantation include alcoholism, chronic renal disease, pulmonary parenchymal disease, continued tobacco use, advanced liver disease and advanced age. Diabetes mellitus is a relative contraindication.

CMV = cytomegalovirus; EBV = Epstein-Barr virus; ESR = erythrocyte sedimentation rate; HIV = human immunodeficiency virus; HLA = human leucocyte antigen.

The history

1. Try to establish the cause of the patient's cardiac failure. In younger patients cardiomyopathy is more likely to be the problem, but nearly half the patients currently undergoing heart transplantation have ischaemic heart disease. Rheumatic valvular heart disease can also affect a younger patient. Combined heart and lung transplantation is occasionally carried out for patients with primary pulmonary hypertension or cystic fibrosis. It may also be the treatment of choice for some forms of congenital heart disease either in childhood or adult life; if pulmonary hypertension is present these patients have to be considered for combined heart and lung transplantation.

   Ask about previous myocardial infarction or angina and whether the patient knows the results of cardiac catheterisation. All patients undergoing a transplant are required to have cardiac catheterisation. There may have been a preoperative cardiac biopsy performed and the patient may be aware of the results of this test. Also ask about previous thoracotomies.

2. Ask about the patient's symptoms before surgery. Obtain an idea of the exercise tolerance and the severity of angina, if present. The patient may know the results of investigations of cardiac function, such as exercise tests and gated blood pool scans, before and after surgery.

3. Ask what treatment the patient was receiving before transplantation—particularly the doses of diuretics, ACE inhibitors and beta-blockers (e.g. carvedilol). Find out whether frequent admissions to hospital were necessary and whether intravenous inotropes had been required. There may have been recurrent ventricular arrhythmias before surgery. Treatment may have been with drugs, especially amiodarone, or an implanted defibrillator and antitachycardia pacemaker. Some patients have undergone previous surgery for arrhythmias. This may include resection of an aneurysm or myocardial resection following ventricular mapping. Occasionally, transplantation is used to treat intractable ventricular arrhythmias.

4. Find out how long it is since a transplant was performed or how long the patient has been on the waiting list. Ask whether there were any problems with the surgery—either technical or involving acute rejection. Find out how long the patient was in hospital and what further admissions to hospital have occurred since the operation. Ask whether a permanent pacemaker was inserted. Some patients awaiting transplant may have been given a ventricular assist device as a bridge to transplant.

5. Endomyocardial biopsies are fairly memorable events and the patient should be able to tell you how often these have been performed and when the last one was obtained. It is now routine to carry these out at weekly intervals for the first 3 weeks after operation, every 2 weeks for the following month, and every 6 months after that for patients whose condition is stable.

6. Find out what drugs the patient is taking currently. Transplant patients should not require antifailure treatment but will, of course, be taking immunosuppressive drugs. Almost all patients are now maintained on cyclosporin, whose dose is determined by its serum level, and prednisone. Cyclosporin is nephrotoxic and causes hypertension. Newer immunosuppressive drugs include mycophenolate, tacrolimus and rapamycin. Diltiazem is often used as a cyclosporin-sparing agent. It dramatically reduces cyclosporin metabolism and therefore the cost of treating patients. Often azathioprine is also prescribed, and the dose is adjusted according to the white cell count. The patient may know of boosts of prednisone that have been given for rejection episodes. Early episodes of rejection are often treated with 1 g of methyl-prednisolone IV for 3 days. Later rejection tends to be milder and may respond to an increase in oral steroids. Severe rejection is often treated with antithymocyte globulin or the murine monoclonal muromonab–CD3. Repetitive rejection may be treated with total lymphoid irradiation or methotrexate. Inquire about complications of immunosuppression (Table 6.8). Patients are often well informed about symptoms suggesting rejection—often these resemble an attack of pericarditis. Many patients are also taking regular antibiotics to prevent *Pneumocystis carinii* infection. Cotrimoxazole bd 3 days a week is a common regimen.

7. Some general questions about the transplant patient's current life are very relevant. Find out how much difference has occurred in the patient's exercise tolerance and whether he or she has been able to go back to work. If the patient is currently an inpatient, find out why he or she has been admitted to hospital on this occasion. Ask about the patient's family and how they have coped with the illness and the transplant itself. Make some discreet inquiries about the patient's finances and whether there have been any problems returning to the transplant hospital for the various investigations required.

Table 6.8 Commonly used immunosuppressants for heart transplant patients		
Drug	**Side-effects**	**Monitoring/avoidance**
Steroids	Cushingoid, diabetes, osteoporosis	Minimal dose
Cyclosporin	Renal impairment, hypertension, neurotoxicity	Blood levels, drug interactions
Mycophenolate	Mild marrow suppression, gastrointestinal upset	Reduce dose, check FBC
Methotrexate	Hepato- and marrow toxicity	FBC
Azathioprine	Hepato- and marrow toxicity, pancreatitis	FBC, liver function tests
FBC = full blood count.		

8. Ask about routine cardiac catheterisation. This is typically performed biannually in patients who have had transplants. Coronary artery intimal proliferation can cause ischaemic heart disease in the transplanted heart. Because the heart has been denervated there is not usually any pain. However, there are now patients in whom re-innervation seems to have occurred and led to symptoms of angina. This allograft arteriopathy is one of the most important problems after transplant. It represents a rejection phenomenon. The condition is usually diffuse but once lesions causing 40% coronary stenosis have occurred the prognosis is quite poor. The 2-year survival rate is only about 50%. The condition is present in 10% of recipients at 1-year post-transplant and 50% at 5 years. Once myocardial infarction has occurred the 2-year survival rate is only 10–20%. Although the disease is a form of rejection, it is still considered important that the patient's cholesterol level be kept as low as possible. Find out if he or she knows what the cholesterol level is and what treatment is being used to keep it low. Intravascular ultrasound is used increasingly to detect subclinical vasculopathy and to study the benefits of various antirejection regimens.

9. Hypertension is another important post-transplant problem. It is associated with the use of cyclosporin. Ask about blood pressure control and treatment.

10. Transplant patients have an increased risk of malignancy. Skin cancers are common. There is also a higher incidence of lymphoproliferative disorders. Post-transplant lymphoproliferative disease (PTLD) is an increasingly recognised complication of the immunosuppression required for organ transplants. The incidence in heart transplant patients is less than that for those with liver transplants but more than that for those with renal transplants. Primary or reactivated Ebstein–Barr virus infection is thought to be the cause. The lesions tend to occur in unusual extranodal sites. Reduction in the amount of immunosuppression will sometimes help but antiviral treatment with acyclovir or interferon may be necessary.

The examination

1. If the transplant has been successful there should not be many signs. A large median sternotomy scar will be present.

2. Look for signs of cardiac failure and pericarditis. Pericarditis can be an indication of rejection.
3. Note the small scars in the neck at the point of introduction of the endomyocardial biopsy forceps.
4. Look for any evidence of Cushing's syndrome from steroid therapy.
5. Examine the chest carefully for signs of infection, examine the mouth for candidiasis, look for infection at intravenous access sites, and look at the temperature chart.

Investigations

1. These depend somewhat on the reason the patient has been admitted to hospital on this occasion. As mentioned above, endomyocardial biopsies are performed routinely and at any suggestion of rejection. Ask about the results of these biopsies.
2. A full blood count may be indicated because of possible infection and to monitor the azathioprine dose.
3. Chest X-ray may show signs of cardiac enlargement, although this is a late sign of rejection. Changes of rejection on the ECG include a reduction in voltage caused by myocardial oedema, or atrial arrhythmias. Sometimes the patient's ECG shows two sets of P waves: one comes from the transplanted heart and one arises from the residual atrium.
4. Recent assessments of myocardial function, including gated blood pool scans and resting or stress echocardiograms, may be available.
5. Routine coronary angiography may have been performed.
6. If there have been problems with possible infection, results of blood, urine and other cultures should be sought.

Management

The discussion should revolve around the patient's current problem or reason for admission. However, there is likely to be time to discuss the management of rejection, infection, cardiac failure or social problems.

1. Rejection may have been suspected because of pleuritic chest pain, deterioration in left ventricular function or ECG changes. It is diagnosed on the basis of a routine biopsy. The usual approach is to give the patient a boost of methylprednisolone—usually 1 g intravenously daily for 3 days followed by a repeat biopsy.
2. Infections occurring as a result of immunosuppression are a major cause of death. Possible episodes of infection should be investigated thoroughly and treated aggressively with appropriate therapy. Opportunistic infections are relatively common as a late complication. Cytomegalovirus, herpes, *P. carinii*, fungal infection, and *Nocardia* and *Toxoplasma* are all more common than in non-immunosuppressed people.
3. Further cardiac failure may be an indication of rejection, which should be treated. Cardiac failure may also be an indication of silent myocardial infarction.
4. Hyperlipidaemia should be sought routinely and treated most vigorously with drugs and diet.

There may be discussion about the patient's prognosis. The 1-year survival rate after transplant is about 90% and the 5-year survival rate 70–80%. The 10-year survival rate approaches 50%.

The discussion of a patient awaiting cardiac transplantation will probably run along similar lines. However, it is important to know how well informed the patient is about what is likely to happen, whether he or she appears to fulfil the criteria for transplantation (see Table 6.7), and whether there appear to be any contraindications. Some patients awaiting transplantation are sick enough to require intravenous inotropes. There may even have been talk about the use of external circulatory assistance devices for use as a bridge to transplant.

Cardiac arrhythmias

The management of some cardiac rhythm disturbances has become complicated. These patients may be in hospital while waiting for diagnostic tests or, in cases of serious arrhythmias, for treatment to become effective.

They sometimes represent diagnostic but more often management problems. Ventricular arrhythmias are a more common reason for admission than supraventricular arrhythmias, but patients with the latter may be awaiting diagnostic or therapeutic procedures. Atrial fibrillation, the most common of the significant cardiac arrhythmias, is unlikely to be the patient's only problem if it appears in a long case.

The history

Ask why the patient is in hospital—all may be revealed without much further effort. Otherwise, the patient may know the name of the arrhythmia or be able to describe symptoms that make the diagnosis likely. If the rhythm problem is a serious and continuing one, the candidate may be fortunate enough to find the patient on an ECG monitor. Possible presenting symptoms include:

1. rapid and irregular palpitations—suggest atrial fibrillation (AF) (Fig 6.6)
2. rapid and regular palpitations, with or without dizziness and perhaps terminated by Valsalva—suggest supraventricular tachycardia (SVT) (Fig 6.7)
3. rapid and regular palpitations with dizziness, syncope or near syncope— suggest ventricular tachycardia (VT), *particularly if there is a history of ischaemic heart disease*
4. syncope with bradycardia or no palpitations—suggests heart block (Fig 6.8)
5. symptoms of AF and episodes of syncope—suggests sick sinus syndrome

---

Figure 6.6   Atrial fibrillation. The ventricular response rate is rapid— between 95 and 160 beats/minute.

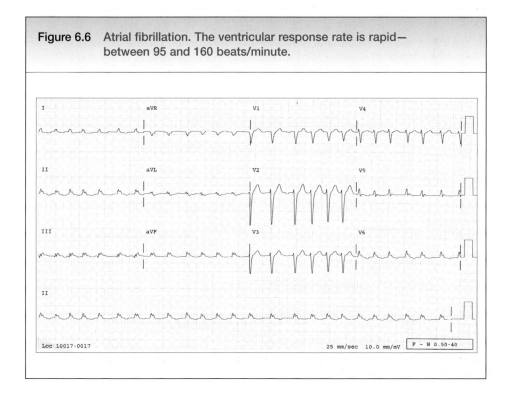

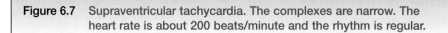

Figure 6.7 Supraventricular tachycardia. The complexes are narrow. The heart rate is about 200 beats/minute and the rhythm is regular.

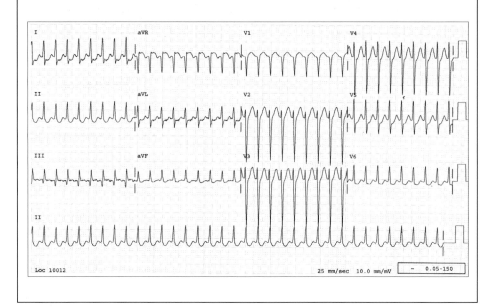

Figure 6.8 Sinus rhythm. First degree heart block. Right bundle branch block (RBBB) and left anterior hemi-block (LAHB). This combination of abnormalities is called *trifascicular block*. It is a sign of significant conduction system disease and, in a patient with recurrent syncope, suggests that intermittent complete heart block may be the cause of the symptoms.

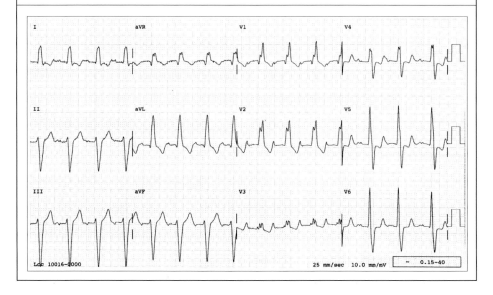

6. a family history of sudden death—suggests the possibility of congenital long QT interval (Fig 6.9), Brugada syndrome or a structural cardiac problem such as hypertrophic cardiomyopathy

7. the occurrence of syncope in association with antiarrhythmic drug treatment—suggests the possibility of proarrhythmia; ask about class 1C drugs and sotalol, perhaps prescribed because of paroxysmal AF, as these drugs may also worsen bradyarrhythmias in patients with sick sinus syndrome.

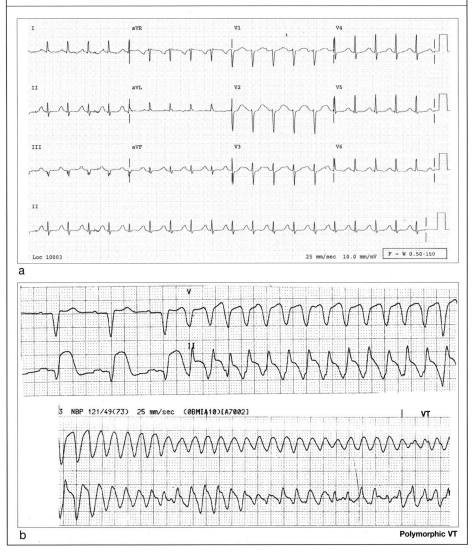

Figure 6.9 (a) Sinus rhythm. The QT interval is prolonged (423 ms) and the corrected QT (QTc) is 460 ms (normal <440 ms). These patients are at risk of syncope or sudden death as a result of the development of polymorphic ventricular tachycardia (VT). (b) Polymorphic VT or *torsade de pointes*. This apparent twisting of the QRS complexes is named after the gold braid on French military uniforms.

Ask now about previous known heart disease (e.g. ischaemic heart disease and VT, aortic stenosis and heart block) and recent cardiac, thoracic or abdominal surgery. Cardiac surgery may be complicated by heart block, and all of the above may precipitate AF. The 'grown-up' congenital heart disease patient may have persisting problems with atrial or ventricular arrhythmias following cardiac surgery in childhood.

Consider the common causes and associations of AF:

1. advancing age (3% of 65 year olds, >6% of people in their 80s)
2. ischaemic heart disease and myocardial infarction
3. mitral valve disease
4. thyrotoxicosis
5. recent thoracic or abdominal surgery
6. atrial septal defect
7. Wolff-Parkinson-White syndrome (Fig 6.10)
8. recent alcoholic binge
9. pulmonary embolism
10. hypertension.

Figure 6.10 Sinus rhythm. Wolff-Parkinson-White (WPW) syndrome. The PR interval is short and delta waves are visible. There are positive delta waves in lead I—seen as a slurred upstroke at the start of the R wave—and negative delta waves in lead III— seen as a slurred Q wave. These patients' ECGs are usually abnormal between their attacks of tachycardia but the *pre-excitation* (delta wave) may occur only intermittently. They are at risk of sudden death or syncope if atrial fibrillation occurs (they are often at increased risk of this arrhythmia) because very rapid ventricular rates may occur if the accessory pathway can conduct at high rates.

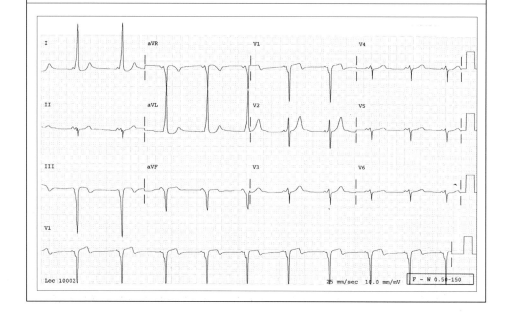

Ask if the rhythm has been paroxysmal and self-limiting, persistent and required cardioversion, or permanent.

Now find out about treatment. Has the patient required intravenous drugs to control the heart? Have these been by infusion or bolus injection? Intravenous adenosine is now the drug treatment of first choice for SVT. Patients may well remember its use. It causes a brief but distressing sensation of impending death. Have physical manoeuvres been tried? What oral drugs have been used in the past and during this admission? Make inquiries about the known side-effects of these drugs.

The investigations the patient has undergone or may be about to undergo can help sort out the diagnosis. Certain tests, such as electrophysiological studies (EPS), are more memorable than others. An EPS with induction of VT may mean that direct current (DC) cardioversion was required; despite sedation and reduced cardiac output, some memory of this may remain. Other procedures may have been entirely therapeutic: for example, DC cardioversion performed electively under general anaesthesia suggests AF or atrial flutter; catheter ablation, often a fairly prolonged procedure, suggests SVT or VT; pacemaker insertion suggests bradycardia; antiarrhythmia surgery suggests VT or, less often now, SVT.

Catheter ablation is now a routine treatment for SVT that does not respond to simple drug treatment. Rarely there may be failure to suppress the arrhythmia, or a complication such as complete heart block or cardiac rupture can occur. Ablation is also very effective for some forms of VT. These include right, and the less common left, ventricular outflow tract tachycardias. These benign forms of VT can cause frequent recurrent episodes of self-limiting VT with a left or right bundle branch block morphology, respectively. They may respond to treatment with verapamil but are otherwise curable with catheter ablation.

Patients with automatic implantable cardioverter-defibrillators (AICDs) can usually provide vast amounts of useful information about their devices and about their arrhythmia.

The examination

Examine the cardiovascular system. Is the patient in sinus rhythm clinically? Look for thoracotomy scars, pacemakers and implanted defibrillators. Look for signs of cardiac failure, valvular heart disease, evidence of recent abdominal surgery, or thyrotoxicosis.

Investigations

These depend on the actual rhythm problem.

1. Resting ECG—look for:
   (a) the current rhythm
   (b) evidence of pre-excitation (Wolff-Parkinson-White syndrome, Lown-Ganong-Levine syndrome)
   (c) heart block
   (d) old infarction
   (e) paced rhythm (ventricular-ventricular inhibited [VVI] or dual chamber—atrial sensing and ventricular pacing or dual chamber pacing)
   (f) long QT interval (increased risk of polymorphic VT—*torsade de pointes*).
2. The examiners may produce previous ECGs or parts of 24-hour Holter monitors. Remember that a broad complex tachycardia should be considered VT unless there is good reason to consider otherwise. There are a number of ECG criteria for distinguishing VT from SVT with aberrant conduction. Findings suggestive of VT include a QRS >0.14 seconds (if a right bundle branch block pattern) or >0.16 seconds (if a left bundle branch block pattern), left axis deviation (between −90° and −180°), atrioventricular (AV) dissociation (with P waves 'marching through' the QRS complexes) and changes from the pre-existing QRS morphology in

pre-existing bundle branch block (but note these rules do not apply in SVT with aberration caused by Wolff-Parkinson-White syndrome). The presence of known ischaemic heart disease, however, is particularly useful. Broad complex tachycardia in a patient with ischaemic heart disease is usually VT (95%).

3. EPS may be used to assess inducibility of atrial and ventricular arrhythmias before and after treatment. It is now used in conjunction with catheter ablation as curative treatment for SVT caused by accessory pathways and for some types of VT. It can also be performed to ablate the AV node or the regions around the four pulmonary veins for patients with intractable and disabling AF.

4. Routine investigations for patients with AF include echocardiography, thyroid function testing, and sometimes exercise testing. Echocardiography may reveal an underlying pathology that is responsible for the AF (e.g. mitral stenosis). It is as important in helping quantify embolic risk. At echocardiography one looks for valve abnormalities, cardiomyopathy, diastolic dysfunction of the left ventricle (especially important in hypertensive patients), left ventricular hypertrophy, atrial size (consider atrial septal defect), mitral valve disease and segmental wall abnormalities consistent with ischaemic heart disease.

5. Tests may be needed because of actual or potential drug side-effects (e.g. liver function or thyroid function tests for patients on amiodarone).

6. Cardiac catheterisation may be needed for patients with ventricular arrhythmias, as they often have an ischaemic substrate.

Management

Much depends on the rhythm abnormality. Arrhythmias that are not life-threatening are usually managed, at least at first, with drugs. Candidates will be expected to have a thorough working knowledge of the common antiarrhythmic drugs, their methods of action, indications and side-effects. Remember that all antiarrhythmic drugs have a potentially dangerous proarrhythmic effect.

The indications for permanent pacing (Table 6.9) and different uses for VVI, VVIR (rate responsive) and DDD (dual chamber) pacers (Figs 6.11, 6.12) should be well understood. A basic understanding of antitachycardia devices and indications for their use (Table 6.10) is also important.

Automatic implanted cardioverter-defibrillators (AICDs) are increasingly used to manage recurrent VT. They are often used in combination with antiarrhythmic drugs of some sort. They are becoming smaller, cheaper (about $25,000) and more complicated. It is now established that they improve mortality rates in selected patients. They are usually the treatment of choice for hypotensive VT or missed sudden death from VF. Drug treatment of these conditions is not very effective. The current models may be implanted without the need for an epicardial patch; leads can be placed intravenously into the vena cava and for pacing purposes into the right ventricle. A subcutaneous patch is only rarely needed as the other electrode for the purposes of defibrillation. The size of the modern devices means that the box has no longer to be implanted in the upper abdomen. They are small enough to be implanted like pacemakers in the chest wall. Implantation takes place under local anaesthetic in the electrophysiology laboratory. The periprocedural mortality rate is less than 1%, compared with over 5% when surgical implantation was required.

The programming of these machines is complicated, but candidates should know that they are usually set to attempt reversion of VT by overdrive pacing (antitachycardia pacing, ATP) before administering a DC shock. Patients are usually but not always aware of the onset of ATP and almost always aware of DC shock administration. Ask how the device has affected the patient's life and confidence, including how often it goes off and whether the box itself causes problems because of its size. Although AICDs can prevent sudden death their presence is often associated

Table 6.9   Indications for permanent pacemaker insertion in adults

Generally agreed indications
1. Intermittent or permanent complete heart block, with:
    (a) symptomatic bradycardia
    (b) cardiac failure
    (c) arrhythmias that require treatment with drugs that slow conduction
    (d) documented asystole of more than 3 seconds or escape rhythm with a rate <40 beats/minute
    (e) confusional states that improve with temporary pacing
2. Intermittent permanent second-degree AV block with symptomatic bradycardia
3. Sinus node dysfunction with symptomatic bradycardia

Less certain indications
1. Asymptomatic complete heart block; heart rate 40 beats/minute or more
2. Symptomatic type 2 second-degree heart block
3. Bifascicular or trifascicular block with syncope of unproven aetiology

Not indicated
1. First-degree heart block
2. Asymptomatic type 1 second-degree heart block

Table 6.10   Indications for implanted cardioverter-defibrillators (ICDs)

Generally agreed indications
1. Confirmed VF or hypotensive VT not related to an acute infarct or severe electrolyte abnormality, but VF/VT not inducible at EPS. This means drug treatment cannot be tested by EPS
2. VF/VT with contraindications to drug treatment (intolerance)
3. Persistently inducible VT/VF despite drug treatment, ablation or surgery
4. Persistent spontaneous VT/VF despite drug treatment
5. Symptomatic long QT syndrome despite drug treatment

Less certain indications
1. Inducible but not spontaneous VT despite other treatment in high-risk patients
2. VT/VF apparently controlled but in a high-risk patient
3. Serial drug testing possible but defibrillator preferred

Not generally indicated
1. Very frequent or incessant VT
2. Reversible cause
3. Recurrent syncope, VT/VF not inducible
4. Poor life-expectancy anyway (e.g. class IV cardiac failure but not a transplant candidate)

EPS = electrophysiology study; LV = left ventricular; VF = ventricular fibrillation; VT = ventricular tachycardia.

Note: Increasingly proven VT or VF in a patient with poor LV function is considered an indication regardless of EPS findings.

Figure 6.11 Atrial sensing and ventricular pacing. This is the ECG of a patient with a dual chamber pacemaker. Normal P waves are followed by an atrioventricular (PR) interval and then a pacing spike, which precedes a wide QRS complex with a left bundle branch block pattern (pacing is from the right ventricular apex).

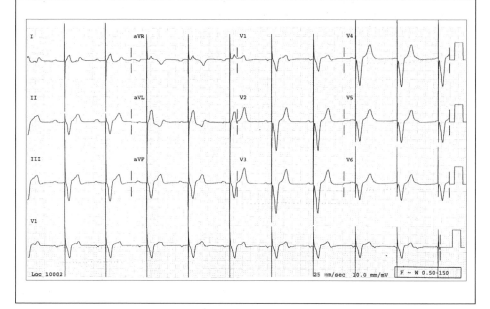

Figure 6.12 Dual chamber pacing. Pacing spikes precede both atrial and ventricular complexes.

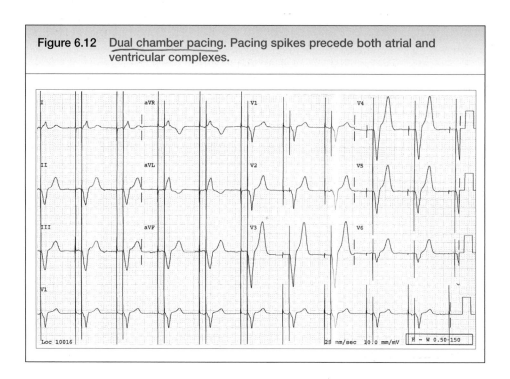

with a feeling of insecurity. Patients often have clear memories of events leading up to activations of the device. They may avoid places where arrhythmias and activations have occurred. They often require repeated explanation and reassurance.

The particular management problems of atrial fibrillation

A sensible approach to the management of AF will be required of candidates by the examiners and the opportunity for them to ask about this common condition will often arise. The principles of management are to:

1. maintain sinus rhythm
2. control the heart rate (if that proves difficult)
3. protect from embolic events.

There is good evidence from recent trials that control of heart rate is at least as satisfactory an approach as that of trying aggressively to maintain sinus rhythm. Nevertheless, patients with paroxysmal AF often find the arrhythmia very disturbing. They should be told at the outset that it may not be possible to keep them in sinus rhythm but that rate control and freedom from embolic episodes can almost be guaranteed. The prophylactic drug treatment of paroxysmal AF involves the use of a class III drug (sotalol or amiodarone) in most cases, but occasionally the class 1C drug, flecainide, can be used if the heart is known to be structurally normal.

Rate control of persistent or paroxysmal AF can be achieved with less toxic drugs. Digoxin is the usual first-line treatment and is usually well tolerated. It is not very effective on its own at controlling the heart rate during exercise. Many patients with chronic AF have persistent dyspnoea during exercise because of inadequate rate control. They benefit from the use of a beta-blocker or one of the non-dihydropyridine calcium channel blockers (diltiazem or verapamil). These can be used with or without digoxin. Control of the heart rate can prevent or reverse the impairment of left ventricular function that is associated with tachycardias (tachycardia-induced cardiomyopathy).

When patients remain unhappy with their symptoms despite rate control, further intervention should be considered. AV nodal ablation is a relatively simple procedure that prevents fibrillation waves reaching the ventricles. The patient then requires an artificial pacemaker. Although atrial systole is lost, the regularisation of the heart rate is usually enough to improve symptoms dramatically. If the patient's AF has been paroxysmal, a dual-chamber pacemaker with a 'mode switch' may be used. When the patient is in sinus rhythm, atrial sensing occurs and the ventricles are paced after an appropriate AV interval. When episodes of AF occur the pacemaker mode switches and paces the ventricle at a steady rate.

DC cardioversion of AF can be a reasonable treatment for the first episode or for patients with infrequent episodes. DC cardioversion is safe in the absence of digoxin toxicity or hypokalaemia but is associated with a risk of embolism if the patient's AF has been present for more than 48 hours. In this case, 1 month's therapeutic anticoagulation with warfarin should be instituted before the procedure and continued for 4 weeks afterwards. An alternative is to perform a transoesophageal echocardiogram to look for left atrial appendage thrombus or spontaneous echocardiograph contrast (a *echogenic swirling pattern of blood flow* sign of slow blood flow). The absence of these means that DC cardioversion is safe but that warfarin must be given for 4 weeks afterwards because there is a persisting risk over this period.

Reversion of AF with drug treatment is difficult. Many episodes terminate spontaneously but drug treatment is given the credit. It is known that digoxin does not increase the reversion rate but the class III drugs and flecainide do improve it somewhat. Sometimes control of the heart rate and awaiting spontaneous reversion can be an option. A decision to go on to DC cardioversion, however, should be made before 48 hours has passed.

Over many years attempts have been made to prevent AF by surgical or catheter ablation techniques. The 'maze' operation aims to divide the atria into separated channels that abolish re-entry circuits large enough to allow AF to occur. It has more recently been replaced by ablation around the pulmonary veins using radiofrequency energy from specially designed catheters. The rationale for this approach is that almost all AF seems to be initiated by extrasystoles arising from this part of the heart. Isolation of this area from the rest of the heart prevents the initiation of AF. The procedure is complicated and time consuming. It is not a practical solution to most AF. Success rates of about 60% are usually quoted. Until recently, an uncommon but severe complication involved the late occurrence of pulmonary vein stenosis. Newer techniques have made this a rare problem.

Protecting patients from embolic events is perhaps the most important aspect of the management of AF. Cerebral embolus is the most feared complication but life-threatening peripheral embolisation (e.g. to the mesenteric bed) can occur. Patients should have this aspect of AF explained to them early on. The risk of embolism is low in people under the age of 60 and without any risk factors (Table 6.11): <0.5% a year. It can be as high as 30% for patients with mitral stenosis.

Table 6.11   Risk factors for embolic events for patients with AF

1. Age >65 years
2. Previous embolic event
3. Mitral valve disease, especially mitral stenosis
4. Cardiac failure
5. Left atrial enlargement >40 mm on echocardiography
6. Hypertension or left ventricular hypertrophy on echocardiography
7. Ischaemic heart disease
8. Diabetes
9. Thyrotoxicosis
10. Thrombus or spontaneous echocardiographic contrast on transoesophageal echocardiography

---

Patients with any of these risk factors should be recommended anticoagulation therapy with warfarin. An assessment of the patient's ability to manage regular blood tests and dosage adjustments is necessary before treatment can begin. Patients are often reluctant to undertake the complexities of treatment but should not be allowed to decline treatment until all the risks of this approach have been carefully explained. The availability of home international normalised ratio (INR) testing machines that use a capillary blood sample has made the use of warfarin more acceptable to some patients (e.g. those who travel frequently). A number of studies have shown that this approach is safe for selected patients. The safe therapeutic range is an INR of between 2 and 2.5.

Find out from the patient how the warfarin is managed and whether he or she knows the last few readings and dosage.

Patients with risk factors remain at risk of stroke even if sinus rhythm has been restored. Those with self-limiting paroxysmal AF are also at risk if episodes are more than a rare event. Aspirin gives some protection to those unwilling or unable to take warfarin. There is no evidence that combination antiplatelet treatment (e.g. with aspirin and clopidogrel) is any more effective than aspirin alone.

The oral antithrombin drug ximelagatran has now been shown in a number of large trials to be at least as effective as warfarin in preventing embolic stoke for AF patients. The drug is taken twice a day and does not need monitoring. Bleeding problems in these comparative trials were <u>less than with warfarin</u>. There was some concern about the development of abnormal liver function tests in a few patients but there is great hope that this drug may replace warfarin in the treatment of non-valvular AF.

Respiratory system

Bronchiectasis

This is a reasonably common subject for a long case and usually poses a management problem. Bronchiectasis is defined as pathological and permanent dilatation of the bronchi. There are associated destructive and inflammatory changes in the walls of the segmental and subsegmental bronchi.

The history

1. Find out when the patient's respiratory problems began. Classically the cough and sputum begin in childhood, although adult onset is becoming more common. Ask about childhood whooping cough or measles. Lower respiratory tract infection with influenza and adenoviruses is an increasingly common cause of the disease. Potentially necrotising bacteria are also a cause if antibiotic treatment is inadequate. These include *Staphylococcus aureus* and *Klebsiella* organisms. The abnormal pulmonary defence mechanisms, or mucus clearance, associated with cystic fibrosis, tuberculosis, immunoglobulin deficiency, human immunodeficiency virus (HIV) infection and primary ciliary dyskinesia (immotile cilia syndrome) make these important causes of the condition. Localised bronchiectasis can occur in association with a space-occupying lesion, which can be endobronchial or external. Symptoms include:
    (a) recurrent haemoptysis
    (b) dyspnoea and wheeze
    (c) chronic sinusitis (70%)
    (d) recurrent pneumonia and pleurisy
    (e) systemic symptoms of weight loss, fever and anorexia
    (f) symptoms of right heart failure—a late event.
2. Recent precipitating causes of admissions to hospital (e.g. infection, haemoptysis).
3. Treatment—physiotherapy, postural drainage, antibiotics (as prophylaxis or treatment), bronchodilators, lung resection.
4. Investigations in the past (e.g. computed tomography [CT] scanning, ciliary function studies, sweat test, bronchograms [memorable!]).
5. Aetiology such as childhood or early adult infections (e.g. pneumonia, measles, whooping cough) (Table 6.12).
6. How the disease interferes with the patient's life (e.g. work).
7. Infertility is usual in men with primary ciliary dyskinesia and is variable in affected women.

The examination

Examine the respiratory system carefully. Particularly note the unpleasant purulent sputum and examine carefully for clubbing and localised crackles and wheezes. Look also for the position of the apex beat (don't miss dextrocardia—Kartagener's syndrome) and for the signs of right heart failure. Consider the complications and look for them. These include:

1. pneumonia
2. pleurisy
3. empyema
4. lung abscess
5. cor pulmonale

Table 6.12 Causes of bronchiectasis

1. Congenital
   (a) cystic fibrosis
   (b) primary ciliary dyskinesia, including the immotile cilia syndrome
   (c) congenital hypogammaglobulinaemia (especially IgA and IgG subclasses)
2. Acquired
   (a) infections in childhood (e.g. pneumonia, measles, whooping cough)
   (b) localised disease (e.g. bronchial adenoma, tuberculosis, foreign body)
   (c) allergic bronchopulmonary aspergillosis (proximal bronchiectasis)
   (d) rheumatoid arthritis, Sjögren's syndrome
   (e) idiopathic (up to 50%)

Note: Lung carcinoma rarely causes bronchiectasis as death tends to intervene first.

---

6. cerebral abscess (very rare)
7. amyloid (rare, but an important topic in the examination).

Investigations

Investigations should include a chest X-ray film (Fig 8.7). This may be normal. It may show 1–2-cm cystic lesions or, more often, streaky infiltration and thickened bronchial walls (tram tracking), especially in the lower lobes. Measure immunoglobulin (IgG, IgM, IgA) levels.

Look at the sputum microscopy result. The common organisms are *Haemophilus influenzae*, *Pseudomonas*, *Escherichia coli*, pneumococcus and *Staph. aureus*. Eosinophilia may indicate allergic bronchopulmonary aspergillosis or asthma. Ventilatory function tests may show a restrictive defect or an obstructive pattern. Arterial blood gas estimations may show mild or moderate hypoxia and, later, respiratory failure—defined as an arterial oxygen tension (PaO_2) <60 mmHg or an arterial carbon dioxide tension ($PaCO_2$) >50 mmHg. High-resolution CT scanning of the chest, which has replaced bronchography, is indicated in most patients to confirm the diagnosis. The extent of the disease is usually generalised. If the bronchiectasis is localised, resection may be indicated as long as the underlying cause is not systemic.

Treatment

The principles of treatment are the facilitation (or maximisation) of clearance of sputum and the treatment of infection with antibiotics and of bronchoconstriction with bronchodilators. Inhaled steroids may be of value if there is bronchial reactivity. Twice-daily postural drainage (20 minutes morning and night) or newer physiotherapy techniques should be recommended. The use of antibiotics during exacerbations is routine and prednisone in tapered doses may be useful. Prophylactic oral or nebulised antibiotics are controversial treatments. Problem pathogens include *Mycobacterium avium* complex (MAC), *Pseudomonas* and *Aspergillus*. Influenza vaccine is advisable for older patients. Treatment of heart failure should go *pari passu* with that of the lung disease. Immunoglobulin deficiency can be treated with monthly intravenous injections of immunoglobulin, which decrease the incidence of infection and the need for hospitalisation. Massive haemoptysis may occur as a result of bronchial wall erosion and the increased vascularity of the bronchial walls. It may respond to bronchial artery embolisation. Smoking cessation is always essential. Surgery should be considered for localised disease to prevent progression or as treatment of intractable haemorrhage. Transplant is occasionally appropriate for end-stage disease.

Lung carcinoma

This is a common disease which candidates often encounter in the examination. It can pose a diagnostic and management problem. Lung carcinoma remains a leading cause of cancer death in men and women. At diagnosis only 20% will have local disease and half will have disseminated disease. The overall 5-year survival rate is less than 15%. The major cell types are set out in Table 6.13. Adenocarcinoma has become more common than squamous cell carcinoma over the last 20 years.

Table 6.13 Carcinoma of the lung—cell types		
Type	**Frequency**	**Overall 5-year survival rate**
Adenocarcinoma	32%	17%
Squamous cell	29%	15%
Small (oat) cell	18%	5%
Large cell	9%	11%
Bronchioalveolar	3%	42%

The history

1. Ask about how the diagnosis was made or suspected—a proportion of patients are asymptomatic and were diagnosed because of a routine chest X-ray or scan.
2. Ask about duration of illness and respiratory symptoms (e.g. haemoptysis, dyspnoea, increasing cough, chest pain).
3. Ask about a history of unresolved pneumonia, pleural effusion or lung abscess.
4. Ask about systemic symptoms (e.g. weight loss).
5. Ask about metastatic and non-metastatic symptoms (Table 6.14).
6. Ask about aetiology:
   (a) smoking and exposure to the cigarette smoke of others (a dose–response relationship—long-term smokers have a 10- to 30-fold risk; discontinuation of smoking reduces the risk over 10–15 years, but the relative risk does not return to 1.0); women have a higher risk for a given level of exposure to cigarette smoke than men (1.5:1); there is a familial association for first-degree relatives
   (b) occupational history (e.g. asbestos exposure, uranium miners); remember, the effect of asbestos plus smoking is synergistic, *not* additive
   (c) chronic scarring (e.g. tuberculosis, scleroderma, pulmonary fibrosis may be associated with adenocarcinoma).
7. Ask about investigations performed, such as chest X-ray changes (the only abnormal finding in 5% of cases), bronchoscopy, sputum cytology, needle biopsy, thoracotomy.
8. Inquire about work and home environment, including the number of dependants, ability to work.
9. Ask about treatment offered and begun.
10. Inquire about the patient's understanding of the condition and the likely prognosis.

Table 6.14   Metastatic and non-metastatic manifestations of lung carcinoma

Local extension
1. Pleural effusion
2. Rib involvement
3. Nerve involvement (e.g. Pancoast's tumour, Horner's syndrome, recurrent laryngeal nerve palsy, diaphragmatic paralysis)
4. Superior vena caval obstruction
5. Pericardial effusion
6. Oesophageal obstruction
7. Tracheal obstruction
8. Lymphangitis

Distant metastases
1. Cervical adenopathy
2. Cerebral, liver or bone metastases

Non-metastatic features
1. Anorexia, weight loss, cachexia, fever
2. Endocrine:
   (a) hypercalcaemia (increased parathyroid hormone occurs usually in squamous cell carcinoma)
   (b) hyponatraemia (antidiuretic hormone—small cell carcinoma)
   (c) ectopic adrenocorticotrophic hormone (ACTH) syndrome (usually small cell carcinoma)
   (d) gynaecomastia (all types—caused by ectopic gonadotrophin secretion)
   (e) carcinoid syndrome (small cell carcinoma)
   (f) insulin-like activity (squamous cell carcinoma)
3. Skeletal (very rare with small cell carcinoma):
   (a) clubbing
   (b) hypertrophic pulmonary osteoarthropathy (may be more common with adenocarcinoma)
4. Neurological:
   (a) Eaton Lambert's syndrome (small cell carcinoma)
   (b) peripheral neuropathy or autonomic neuropathy
   (c) subacute cerebellar degeneration
   (d) polymyositis/dermatomyositis
   (e) cortical degeneration with dementia
   (f) acute transverse myelopathy
5. Haematological:
   (a) migrating venous thrombophlebitis, arterial thrombosis
   (b) diffuse intravascular coagulation
   (c) anaemia, leukoerythroblastosis, red cell aplasia, polycythaemia, eosinophilia
6. Skin:
   e.g. acanthosis nigricans, fibrinolytic purpura, scleroderma (alveolar cell carcinoma)
7. Renal:
   e.g. nephrotic syndrome (owing to membranous glomerulonephritis)
8. Opportunistic infections (most often in those treated with chemotherapy)

The examination

Finger clubbing is a most important sign (see Table 8.10). This is very rare in small cell carcinoma. Chest signs will vary—listen carefully for a fixed inspiratory wheeze over a large bronchus. Recurrent laryngeal nerve palsy may have caused hoarseness and phrenic nerve paralysis may have caused an elevation of a hemidiaphragm. An apical tumour may be responsible for Pancoast's syndrome (C8, T1 thoracic nerve destruction or compression, or Horner's syndrome, or both. Look for metastatic (e.g. supraclavicular lymphadenopathy and hepatomegaly) and non-metastatic manifestations, especially the neurological and endocrinological changes (Table 6.14).

Investigations

Screening of high-risk patients with X-ray or CT scanning may lead to an early diagnosis but has not been shown to affect survival.

The diagnosis may be difficult, even when suspected. Sputum cytology may be helpful in centrally located lesions but fibreoptic bronchoscopy is now more often done first. The chest X-ray may suggest the cell type: for example, peripheral nodule—adenocarcinoma, central lesion with obstructive pneumonitis—squamous, mediastinal or hilar mass—small cell, or alveolar infiltrate—bronchoalveolar cell. A suspect shadow on the chest X-ray film should be investigated by fibreoptic bronchoscopy and biopsy or fine-needle aspiration. Bronchial brushings and washings, taken at bronchoscopy, should also be sent for cytological examination but have a lower yield than biopsy.

For peripheral lesions, especially those less than 2 cm in size, transthoracic fine-needle biopsy with CT guidance is very useful, but complications (e.g. pneumothorax, significant bleeding) can occur. In patients with a malignant pleural effusion, thoracocentesis and pleural biopsy provide a high diagnostic yield (see Table 8.11). Other investigations may need to include bone marrow biopsy, mediastinoscopy and thoracotomy. Video-assisted thoracoscopy has replaced open biopsy in many centres.

Other possible causes (e.g. of a coin lesion) must be excluded. For this purpose CT is helpful; demonstration of central or lamellar calcification usually indicates that a coin lesion is benign. Follow-up scans to confirm a lesion is unchanged are helpful. Positron emission tomography (PET) scans may be of value in these cases.

Once the diagnosis is made and the cell type identified, further investigations may be indicated to stage the disease. Symptoms and signs that suggest central nervous system, liver, bone, chest wall or mediastinal involvement need to be sought carefully. Full blood count (Table 6.15), serum calcium and liver function tests may suggest tumour spread. CT scanning of the chest and abdomen with contrast is an important aid in determining whether disease is localised. In small cell carcinoma, stage the disease into: limited disease (lung primary, ipsilateral and contralateral hilar, mediastinal and supraclavicular nodes) or extensive disease—70% of patients (contralateral lung, distant metastases).

Non-small cell carcinoma is staged according to the tumour node metastases (TNM) international staging system (Table 6.16).

Assessment for resectability should include respiratory function tests. If the forced expiratory volume (FEV_1) is 1.5 L or more, this indicates that the patient could tolerate a pneumonectomy (a postoperative FEV_1 of 1 L or more is usually considered the minimum that will be tolerated). Otherwise, a patient who can climb three flights of stairs is usually considered well enough to tolerate surgery.

Treatment

Small cell carcinomas are only occasionally resected as they have usually metastasised at the time of diagnosis. In limited disease, chemotherapy and concurrent radiotherapy improve the prognosis. Untreated, the median survival is only about 4 months. Treatment often includes etoposide and cisplatin or carboplatin. Prophylactic cranial

Table 6.15 Full blood count and liver function tests from a female patient with carcinoma of the lung

Parameter	Value	Normal value
Haemoglobin	84 g/L	115–165 g/L (female)
Mean corpuscular volume (MCV)	95 fL	80–100 fL
White cell count (WCC)	4.0×10^9/L	$4.5–13.5 \times 10^9$/L
Platelets	95×10^9/L	$150–400 \times 10^9$/L
Erythrocyte sedimentation rate (ESR)	70 mm/h	3–19 mm/h (female <50 years)
Bilirubin	84 mmol/L	<20 mmol/L (total)
Aspartate aminotransferase (AST)	57 U/L	<40 U/L
Alanine aminotransferase (ALT)	50 U/L	<35 U/L
Lactate dehydrogenase (LDH)	780 U/L	110–230 U/L
Protein	60 g/L	62–80 g/L (total)
Albumin	33 g/L	32–45 g/L

Blood film: normochromic red cells, poikilocytosis, tear drop cells. Some nucleated red cells (normoblasts) and myeloid cells (metamyelocytes and myelocytes). Some rouleaux formation.

Comment: The combination of normochromic anaemia and the presence of marrow precursors in the peripheral blood is called a leukoerythroblastic reaction. It is typical of bone marrow infiltration by carcinoma or fibrosis. The abnormal liver function tests are non-specific but suggest liver involvement in this setting. The elevated LDH level probably indicates liver damage but can also occur when there is haemolysis.

Table 6.16 TNM international staging system for carcinoma of the lung

Stage	TNM			5-year survival rate	Management
IA	T1	N0	M0	61%	Surgery
IB	T2	N0	M0	38%	Surgery
IIA	T1	N1	M0	34%	Surgery ± radiotherapy or chemotherapy
IIB	T2	N2	M0	24%	Surgery ± radiotherapy or chemotherapy
IIIA	T3	N1	M0	9%	Surgery + chemotherapy
	T1–3	N2	M0	13%	
IIIB	T4	N0–2	M0	9%	
	T1–4	N3	M0	3%	Chemotherapy or palliation
IV			M1	1%	Chemotherapy or palliation

T0 = no tumour; T1–T3 = ascending degrees of increase in tumour size and involvement; N0 = no lymph nodes; N1–4 = ascending degrees of nodal involvement; M0 = no metastases; M1–4 = ascending degrees of metastatic involvement.

irradiation may be given to patients with complete responses. There is a risk of leukaemia, central nervous system metastases, dementia and second primary malignancies with treatment. Limited small cell carcinoma has a median survival with treatment of 11–18 months; 10–20% are disease-free at 2 years. Extensive small cell carcinoma has a median survival of 6–12 months with therapy.

Non-small cell carcinomas may be resectable—unless there is tumour spread to the contralateral lung or outside the thorax, or there is significant cardiopulmonary disease. The most important prognostic factor is the stage of disease. Staging usually involves bronchoscopy and CT scanning of the chest, abdomen and brain, as well as a physiological assessment of the patient's fitness for surgery, from both the point of view of lung function and general health. One-third of these patients have disease sufficiently localised for an attempt at resection. Radiotherapy with 'curative intent' may be offered to these patients if they refuse surgery or are unfit for surgery for other reasons. About 6% are alive after 5 years. Adjuvant chemotherapy is not routine for surgical patients but regimens including cisplatin may provide a small survival advantage. Median survival is only a few months in patients with intracranial metastases or bone involvement. Combination chemotherapy is sometimes appropriate. Survival benefit is only 1 or 2 months.

The average 5-year survival rate for all types of carcinoma of the lung is about 15%.

Airway obstruction as a result of carcinoma may be relieved by using Nd-YAG laser or brachytherapy for palliation.

Chronic obstructive pulmonary disease (chronic airflow limitation)

This general term is usually applied to patients with chronic bronchitis and emphysema. Although these two conditions are different, they usually occur together. Chronic obstructive pulmonary disease (COPD) is common and presents major management problems. However, in the examination it is unusual for it to be the patient's only medical problem. The vast majority of patients with COPD are or have been smokers. However, only about one-fifth of smokers experience a rapid enough decline in FEV_1 ever to develop COPD.

The history

1. Ask about symptoms, such as cough and sputum, dyspnoea, wheeze, impaired exercise tolerance, ankle oedema and weight loss. Remember that the diagnosis of chronic bronchitis is made largely from the history.
2. Ask about precipitating causes of disease exacerbation, such as an upper respiratory tract infection, pneumonia, omission of drugs, symptoms of right ventricular failure, resumption of smoking, pneumothorax, sleep apnoea, oropharyngeal aspiration and gastro-oesophageal reflux disease.
3. Inquire about smoking habit. Ask about number of cigarettes smoked per day and length of use (10 packet years of smoking is usually a prerequisite) and exposure to other people's cigarette smoke—passive smoking. Absence of a smoking history weighs heavily against the diagnosis unless chronic asthma or alpha$_1$-antitrypsin deficiency is present.
4. Ask about occupational history. This may be important, particularly as an additive feature if the patient has pneumoconiosis or has been exposed to toluene in plastics factories.
5. Ask about medications, especially steroids.
6. Inquire about management at home and work, and the social effects of the disease. Determine exercise tolerance. Ask about financial problems associated with chronic illness and symptoms of depression caused by chronic disability and loss of self-esteem.

7. Ask about family history, such as alpha$_1$-antitrypsin deficiency causing emphysema (autosomal codominant inheritance; mild deficiency, usually associated with the ZZ allele, rarely leads to emphysema in non-smokers but is responsible for 2% of cases of emphysema in smokers).

The examination

Examine the respiratory system carefully. The examination may be normal until airways obstruction is moderately severe. Look particularly for:

1. pursed lip breathing (prolongs the expiratory time and may limit over-inflation) and use of accessory muscles
2. cyanosis and polycythaemia (*Note*: clubbing does not occur unless another disease such as carcinoma has supervened)
3. intercostal recession
4. prolonged forced expiratory time (reduced in both obstructive and restrictive lung disease)
5. tracheal tug
6. reduced diaphragmatic movements, over-inflation, reduced chest wall movement and expansion
7. reduced breath sounds with or without wheezes (rhonchi) and coarse inspiratory crackles
8. sputum
9. signs of right heart failure
10. signs of cachexia, in patients with advanced disease (this is probably related to the increase in tumour necrosis factor alpha associated with chronic hypoxia rather than to the increased work of breathing)
11. side-effects of treatment (e.g. tremor as a result of the use of beta-agonists, or the various changes caused by steroids).

Investigations

1. Chest X-ray film—look for signs of hyperinflation (flat diaphragms and a vertical heart shadow) and cor pulmonale, and exclude pneumonia. Radiolucent bullae may be visible; they are very specific for emphysema. The X-ray may be normal if the patient has mild disease. High resolution CT of the chest is more often performed and is more specific for emphysema.
2. Ventilatory function tests—look for a considerable reduction of the FEV$_1$/FVC (forced vital capacity) ratio. A normal FEV$_1$ excludes the condition. The amount of reversibility should be tested with bronchodilators. An increase in FEV$_1$ or FVC of more than 15% and of at least 200 mL is considered significant. Complete or almost complete reversibility means that the diagnosis is asthma rather than COPD. Some asthmatics smoke and have both conditions; many smokers claim to have asthma but have only COPD. Vital capacity or total lung capacity may be falsely decreased if measured by gas dilution techniques because of the non-homogeneity of ventilation in COPD. The diffusing capacity for carbon monoxide is reduced in emphysema—a value of <50% is associated with exertion-induced hypoxia.
3. Arterial blood gas levels—look for respiratory failure at rest. The demonstration of significant hypoxia (usually a PaO_2 of <55 mmHg, or of <59 mmHg if the patient has cor pulmonale) is required for the prescription of home oxygen treatment.
4. Haemoglobin value—look for polycythaemia.
5. Sputum culture, which will usually grow *Haemophilus influenzae*, *Streptococcus pneumoniae* or *Moraxella catarrhalis* during exacerbations *and* remissions.
6. Electrocardiogram (ECG)—look for signs of right ventricular hypertrophy.

7. Alpha$_1$-antitrypsin measurement is now generally recommended. It should particularly be considered if the patient has never smoked or has associated bronchiectasis, cirrhosis or basilar emphysema.
8. Assessment of nutrition—body mass index (BMI = weight in kg/height in cm^2), body fat, grip strength, serum albumin, calcium and phosphate levels.
9. Exercise testing—to assess the need for ambulatory oxygen therapy and the degree of disability if there are discrepancies.

Differential diagnosis

1. Asthma
2. Bronchiectasis

   Features suggesting asthma:

1. non-smoking patient
2. onset in childhood
3. family history of allergy
4. episodic attacks and also nocturnal symptoms
5. a rapid response to treatment, especially steroids
6. eosinophilia in the sputum
7. atopic diathesis
8. reversibility of obstruction.

   Features suggesting bronchiectasis:

1. daily sputum production with or without haemoptysis
2. onset in childhood
3. recurrent chest infection
4. clubbing.

Treatment

1. Stop smoking. This decreases sputum production and bronchospasm, and may reduce the rate of decline in lung function to that of a non-smoker. It is associated with survival benefit. The candidate should have an approach to the treatment of nicotine addiction. This may involve the temporary use of nicotine substitutes, psychological counselling and encouragement and the use of drugs such as bupropion.
2. Antibiotics to shorten exacerbations (long-term chemoprophylaxis is indicated if there are four or more episodes a year), such as amoxycillin or doxycycline given as a course at home at the first sign of purulent sputum. Remember that 25% of *H. influenzae* and 75% of *M. catarrhalis* infections are ampicillin-resistant.
3. Regular bronchodilators. Beta$_2$-agonists from metered dose inhalers form the basis of treatment. A small change in FEV$_1$ and FVC may produce considerable subjective improvement. Some patients find the inhaler devices difficult to use. Candidates should have a strategy to ensure effective use of the best device for a particular patient. Long-acting drugs, such as salmeterol, provide longer acting bronchodilatation and are at least more convenient. Oral theophylline derivatives may have an additive effect with beta$_2$-agonists, perhaps because they improve respiratory muscle function. They are much less often prescribed now, partly because they cause oesophageal reflux, cardiac arrhythmias, nausea and insomnia, and partly because they are not very effective. The addition of ipratropium may be of benefit even if the patient has not responded to beta$_2$-agonists. The new long-acting anticholinergic drug, triotropium, is replacing ipratropium, and may be a first-line option. Inhaled steroids are probably not helpful. Antitussives and mucolytics are controversial but may be useful to prevent exacerbations.
4. Pursed lip breathing and postural changes may be of value. Maintain adequate hydration.

5. Steroid use may be effective in an acute exacerbation and as a way of excluding asthma if there is persisting doubt. A trial of high doses for 2 weeks may be beneficial when bronchodilators are insufficient. Maintenance steroid treatment should be given only if a short course has been shown objectively to be effective (i.e. improved respiratory function test results). Use the lowest dose possible. The associated weight gain, loss of muscle strength and osteoporosis may make things worse.

6. Annual influenza vaccine and 5-yearly pneumococcal vaccine are useful. Routine prophylactic antibiotics are not.

7. Pulmonary rehabilitation programs have been demonstrated in randomised controlled trials to improve symptoms and quality of life, but not to prolong life. Exercise and weight reduction increase the patients' well-being, but not their lung function.

8. Domiciliary oxygen. This is indicated for patients with a PaO_2 of <55 mmHg, or cor pulmonale and a PaO_2 of <59 mmHg. There is evidence that mortality rates are decreased by the use of domiciliary low-flow oxygen given for 19 hours per day (especially during sleep). This may work by reducing the progression of pulmonary hypertension. Find out what type of oxygen supplementation the patient uses (e.g. concentrator, cylinders) and how this is managed with regard to convenience and cost.

9. Treatment of cor pulmonale. Heart failure is likely to improve with successful treatment of the lung disease. Spironolactone and diuretics may be useful.

10. Alpha$_1$-antitrypsin deficiency can be treated by replenishing the missing antiprotease, which re-establishes antineutrophil elastase protection for the lower lung zones. An intravenous preparation can be administered weekly or monthly. This expensive treatment is only indicated if alpha$_1$-antitrypsin levels are below 11 µmol/L. The clinical benefit of this treatment is not established.

11. Lung transplantation is an option for younger (<65 years) patients with end-stage disease and without serious comorbidity who have not had previous thoracic surgery. The 1-year survival rate is over 80% for this group.

12. Lung reduction surgery is an option for some severely symptomatic patients who have stopped smoking. Thorascopic removal of the worst lung segments gives symptomatic improvement to many patients. The procedure remains controversial, at least partly because lung function continues to decline. Symptomatic benefit may be lost within a year and accelerated decline in lung function may occur. Pulmonary hypertension is a contraindication and air leaks from the stapled lung are the most important postoperative problem. This operation is combined with an intensive rehabilitation and exercise program, which may in itself account for some of the postoperative improvement.

13. The use of positive pressure ventilation (continuous positive airways pressure [CPAP]) is a possible option for long-term management.

14. The management of severe exacerbations is difficult, particularly when these are associated with severe carbon dioxide retention and a reduced level of consciousness. Steroids and theophylline are both used commonly for these patients. Evidence for their effectiveness is not strong. The decision about whether or not to try mechanical ventilation is a difficult one. Ventilation via a mask may improve things without the need for intubation. Intensive care units will usually require some evidence of a potentially reversible problem before allowing intubation. The patient's own wishes are important and should be obtained before he or she is too sick to make a decision.

Sleep apnoea

This is an increasingly recognised clinical syndrome that should be suspected in patients who have obesity, hypertension, fatigue, excessive snoring or unexplained respiratory failure. Obstructive sleep apnoea is a common cause of sleep disturbance but by no means the only explanation for it. Sleep apnoea patients commonly have some combination of these symptoms.

The history

1. Classically, in obstructive sleep apnoea, patients or anyone in the house will describe a history of loud snoring at night, associated with multiple periods of cessation of respiratory movement and waking and gasping for breath. Apnoeas of more than 10 seconds are considered significant but for patients with this condition, pauses of up to 2 or 3 minutes can occur, and of 30 seconds are common. Ask the patient if there have been problems with excessive daytime sleepiness and with working during the day. Inquire whether the patient drinks alcohol and, if so, how much. Alcohol consumption is a common exacerbating factor. Remember, though, that the majority of people who snore do not have sleep apnoea and brief apnoeas not associated with signs of arousal are normal for many people.
2. Ask whether there is a history of hypertension and whether this has been treated (50% of these patients have hypertension). Find out whether the patient has had angina or arrhythmias at night. Both of these may be precipitated by the hypoxia associated with apnoea. Heartburn and non-cardiac chest pain caused by gastro-oesophageal reflux are also common.
3. Inquire about medications, such as hypnotics, that may have been prescribed for poor sleeping but actually aggravate sleep apnoea.
4. Ask about a previous diagnosis of COPD or symptoms of heart failure. The recurrent increase in afterload that occurs during apnoeic episodes can precipitate or exacerbate left ventricular failure. Fewer than 10% of patients develop right heart failure and significant pulmonary hypertension.
5. Ask about a history of tonsillar enlargement or throat surgery. In a few sleep apnoea patients there is a clear anatomical cause for the obstruction.
6. In the absence of excessive snoring, central sleep apnoea needs to be considered for a patient with the other symptoms.
7. Ask about symptoms suggestive of narcolepsy rather than sleep apnoea. The sudden sleep attacks of narcolepsy can occur at any time, including during meals, conversation or driving. These patients may also report sudden loss of muscle tone from emotion (e.g. laughter). The result is the unexpected dropping of an object or sudden buckling at the knees and falling down; here cataplexy should be considered. Cataplexy is usually associated with narcolepsy although it may precede narcolepsy by several years.
8. Ask about symptoms of the restless legs syndrome, which may also lead to daytime sleepiness. The use of diuretics or insulin may also predispose patients to inadequate sleep and should not be confused with sleep apnoea.
9. Ask whether the patient drives a motor car and whether the risks of driving have been discussed. Also ask whether it has been recommended that the anaesthetist be informed of the patient's sleep apnoea before any administration of an anaesthetic.
10. Find out how this chronic condition has affected the patient's family and work.

The examination

Assess the BMI but remember that up to 50% of patients with obstructive sleep apnoea are not obese, and most patients with central sleep apnoea are not obese. Respiratory examination is usually normal. Blood pressure should be measured and the fundi examined for signs of hypertension. The cardiovascular system should be examined carefully for evidence of pulmonary hypertension. Inspect the head and neck for signs of uvular enlargement and macroglossia or tonsillar hypertrophy. Look at the neck circumference. Perform a neurological examination to look for signs of autonomic neuropathy (e.g. diabetes, Shy-Drager syndrome), brain stem lesions or spinal cord disease (e.g. tumour, demyelination), which can cause central sleep apnoea. Also examine the patient for neurological causes of obstructive sleep apnoea, such as myasthenia gravis or muscular dystrophy. Look for signs of hypothyroidism or acromegaly.

Investigations

Consider sleep study monitoring (polysomnography) with the electroencephalogram, chin electromyogram, electro-ocular monitoring (to detect rapid eye movement [REM] sleep), oximetry, $PaCO_2$ monitoring and, if indicated, ECG monitoring (for arrhythmias). For a definitive diagnosis, the apnoeic spells must be 10 seconds or longer in duration and at least five per hour must be recorded over several hours. The apnoea hypopnoea index (AHI) is the total number of episodes of apnoea or hypopnoea per night divided by the number of hours of sleep. A value greater than 5 is considered abnormal but is probably not diagnostic in the absence of symptoms. For patients with typical features of the condition home PaO_2 monitoring overnight may be an option. A positive test (several significant desaturation episodes per hour) is enough evidence to justify treatment. A negative test, however, does not exclude the diagnosis. Narcolepsy can also be diagnosed by a sleep study. Hypothyroidism should be excluded with thyroid function tests. Echocardiography may be indicated to enable estimation of pulmonary artery pressures and to assess right ventricular function.

Treatment

If the patient has hypothyroidism, thyroid hormone replacement may reverse sleep apnoea. Concomitant diseases such as cardiac failure, hypertension or asthma need to be treated vigorously. Nasal decongestants may be helpful. Weight loss is of value but may be difficult to achieve. Respiratory depressants, such as tranquillisers, should be withdrawn.

CPAP is of value for long-term treatment of irreversible obstructive sleep apnoea. These devices are not always well tolerated. Nasal CPAP is effective in the majority of patients who can adjust to it. The devices are improving steadily in comfort and portability.

Surgical correction of upper airways narrowing caused by polyps, enlarged tonsils or macroglossia can lead to significant improvement. Excision of soft tissue in the oropharynx is of value for some patients.

If there has been a recent stroke, observation may be all that is required, as respiratory function may improve with time. Patients with central sleep apnoea can often be successfully treated with bilevel positive airways pressure (BiPAP) ventilation.

Pulmonary fibrosis

Infiltrative lung disease has a prolonged course, so patients are often available for the examinations. Discovering the aetiology may be difficult.

The history

The diagnosis may not be obvious until you examine the patient, at which stage you may have to ask further questions.
1. Presenting respiratory symptoms (e.g. dry cough, dyspnoea, lethargy, malaise).
2. Does the patient know the cause of the respiratory symptoms?
3. Systemic symptoms (e.g. weight loss, fatigue, fever, rash and arthralgia, which may indicate a systemic disease, particularly a connective tissue disease or sarcoidosis; Table 6.17).
4. Drug use—cardiac (amiodarone, hydralazine, procainamide); rheumatological (methotrexate, D-penicillamine); chemotherapeutic (busulphan, bleomycin,

cyclophosphamide); others (nitrofurantoin, bromocriptine). The majority of patients are, or have been, smokers.

5. A detailed occupational history, such as exposure to mineral dust (silicosis, asbestosis, coal miner's pneumoconiosis), chemical fumes (nitrogen dioxide, chlorine, ammonia) or organic dusts (Table 6.18).
6. Any history of radiotherapy.
7. History of extrinsic allergic alveolitis (e.g. bird fancier's lung, humidifier lung, farmer's lung).
8. Infections (e.g. miliary tuberculosis).
9. Investigations (e.g. high-resolution CT of the thorax, lung biopsy or bronchial lavage).
10. Treatment, if any.
11. Social problems as a result of the chronic disability.

Table 6.17 Fibrotic and granulomatous lung disease

Connective tissue diseases causing fibrosis
1. Rheumatoid arthritis
2. Systemic lupus erythematosus
3. Scleroderma
4. Polymyositis and dermatomyositis
5. Sjögren's syndrome
6. Polyarteritis nodosa (rare)

Causes of granulomatous lung disease on lung biopsy
1. Sarcoidosis
2. Tuberculosis
3. Chronic berylliosis
4. Extrinsic allergic alveolitis

Table 6.18 Asbestos and the lung

Heavy exposure associated with:
1. Asbestosis
2. Bronchial carcinoma

Trivial exposure associated with:
1. Pleural fibrosis and plaques
2. Mesothelioma after a latent period of 30–40 years

The examination

Clubbing, cyanosis and crackles (fine, late, inspiratory) make the diagnosis likely. Look for signs of associated systemic disease, as well as sarcoidosis and connective tissue disease. Assess the severity of the disease (signs of pulmonary hypertension) and for signs of drug side-effects (especially steroids).

Investigations

The goals of investigations are to find the aetiology, establish the severity of the disease and to look for signs of active inflammation. If active inflammation is present, the condition may respond to immunotherapy (steroids or cyclophosphamide). If established fibrosis is present, such treatment is unlikely to help.

Chest radiography is the initial investigation but may be normal (Fig 8.7). High-resolution CT of the thorax is the investigation of choice. It is probably the most sensitive non-invasive test. The changes of pulmonary fibrosis are characteristic. Note whether there is a localised or diffuse abnormality or progressive massive fibrosis (caused by silicosis and coal miner's lung).

Pulmonary function tests will reveal a restrictive pattern, with reduction of lung volumes and reduced transfer factor. Blood gas levels will show hypoxia with a normal or low $PaCO_2$. The erythrocyte sedimentation rate (ESR) is often raised. There may be hypergammaglobulinaemia and a raised lactate dehydrogenase (LDH) level. Eosinophilia may be a useful clue (Table 6.19). Serological testing for connective tissue diseases is routine.

Table 6.19   Causes of pulmonary infiltrate and eosinophilia (PIE)

Mnemonic: PLATE
P — Prolonged pulmonary eosinophilia—this may be caused by: drugs (e.g. sulfonamides, sulfasalazine, salicylates, nitrofurantoin, penicillin, isoniazid, methotrexate, carbamazepine, imipramine, L-tryptophan); parasites (e.g. *Ascaris*); idiopathic
L — Loeffler's syndrome (benign and acute)
A — Allergic bronchopulmonary aspergillosis (always associated with asthma)
T — Tropical (e.g. microfilaria)
E — Eosinophilic pneumonia and vasculitis (e.g. polyarteritis nodosa, Wegener's granulomatosis)

Bronchoalveolar lavage and transbronchial lung biopsy can be performed—it is suggested that fibrosis associated with a lavage showing a predominance of polymorphonuclear cells is less responsive to treatment. Lymphocytosis on lavage suggests drug-induced or granulomatous disease. A positive gallium-67 lung scan may also indicate disease activity. Lung clearance studies using pertechnate may also be helpful (rapid clearance suggests active alveolitis). Diagnoses likely to be made by transbronchial lung biopsy include sarcoidosis and lymphangitic spread of carcinoma. Open lung biopsy or video-assisted thoracoscopic biopsy may be required to confirm the presence of idiopathic pulmonary fibrosis but only if there is clinical uncertainty and the test could change treatment.

Treatment

This depends on the cause (Table 6.20). Remove exposure if appropriate. Treatment will not reverse established fibrosis. Steroids may help in diffuse fibrosing alveolitis, chemical injuries, hypersensitivity pneumonias, sarcoidosis, histiocytosis X and connective tissue disease. There is no evidence that they improve survival in these conditions. They are of no value in dust diseases. Treatment with prednisolone is usually begun at 1 mg/kg/day and reduced to half this dose after 4–12 weeks. Follow-up with measurement of spirometry, lung volumes and transfer factor is important to document response to treatment. Consider maintenance steroids in lower dose for

---

Table 6.20   Causes of pulmonary fibrosis

Upper lobe (SCHAT)
S — Silicosis (progressive massive fibrosis); sarcoidosis
C — Coal worker's pneumoconiosis (progressive massive fibrosis)
H — Histiocytosis X
A — Ankylosing spondylitis; allergic bronchopulmonary aspergillosis (allergic alveolitis may affect the upper or lower lobes)
T — Tuberculosis

Lower lobe (RASHO)
R — Rheumatoid arthritis
A — Asbestosis
S — Scleroderma
H — Hamman-Rich syndrome and other forms of idiopathic pulmonary fibrosis (i.e. diffuse fibrosing alveolitis)
O — Other, such as radiation, drugs (e.g. busulphan, bleomycin, nitrofurantoin, hydralazine, methotrexate, amiodarone)

---

patients who are improving or stabilised. Immunosuppressive agents and especially cyclophosphamide may sometimes be of benefit and can be used in combination with low-dose steroids. Colchicine in doses of 0.6 mg daily has been shown to improve some patients. It inhibits macrophage production of fibroblast growth factors.

General measures, such as administration of pneumococcal and influenza vaccines, may be indicated. Home oxygen therapy may provide symptomatic relief for hypoxaemic patients. Unilateral lung transplantation may be considered for some patients in the final stage of their disease.

Pulmonary hypertension

Many of the patients with this chronic and often severe illness will have raised pulmonary artery pressures as a result of a cardiac or respiratory illness. The patient may or may not be aware of this complication of his or her underlying disease, but it is essential for the candidate to know when to look for it. Idiopathic (primary) pulmonary hypertension (IPH) is a rare but important condition, which is diagnosed when other causes of pulmonary hypertension have been excluded. By definition, pulmonary hypertension is present when the mean pulmonary artery pressure (PAP) exceeds 25 mmHg at rest or 30 mmHg during exercise.

The classification of pulmonary hypertension has been revised recently. The Venice classification was released in 2003 and the term 'primary pulmonary hypertension' has been replaced with 'idiopathic pulmonary hypertension' (Table 6.21).

The history

1. Symptoms are usually non-specific but often severe. As usual, begin by asking if the patient knows what is wrong and the reason for the admission, or visit, to hospital.
2. If pulmonary hypertension seems a possibility, ask about the possible causes (see Table 6.21). Remember to ask specifically about appetite-suppressing drugs. The use of fenfluramine and phenermine in combination and for long periods has been associated with the greatest risk.

Table 6.21   The Venice classification for pulmonary hypertension 2003

1. Pulmonary arterial hypertension (PAH):
   1.1   Idiopathic (IPAH)
   1.2   Familial (FPAH)
   1.3   Associated with (APAH):
      1.3.1   Collagen vascular disease
      1.3.2   Congenital systemic-to-pulmonary shunts
      1.3.3   Portal hypertension
      1.3.4   HIV infection
      1.3.5   Drugs and toxins
      1.3.6   Other (thyroid disorders, glycogen storage disease, Gaucher's disease, hereditary haemorrhagic telangiectasia, haemoglobinopathies, myeloproliferative disorders, splenectomy)
   1.4   Associated with significant venous or capillary involvement:
      1.4.1   Pulmonary veno-occlusive disease (PVOD)
      1.4.2   Pulmonary capillary haemangiomatosis (PCH)
   1.5   Persistent pulmonary hypertension of the newborn
2. Pulmonary hypertension with left heart disease:
   2.1   Left-sided atrial or ventricular heart disease
   2.2   Left-sided valvular heart disease
3. Pulmonary hypertension associated with lung diseases and/or hypoxaemia:
   3.1   Chronic obstructive pulmonary disease
   3.2   Interstitial lung disease
   3.3   Sleep-disordered breathing
   3.4   Alveolar hypoventilation disorders
   3.5   Chronic exposure to high altitude
   3.6   Developmental abnormalities
4. Pulmonary hypertension as a result of chronic thrombotic and/or embolic disease:
   4.1   Thromboembolic obstruction of proximal pulmonary arteries
   4.2   Thromboembolic obstruction of distal pulmonary arteries
   4.3   Non-thrombotic pulmonary embolism (tumour, parasites, foreign material)
5. Miscellaneous—sarcoidosis, histiocytosis X, lymphangiomatosis, compression of pulmonary vessels (adenopathy, fibrosing mediastinitis)

---

3. If the patient has an illness that could be a cause, ask detailed questions about that condition, its severity and chronicity. There may be a family history in cases of IPH (6%; autosomal dominant condition with incomplete penetrance, 20–80%). The majority of familial cases are associated with a mutation on the *BMPR2* gene.

4. Find out how symptomatic the patient is. Idiopathic and secondary pulmonary hypertension cause dyspnoea. Almost all patients have dyspnoea at the time of diagnosis. Other less common symptoms include fatigue, chest pain, syncope and oedema. Cough and haemoptysis can be present. Ask about symptoms of connective tissue diseases and especially about scleroderma. Try to work out the patient's functional class (p 56) (New York Heart Association [NYHA] I–IV, often called the NYHA-WHO class when related to pulmonary hypertension).

5. Ask about previous or planned investigations. These may relate to the underlying condition, for example, respiratory function tests or scans, echocardiography (often transoesophageal echocardiography) or cardiac catheterisation. The patient who

presents with symptoms and signs of pulmonary hypertension needs a number of investigations before IPH can be diagnosed.

6. What general treatment has been recommended? This may be for the underlying cardiac or respiratory condition or for thrombosis. There may be a history of cardiac surgery in childhood for congenital heart disease. Oxygen supplementation is often prescribed. Find out how this is administered (e.g. via nasal prongs or a mask), for how many hours a day and whether it comes from a concentrator or oxygen tanks. Oxygen is very expensive unless subsidised. Ask about cost and the inconvenience of the treatment with regard to portability and noise (oxygen concentrators are noisy and use a lot of electricity). Has the treatment been helpful?

7. What drugs is the patient taking? Heparin and then warfarin are routine for pulmonary embolism but warfarin is also used for most patients with IPH because of the risk of in situ thrombosis in the pulmonary arteries. Bronchodilators and steroids may have been prescribed for lung disease. Vasodilators are the usual treatment for primary pulmonary hypertension. The possibility of heart or lung transplant, or both, may have been raised with the patient. The patient may be on a therapeutic trial or taking one of the newer agents, such as bosentan, sildenafil or the inhaled prostacyclin analogue iloprost. Patients involved in trials or taking new drugs are often very well informed about what is going on.

8. As with any chronic and possibly debilitating condition, questions about the patient's ability to work and manage the activities of daily living need to be detailed and comprehensive.

The examination

Try to assess the severity of the patient's dyspnoea as he or she undresses or by asking him or her to walk around the room. Perform a thorough respiratory and cardiac examination. Look for signs of chronic lung disease and of congenital heart disease, and for the specific signs of pulmonary hypertension and right heart failure.

Investigations

Investigations are directed at finding an underlying reason for pulmonary hypertension—IPH is a diagnosis of exclusion—and at assessing its severity and potential reversibility. These include:

1. Chest X-ray—abnormal in 90% of IPH patients (may show pulmonary fibrosis or an abnormal cardiac silhouette—right ventricular dilatation; there may be large proximal pulmonary arteries that appear 'pruned' in the periphery, the right ventricle may appear enlarged on the lateral film.) (see Fig 9.4).

2. Respiratory function tests (normal, restrictive or obstructive pattern). Moderate pulmonary hypertension itself is associated with a reduction in the diffusion capacity for carbon monoxide (DLCO) to about 50% of predicted.

3. ECG—signs of right heart strain or hypertrophy are present in up to 90% of patients (Fig 6.13).

4. Blood gases—hypercapnia in hypoventilation syndromes but hypocapnia is more common in IPH because of increased alveolar ventilation. Mild hypoxia in IPH, but more severe when pulmonary hypertension is secondary to lung disease.

5. CT pulmonary angiogram or ventilation–perfusion (V/Q) scan and Doppler venograms (deep venous thrombosis and pulmonary embolism—assessment of extent of involvement of the pulmonary bed). High-resolution CT of the lungs looking for interstitial lung disease.

6. Six-minute walking test—predicts survival and correlates with NYHA-WHO class. Reduction in arterial oxygen concentration of >10% during this test predicts almost threefold mortality risk over 29 months. Patients unable to manage 332 m in 6 minutes also have an adverse prognosis.

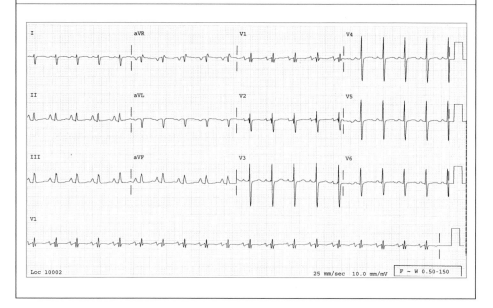

Fig 6.13 ECG of a patient with idiopathic pulmonary hypertension. Note 'P' pulmonale, right axis, right ventricular hypertrophy and strain, and sinus tachycardia.

7. Transthoracic or transoesophageal echocardiogram (Fig 6.14). A transthoracic echocardiogram will usually enable left ventricular failure or severe mitral valve disease to be excluded. One or both will enable the assessment of known congenital heart disease, the detection of a left to right (or reversed) shunting (Eisenmenger's syndrome) and measurement, in many cases, of pulmonary artery pressures. The presence of tricuspid regurgitation (common in normal people and almost universal in the presence of raised right ventricular pressures) enables estimation of right ventricular and therefore of pulmonary artery pressures in many patients. The pressure difference across the tricuspid valve can be calculated if the velocity of the regurgitant jet is measured by Doppler. Right atrial pressures are usually close to 5 mmHg, the right ventricular pressure can be estimated by adding 5 to the pressure difference across the tricuspid valve. The normal right ventricular and pulmonary artery systolic pressure is 20–25 mmHg. Assessment of pulmonary artery ejection characteristics can also be used to estimate pulmonary artery pressures. Right ventricular size and function can be assessed. Right ventricular dilatation and abnormal septal motion are useful signs of pulmonary hypertension. The right ventricle appears abnormal on echocardiograms in over 90% of people with pulmonary hypertension.
8. Catheterisation of the right heart is an essential investigation. It is the gold standard and should also be performed if other tests have not been definitive. It is usually performed with a multiple lumen flotation catheter and enables direct measurement of the right heart pressures. Left to right shunting can be detected by the collection of blood samples from the venae cavae, right atrium, right ventricle and pulmonary artery. A 'step-up' in the blood oxygen saturation indicates a shunt. The size of the shunt can be calculated if the cardiac output is measured by thermodilution. Measurement of the pulmonary artery wedge pressure enables the detection of mitral stenosis or the very rare pulmonary veno-occlusive disease. By definition,

Fig 6.14   Echocardiography report in a patient with pulmonary hypertension.

Echocardiography Report

Reason for study
?Pulmonary hypertension

Study quality: Good   <u>Satisfactory</u>   Poor

RV_____32____ (mm) (N 10–26)
Sept._____8_____ (mm) (N 7–11)
LVEDD___51____ (mm) (N 36–56)
LVESD___30____ (mm) (N 20–40)
LVPW____10____ (mm) (N 7–11)
Aorta____22____ (mm) (N 20–35)
LA_____36____ (mm) (N 24–40)
FS_____41____ % (N 27–40)
EF_____72____ % (N 55–70)

Valves

Mitral	Mild MR
Tricus.	Moderate TR
Aortic	Appears normal
Pulm.	Appears normal

Doppler—2D
The right ventricle is dilated. There is paradoxical septal motion.
   The LV is not dilated. The cardiac valves appear normal. The main pulmonary artery was not dilated. No ASD was seen.

Doppler—colour flow mapping
Moderate tricuspid regurgitation was detected. The TR flow velocity was 4 m/s. Estimated RV pressure 70 mmHg. Mild MR is present. No ASD flow or intracardiac shunting was detected.

Conclusions
Severe pulmonary hypertension. RV dilated, abnormal septal motion. No intracardiac shunting detected.

Comment
The most important signs of pulmonary hypertension on 2D echocardiographs are RV dilatation and abnormal septal motion. The septum normally behaves as part of the left ventricle and contracts inwards, towards the lateral wall of the left ventricle. Significant increases in RV pressure cause the septum to move away from the left ventricle during systole. Measurement of the velocity of the regurgitant tricuspid valve jet enables estimation of RV pressures. It is difficult to exclude an ASD on a transthoracic echocardiogram unless it is of very good quality. A transoesophageal echocardiograph may be required if there is any doubt about the cause of pulmonary hypertension.

Key
ASD = atrial septal defect; EF = ejection fraction; FS = fractional shortening; LA = left atrium; LVEDD = left ventricular end-diastolic dimension; LVESD = left ventricular end-systolic dimension; LVPW = left ventricular posterior wall;
MR = mitral regurgitation; Pulm. = pulmonary; RV = right ventricle; Sept. = septal thickness; TR = tricuspid regurgitation; Tricus. = tricuspid.

IPH means the pulmonary capillary wedge pressure is <18 mmHg (i.e. the raised pulmonary pressures are not secondary to left ventricular failure). Pulmonary vascular resistance can be calculated using the cardiac output, pulmonary artery pressure and pulmonary artery wedge pressure measurements. The formula is:

$$\text{Pulmonary vascular resistance} = \frac{\text{pulmonary artery pressure} - \text{pulmonary artery wedge pressure}}{\text{cardiac output}}$$

This gives a result in mmHg/L/min or Wood units. The normal is 1.7 mmHg/L/min. Assessment of the response to vasodilators should be performed for all these patients. It is used to direct treatment. The usual agents are epoprostenol (a derivative of prostacyclin), adenosine or inhaled nitric oxide. A positive test is defined as a reduction of pulmonary artery pressure of >10 mmHg to an absolute value <40 mmHg, without a fall in cardiac output. Only about 15% of IPH patients have a positive test.

Treatment

Treatment of pulmonary hypertension that is secondary to an underlying respiratory or cardiac condition begins with the attempt to optimise treatment or fix the underlying condition.

1. COPD: bronchodilators, steroids, continuous oxygen.
2. Pulmonary fibrosis: oxygen. Aggressive treatment of an underlying connective tissue disease may halt or slow progression of the pulmonary pressures.
3. Pulmonary embolus: anticoagulation, vena caval filter and occasionally pulmonary embolectomy.
4. Mitral stenosis: valvotomy or replacement.
5. Mitral regurgitation: repair or replacement if left ventricular function remains reasonable.
6. Atrial septal defect: surgery or, if suitable, closure in the catheter laboratory (e.g. with an Amplatzer closure device). There must be evidence of reversibility of the pulmonary pressure if it is close to systemic.
7. Eisenmenger's syndrome: repair of the defect responsible for the shunt is not usually possible once reversal of shunting has occurred. Consider heart and lung transplant if conservative treatment (diuretics, digoxin and sometimes angiotensin-converting enzyme [ACE] inhibitors) has failed.

General measures include continuous oxygen, diuretics, digoxin and aldactone for problems with right heart failure. Vasodilators of the sort used for primary pulmonary hypertension may be tried but only if the pulmonary pressures have been shown to respond to treatment during cardiac catheterisation.

Idiopathic (primary) pulmonary hypertension

Treatment of this progressive and debilitating condition involves the general measures outlined above. Vasodilators are only indicated for the minority of patients who have responded to them during right heart catheterisation. Nifedipine is perhaps the most used drug. Doses should be titrated upwards as far as 240 mg if possible. If there is a resting tachycardia, diltiazem should be used in doses of up to 720 mg/day. Many patients will not tolerate very large doses because of the development of systemic hypotension.

Only a proportion of patients who respond acutely to vasodilator treatment (about half) will remain longer term responders.

Bosentan has recently been approved for use for these patients. This drug is an endothelin receptor antagonist. Endothelin-1 is a potent vasoconstrictor whose levels have been shown to be elevated in patients with primary pulmonary hypertension.

Modest improvements in functional capacity and pulmonary artery pressures have been demonstrated after treatment of IPH patients and those with underlying connective tissue disease. The drug is only available for patients with class III symptoms, a right atrial pressure of >8 mmHg and who fail to respond clinically, or at right heart catheterisation, to vasodilators. Its side-effects include teratogenicity, an increase in liver enzyme levels and possibly male infertility.

Prostacyclin analogues, such as iloprost, which are taken by inhalation, can be effective but are very expensive for the patient. Continuous intravenous epoprostenol is available in some countries and has been shown to improve symptoms and prognosis in a number of small randomised trials for IPH patients at least.

Sildenafil (a phosphodiesterase inhibitor) is the most recent vasodilator to become fashionable for IPH. It is not approved for this purpose in Australia. It must not be used in combination with nitrates because of the risk of severe and prolonged hypotension.

Warfarin is usually recommended because of the demonstrated risk of the formation of in situ thrombus in the pulmonary arteries.

Suitable patients (severe unresponsive disease, right heart failure, young patient) should be considered for transplant. Successful outcomes have been shown with heart–lung, double lung or single lung transplants. IPH has not been found to recur in the transplanted lung. The prognosis depends on the NYHA-WHO functional class: class I–II, 6 years; class III, 2.5 years, class IV, 6 months.

Sarcoidosis

This chronic, systemic, granulomatous disease is relatively common and patients occasionally require admission to hospital for investigation or treatment. It is an unusual lung disease in that it is less common in smokers. Although most patients present between the ages of 20 and 40 years, children and elderly people are sometimes affected. There are cases of familial sarcoidosis. The disorder results from an exaggerated T-helper lymphocyte response that occurs for unknown reasons and is responsible for granuloma formation and fibrosis.

The history

1. Ask whether the patient is in hospital and why. He or she may already know the diagnosis and be in hospital for further investigations or treatment, or the diagnosis may be suspected because of lymphadenopathy or changes on chest X-ray (most patients present with asymptomatic hilar adenopathy).
2. Ask about acute or subacute symptoms, as sarcoidosis develops in this way in about one-third of cases. The patient may have fever, weight loss, loss of appetite and malaise. The occurrence of erythema nodosum, joint symptoms and bilateral hilar adenopathy on chest X-ray suggests an acute presentation. A combination of fever, facial nerve palsy, parotid enlargement and anterior uveitis may occur.
3. Symptoms suggesting a more insidious onset include persistent cough and dyspnoea. If the patient has chronic sarcoidosis, it is still important to find out how he or she originally presented as the insidious onset is more often associated with chronic sarcoidosis and the development of damage to the lungs (up to 15% develop progressive pulmonary fibrosis) and other organs.
4. Ask about skin eruptions (e.g. erythema nodosum, plaques, maculopapular lesions and subcutaneous nodules). Erythema nodosum, fever and migratory polyarthralgias, when found in combination with hilar lymphadenopathy, may indicate Lofgren's syndrome.
5. Eye symptoms occur in about one-quarter of patients. The patient may have noticed blurred vision, excess tears and light sensitivity as a result of uveitis. Involvement of the lacrimal glands can cause the sicca syndrome, resulting in dry, sore eyes.

6. Ask about nasal stuffiness, as the nasal mucosa is involved in about one-fifth of patients. Occasionally a hoarse voice or even stridor may result from sarcoid involving the larynx.
7. Renal involvement is uncommon but occasionally nephrolithiasis can result because of hypercalcaemia.
8. Ask about neurological symptoms—facial nerve palsy is the most common manifestation but psychiatric disturbances and fits may occur.
9. Almost half the patients at some time in the course of the disease have arthralgia; even frank arthritis can occur.
10. The patient may be aware of cardiac abnormalities. Conduction problems, including complete heart block and ventricular arrhythmias, occur in about 5% of patients.
11. If the patient is a woman, ask about pregnancies. Sarcoidosis tends to abate in pregnancy but then flare up in the postpartum period.
12. Inquire about gastrointestinal symptoms (e.g. dysphagia from hilar adenopathy), although these are very rare. Liver involvement is common but rarely causes symptoms. The patient may know about abnormal liver function tests (usually a cholestatic picture).
13. Ask how the diagnosis was made. Specifically determine whether a lymph node biopsy or closed or open lung biopsy has been performed. Sometimes a skin or conjunctival biopsy may have been obtained to make the diagnosis. Bronchial or transbronchial lung biopsies are used to make the diagnosis in most cases. Occasionally, mediastinoscopy with lymph node biopsy is needed to make the diagnosis. The CT scan has a characteristic appearance and may have been the only investigation performed, although in most cases the diagnosis is confirmed by biopsy.
14. Ask about treatment. Find out whether the patient has been receiving steroids and what dose is currently being taken. Various other treatments may have been tried, including non-steroidal anti-inflammatory drugs (NSAIDs), cyclosporin and cyclophosphamide.

The examination

Begin with the examination of the skin. You might be lucky enough to find erythema nodosum. These raised red or purple lesions are most commonly found on the lower limbs. They resolve spontaneously after 3 or 4 weeks. Look at the face, back and extremities for maculopapular eruptions. These are elevated spots less than 1 cm in diameter which have a waxy, flat top. There may also be lupus pernio on the face. These are purple swollen nodules with a shiny surface, which affect particularly the nose, cheeks, lids and ears. They may make the nose appear bulbous; occasionally the mucosa of the nose may be involved, and the underlying bone can be destroyed. Lupus pernio sometimes also involves the fingers and knees. Pink nodules may be found in old scars.

Examine the eyes for signs of uveitis (p 286). Yellow conjunctival nodules may be present. Examine the fundi for papilloedema. Feel the parotids. Uveoparotid fever presents with uveitis, parotid swelling and seventh cranial nerve palsy.

Next examine the respiratory system (p 249). Most commonly, physical examination of the chest reveals no abnormality. Look particularly for signs of interstitial lung disease; basal end-inspiratory crackles may be present. Pleural effusions occur rarely.

Next examine all the lymph nodes. Lymphadenopathy is sometimes generalised. Now examine the abdomen for hepatomegaly (20%) and splenomegaly (up to 40%).

Examine the joints for signs of arthritis, which is almost always non-deforming.

Examine the nervous system. Look particularly for facial nerve palsy.

Feel the pulse (heart block or arrhythmia) and look for signs of right ventricular failure or cardiomyopathy.

Investigations

A full blood count may reveal lymphocytopenia and sometimes eosinophilia. The ESR is often raised. There may be hyperglobulinaemia. The ACE level is raised in about two-thirds of patients with active sarcoidosis but unfortunately is also sometimes elevated (5%) in healthy persons or those with primary biliary cirrhosis, leprosy, atypical mycobacterial infection, miliary tuberculosis, silicosis, acute histoplasmosis and hyperparathyroidism. Hypercalcaemia and, more commonly, hypercalciuria may be present.

The chest X-ray is usually abnormal (Table 6.22) and the changes can be classified into three stages.

Stage 1   Bilateral hilar lymphadenopathy alone
Stage 2   Bilateral hilar lymphadenopathy and pulmonary infiltration
Stage 3   Pulmonary infiltration without hilar lymphadenopathy

Table 6.22   Chest X-ray changes in sarcoidosis
1. Hilar lymphadenopathy—up to 90% 2. Paratracheal lymphadenopathy—less than 80% 3. Reticulonodular changes—70% 4. Peripheral nodules—less than 5% 5. Cavitation—less than 5% 6. Pleural effusion—less than 5% 7. Linear atelectasis—less than 1%

Patients with stage 1 X-rays are considered to have an acute reversible form of the disease, whereas the other stages tend to be more chronic. The chest X-ray may show paratracheal lymphadenopathy; cavitation and pleural effusions are rare. Cavities may become colonised with *Aspergillus*. CT scans of the chest may show a ground-glass appearance when active alveolitis is present. Always think about excluding tuberculosis and histoplasmosis.

If there is parenchymal granulomatous involvement, respiratory function tests reveal the changes that are typical of interstitial lung disease, with reduced lung volumes and diffusing capacity but a normal FEV_1/FVC ratio. Occasionally, a mixed pattern of obstruction and restriction is seen. Blood gas estimations may show mild hypoxaemia.

A gallium-67 lung scan usually shows a pattern of diffuse uptake but is of little diagnostic value. Enlarged nodes also tend to show up on the scans.

Bronchoscopy with transbronchial biopsy will usually establish the pathological diagnosis. Bronchioalveolar lavage will show an increase in the number of $CD4^+$ T-helper lymphocytes. However, this is not diagnostic of the condition. Biopsy of lymph nodes, skin or liver may be diagnostic. The non-caseating granulomas found in sarcoidosis are non-specific; they are also found in berylliosis, leprosy, hypersensitivity pneumonitis and granulomatous infection, and in lymph nodes that drain adjacent carcinomas.

Treatment

Indications for treatment are lack of resolution of active pulmonary sarcoidosis with increasing symptoms or worsening lung function, neurological, renal or cardiac complications, major eye disease, and occasionally severe systemic symptoms (e.g. fever and weight loss). The drug of choice is prednisolone. This is begun in high dose (1 mg/kg) for up to 6 weeks and then tapered over the following few months. Treatment is continued for 12 months. The prognosis is good. About 50% of patients develop some permanent organ damage but, in most, this is mild.

Cystic fibrosis

The survival of children with cystic fibrosis into adult life is now common. Over 50% of patients now reach the age of 30 years and the prognosis is improving all the time. Although paediatricians are often reluctant to give these patients up, they are increasingly coming under the care of adult physicians. A small number of cases are diagnosed in adult life. They, unfortunately, tend to spend long periods in hospital and are thus readily available for clinical examinations.

Cystic fibrosis is a common, serious, congenital inherited defect in Caucasian people. It has an autosomal recessive inheritance and the gene has been identified. The mutation is in the cystic fibrosis transmembrane conductance regulator protein gene on chromosome 7. The trait is present in about 1 in 25 Caucasians, and 1 in 2000 has the condition. It is very rare in other races. It is a chronic disease that can affect the lungs, pancreas, bowel, liver and sweat glands.

The history

1. Ask about presentation:
   (a) the age at diagnosis—milder forms are sometimes not diagnosed until adult life
   (b) the presenting symptoms—the patient may have been told that he or she had meconium ileus as a baby or recurrent respiratory infections in early life; failure to thrive may suggest the diagnosis
   (c) pulmonary symptoms—cough and sputum, haemoptysis, wheeze, dyspnoea
   (d) nasal polyps and sinusitis—relatively common
   (e) gastrointestinal symptoms—problems maintaining weight, diarrhoea and steatorrhoea (pancreatic malabsorption); constipation and abdominal distension and bowel obstruction (defective water excretion into the bowel)
   (f) heat exhaustion in hot weather—patients with cystic fibrosis can lose large amounts of salt in their sweat, which sometimes causes problems, particularly in the tropics
   (g) cardiac symptoms—the patient may know of cardiac involvement (cor pulmonale is a late development)
   (h) jaundice and variceal bleeding—focal biliary cirrhosis and portal hypertension occur occasionally
   (i) diabetes mellitus occurs in 10% of patients with cystic fibrosis.
2. Ask about diagnosis. The patient may know whether a sweat test was performed. Collection of sweat and measurement of the chloride concentration is still the accepted method of diagnosing the condition. A sweat chloride concentration of more than 70 mmol/L suggests cystic fibrosis in an adult. Otherwise, a combination of respiratory and malabsorptive problems may be considered enough to make the diagnosis. A list of the major and minor diagnostic criteria is presented in Table 6.23. DNA markers are likely to be used increasingly in the diagnosis. At the moment this is difficult because there are a large number (over 1200) of abnormal genotypes that can result in the disease. Screening for the commonest mutations is especially helpful for those patients who have the clinical syndrome but a negative sweat test (1–2%).
3. Ask about family history—the autosomal recessive inheritance means siblings and other close relatives may be affected.

Table 6.23 **Diagnosis of cystic fibrosis**

Major criteria
1. Elevated chloride sweat test (98%)—pilocarpine iontophoresis on 100 mg of sweat
   >70 mmol/L diagnostic in adults
   >60 mmol/L diagnostic in children
   50–60 mmol/L suggestive
   <50 mmol/L normal
2. Azoospermia in males (95%)
3. Family history of cystic fibrosis (70%)

Minor criteria
1. Nasal polyps (relatively uncommon)
2. Meconium ileus equivalent (distal bowel obstruction from inspissated secretions)
3. Rectal prolapse
4. Focal biliary cirrhosis
5. Diabetes mellitus (uncommon)

4. Ask about treatment. Pulmonary disease is the main determinant of mortality. Aggressive treatment of the pulmonary complications has had the greatest effect on improvement in life expectancy. The patients are usually well aware of this and are largely responsible for their own treatment. The condition is a chronic suppurative progressive one causing bronchiolitis, bronchitis, pneumonia and eventually bronchiectasis. The pathology is probably the result of the formation of viscous mucous plugs, which lead to distal infection and lung damage. The mainstay of treatment is physiotherapy, which the patient, with help from the family and a physiotherapist, will perform. Ask about deep breathing, percussion, postural drainage, the use of a flutter valve and the forced expiratory technique called 'huffing'. Mucolytic drugs are of doubtful benefit and may even be harmful. The patient should also know what antibiotics have been used and whether continuously or intermittently. Nebulised bronchodilators and antibiotics are commonly prescribed. *Staph. aureus* and *Pseudomonas aeruginosa* are common pathogens because of their ability to grow on the abnormal bronchial mucus of cystic fibrotic lungs. Ask whether treatment for complications, such as pneumothorax, haemoptysis or cor pulmonale, has been required. Minor haemoptysis, where less than 250 mL of blood is lost, occurs in about 60% of patients. Major haemoptysis occurs in about 7% of patients and bronchial artery embolisation may be required. Cor pulmonale may require treatment with diuretics, aldactone and possibly vasodilators but aggressive treatment of the lung disease and supplementary oxygen are more important in the long and medium terms. Pleurodesis used to be the treatment of choice for recurrent pneumothorax, but this results in a contraindication to lung transplantation.

   Macrolide antibiotics, especially azithromycin, are being used because of their anti–inflammatory properties.
5. Inquire about gastrointestinal symptoms. These tend to be less of a problem but malabsorption may make weight gain very difficult for these patients. Ask what pancreatic enzyme replacement the patient uses and how often.
6. Ask about the number of admissions to hospital over the past 12 months and the length of each stay. There is some evidence that routine admission to hospital three or four times a year for intensive physiotherapy and nebulised antibiotics and bronchodilators will be beneficial.

7. Inquire about social support. Ask whether the patient knows about or belongs to the local cystic fibrosis association and whether he or she has been in touch with other affected patients. Try to find out tactfully whether the patient understands the inheritance of the disease; male patients may know that azoospermia is usually present (95%). Eighty per cent of women are fertile and pregnancy and breast-feeding are often successful. Find out in some detail how a young adult copes with this debilitating and life-shortening disease.

The examination

Look at the patient's size and physique. Muscle bulk is considered a good indicator of the severity and prognosis in a particular patient. Measure the patient's height and weight.

Ask the patient to cough. Listen for a loose cough and examine any sputum for the degree of purulence. Now examine the respiratory system carefully. Note clubbing, which is present in the majority of patients. Look for abnormal chest wall development. Estimate forced expiratory time and examine the chest, listening particularly for crackles, wheezes and reduced breath sounds.

Examine the heart for signs of cor pulmonale and right ventricular failure.

Examine the abdomen for signs of faecal loading, especially in the right iliac fossa.

Investigations

Sputum culture is most important. Colonisation with *H. influenzae* and *Staph. aureus* tends to occur in young patients, and this is often followed by nosocomial *E. coli* and *Proteus* spp. By the age of 10 years, *Pseudomonas* is the main pathogen in most patients, but usually it does not cause systemic infection.

A full blood count should be asked for to look for anaemia, which may be caused by malabsorption or chronic disease; the white cell count may indicate acute infection. Polycythaemia is rare despite chronic hypoxia. The electrolyte levels and liver function tests should be looked at. There may be evidence of deficiencies of fat-soluble vitamins (A, D, E and K). The creatinine level should be known before aminoglycosides are used.

The chest X-ray should be looked at carefully and should be compared with previous films if these are available. Increased lung markings are present in 98% of patients. These occur particularly in the upper lobes. Cystic bronchiectatic changes occur in over 60% of patients. Mucous plugs may be seen in one-third and atelectasis occurs in just over 10% of patients. Look also for pneumothorax and pleural changes at the site of previous pneumothoraces or pleurodesis. Chest CT is not routine but may help define focal areas of bronchiectasis that are amenable to resection. Spirometry readings may fluctuate because of airway inflammation. An FEV_1 that is persistently less than 38% indicates a poor prognosis.

Management

Intensive and repetitive physiotherapy is the mainstay of treatment. You should try to form an idea of the patient's ability to cope with the illness as so much of the management depends on him or her. Intravenous antibiotics may be indicated for acute exacerbations of pulmonary disease if these are severe or fail to respond to oral antibiotic treatment. Intravenous options include tobramycin and ceftazimide for *Pseudomonas*. The chronic use of antibiotics is controversial. Inhaled tobramycin seems useful and bronchodilators can help airway clearance.

Malabsorption may require aggressive treatment with pancreatic enzyme supplements and frequent small meals as well as vitamin supplements. Double lung transplantation and sometimes combined heart and lung transplantation is now an accepted, although still uncommon, treatment in patients with advanced disease. Cystic fibrosis does not recur in the transplanted lung. Human recombinant DNAase seems effective in degrading the concentration of DNA in sputum, reducing sputum viscosity, and in improving the patient's ability to clear pulmonary secretions. Gene therapy may be the treatment of choice in the future.

Tuberculosis (TB)

The increased incidence of pulmonary TB over the past 10 years and its association with HIV infection have made it a possible long case. Protection from *Mycobacterium tuberculosis* is via cell-mediated immunity involving CD4$^+$ T-helper lymphocytes. The defects of these cells in number and effectiveness, which is characteristic of HIV infection, explains this susceptibility. It may be a difficult diagnostic or management problem, or both. It also has important social and public health implications.

The history

The patient is likely to know that the diagnosis has been made or is suspected.

1. Find out whether the patient is a recent immigrant and, if so, from where.
2. Ask whether there has been a previous diagnosis of any other serious medical problem that might interfere with cell-mediated immunity, such as malnutrition, alcoholism or HIV infection.
3. How has the diagnosis been made, and how long ago?
4. Ask about some of the important symptoms—weight loss, sweats and fever, cough with purulent and blood-stained sputum, and pleuritic chest pain from pleural lesions or uncontrolled coughing.
5. What investigations have been performed or are planned? TB may have been suspected after a chest X-ray was performed because of respiratory symptoms or as a routine screening test. The patient may remember having to give early morning sputum specimens on a number of occasions, or having had a bronchocospy with washings, if sputum was not being produced. Bronchoscopy may have been performed to exclude other causes of an abnormal chest X-ray, such as carcinoma of the lung. A tuberculin (Mantoux) skin test may have been performed as a screening test or to support the diagnosis where cultures have been negative. A positive tuberculin test is much less significant if the patient has received bacille Calmette-Guérin (BCG) vaccination in the past.
6. What treatment regimen is the patient receiving? Considerable detail must be sought about the drugs themselves—doses, if known, how long treatment will continue, how the drugs are administered (supervised or unsupervised) and what side-effects have occurred (Table 6.24). Remember that rifampicin and rifabutin colour body fluids, including urine, orange.
7. What effect has this serious and chronic disease had on the patient's life? Has he or she been able to work or go to school? Do his or her friends and workmates know the diagnosis? Does the patient's occupation involve a public health risk?
8. How has the problem been handled from a public health aspect? What screening has been done on the patient's family and friends? Are any of the family also being treated?

The examination

Early in the course of the illness there may be no specific signs. Of those patients without HIV infection who have TB, 80% have only pulmonary disease. However, the majority of patients with HIV and TB have extrapulmonary and pulmonary disease.

Note the general appearance of the patient. Look for wasting and cachexia that may be associated with the cause of the TB (HIV, alcoholism) or may be a result of the disease (which is also known as consumption for this reason).

Examine the lungs for signs of the aggressive primary infection that can occur in immunocompromised patients (especially children). These include a pleural effusion or tuberculous empyema, and lobar collapse (as a result of lymphadenopathy and bronchial obstruction).

Post-primary disease is more common in adults. There is almost always a loose cough and often haemoptysis. There may be no abnormal findings but one should look especially for upper lobe signs, including coarse crackles and wheezes owing to partial bronchial obstruction caused by lymphadenopathy, and the rare amphoric breath sounds that occur over a cavity.

Extrapulmonary disease most commonly involves the lymph nodes (especially in HIV patients). Examine all the palpable lymph node groups. The most often affected are the cervical and supraclavicular. There is usually painless swelling. Involvement of the genitourinary tract can be associated with haematuria and tenderness over the flanks. The bones are involved in a small number of cases. The lumbar spine (Pott's disease), hips and knees are affected most. Collapse of the vertebral bodies may cause kyphosis and even paraplegia. Tuberculous pericarditis can cause symptoms and signs of pericarditis, and occasionally tamponade. Abdominal TB can cause various gastro-intestinal signs. There may be a palpable abdominal mass. Severe abdominal tenderness suggests tuberculous peritonitis.

Investigations

The diagnosis depends on microscopy of a specimen that shows mycobacteria (e.g. send three sputum specimens on separate days, followed by confirmation by culture of the organism). Traditionally, specimens of sputum or gastric or bronchial washings, or a lymph node biopsy, are stained with the Ziehl-Neelsen stain. Modern laboratories are more likely to use auramine-rhodamine stains and fluorescence microscopy. Culture of the organism takes about 6 weeks but is needed for the definitive diagnosis. These organisms should then be tested for sensitivity to the main antituberculous drugs. This takes up to 8 more weeks. Polymerase chain reaction (PCR) testing can now provide rapid identification of *M. tuberculosis* but is not available everywhere and does not distinguish viable and non-viable organisms.

A chest X-ray showing the typical pattern of infiltrates and cavities in the upper lobe strongly suggests the diagnosis, but many other patterns are consistent with TB.

Tuberculin testing is useful for screening. The test may be negative in severe disease (e.g. in up to 50% of cases of miliary TB).

Biopsies of the pleura, lymph nodes or bone marrow may be needed. Bron-choscopy is sometimes necessary to exclude other causes of X-ray changes.

HIV patients may have TB despite a completely normal chest X-ray. They may also have less typical chest X-ray findings—often lower lobe changes without cavities. They are more likely to have infection with other mycobacteria, such as MAC.

Remember that the diagnosis can be made even when the organism is not isolated.

Treatment

There are four first-line drugs for the treatment of TB: isoniazid, rifampicin, etham-butol and pyrazinamide. These are all given orally. Second-line drugs tend to be more toxic and are used only for organisms resistant to the first-line drugs. They include streptomycin, quinolone, kanamycin and amikacin (parenteral) and cycloserine, ethionamide and PAS (para-aminosalicylic acid). The initial isolate should undergo drug susceptibility testing, especially if treatment seems to have failed or there is a relapse of symptoms.

Treatment begins with a combination regimen of three drugs (usually isoniazid, rifampicin and pyrazinamide) for 2 months. A fourth drug (usually ethambutol) is often given until the organism's sensitivities are available. The aim here is to kill the majority of the organisms, improve the patient's symptoms and render him or her non-infectious. This is followed by 4 months of treatment with two drugs (isoniazid and rifampicin).

Adherence to the full course of treatment is very important but difficult to ensure. Complicated public health arrangements, with monitoring of compliance, may be needed to enforce treatment. Direct observed treatment (DOT) is insisted on by public health authorities if compliance seems doubtful. These patients present as required to be observed taking their treatment. The response to treatment is monitored by repeat sputum cultures until they become negative. Persisting positive cultures after 3 months suggest resistance of the organism or non-compliance on the part of the patient. Patients are probably not an infectious risk if no sputum is produced or if the sputum is consistently acid fast bacilli (AFB) negative. Patients need to be aware of the most important side-effects of treatment, which include hepatitis (up to 5% in general populations and 30% in HIV patients), deafness and visual disturbance (Table 6.24).

Small increases in the transaminases (to three times normal) are no cause for alarm and are poor predictors of significant hepatotoxicity. Treatment should be reviewed immediately if jaundice develops.

Multiple drug resistance is increasingly common. It should be expected if the infection was acquired from a patient with a known resistant organism or if the infection was acquired in parts of Asia or South America. The addition of fluoro-quinolone to the regimen should be considered while resistance studies are underway.

Prevention of infection by vaccination with BCG is not widely practised in Australia. Its effectiveness is uncertain. It negates the usefulness of later Mantoux testing. Patients with exposure to TB (especially household contacts) or in a high-risk group (HIV infected, diabetes, prolonged steroid treatment, end-stage renal disease) and a positive tuberculin test are candidates for chemical prophylaxis with isoniazid (5 mg/kg/day for 6–12 months). Treatment of children is especially important in these circumstances. This reduces the chance of the development of open TB by 90%.

Table 6.24   Common antituberculous drugs and their side-effects

Drug	Main side-effects	Usual dose/day
Rifampicin	Hepatitis, flu-like illness	600 mg
Isoniazid	Hepatitis, fever, peripheral neuropathy	300 mg (reduced to 2 or 3 doses a week in renal failure)
Streptomycin	Ototoxicity, renal impairment	1 g (not safe in pregnancy)
Ethambutol	Optic neuritis	15 mg/kg
Pyrazinamide	Hepatitis	1.5–2 g
PAS	Hepatitis, diarrhoea, hypersensitivity	12 g

PAS = para-aminosalicylic acid.

Screening of contacts and of high-risk patients (e.g. HIV patients) with tuberculin testing is an important public health measure.

Lung transplant

Although this is an uncommon procedure, patients have chronic management problems that make them very suitable long cases. The examiners will have the opportunity to ask questions about the patient's underlying pulmonary problem, the general indications for lung transplant, issues of management of the complications of transplant and, of course, the types of social problems associated with a severe chronic illness. Occasionally, patients who are being assessed for possible transplant may be suitable for the clinical examinations.

The history

1. Find out why the patient is in hospital (it may just be for the clinical examinations).
2. Obtain some basic information about the transplant: how long ago, how many lungs were transplanted and was the heart also originally someone else's.
3. What was the original lung disease? Emphysema (including that caused by alpha$_1$-antitrypsin deficiency) is the most common indication, accounting for about half the unilateral and a third of the bilateral transplants. Primary pulmonary hypertension, cystic fibrosis and Eisenmenger's syndrome are the main indications for heart/lung transplants.
4. How successful has the procedure been from the patient's point of view?
5. What important complications can the patient remember? Ask about known rejection episodes and how they were managed. Have there been difficult infections? The patient may know what organisms have been detected. Stenosis of a bronchial anastomosis site is an occasional early problem. This is often treated with dilatation and stenting.
6. What medications is the patient taking? If necessary, prompt for prednisolone, cyclosporin, mycophenolate, azathioprine and tacrolimus.
7. If the patient is being assessed for transplant, try to find out if the patient fits the current guidelines for transplant (Tables 6.25 and 6.26). In general, suitable patients are sick enough to require the operation but not too sick to present an intolerable operative risk.
8. How has the patient coped with the procedure, its complications and the immunosuppressants?

Table 6.25 Age criteria for lung transplant			
	Unilateral	**Bilateral**	**Heart/lung**
Age (years)	<65	<60	<55

The examination

Perform a thorough respiratory examination. Look especially for thoracotomy scars and attempt an assessment of the patient's functional capacity (e.g. look for signs of breathlessness while he or she is undressing and, if the room is big enough, get the patient to walk backwards and forwards). Listen for end-inspiratory pops and squeaks (bronchiolitis obliterans at an advanced stage can be associated with the development of

Table 6.26   Indications and contraindications for lung transplant

Indications	Contraindications
COPD—FEV_1 <25% predicted, $Paco_2$ >55 mmHg	**Relative**
Cystic fibrosis, bronchiectasis— FEV_1 <30% or complications (e.g. cachexia, severe haemoptysis) or $Paco_2$ >50 mmHg, Pao_2 <55 mmHg	Diabetes
	Osteoporosis
	Alcohol excess
	Still smoking
	Likely compliance problems
	Atypical mycobacterial colonisation of lungs
Pulmonary fibrosis—progressive symptoms, VC, DLCO <60%	Weight >130% of ideal or < 70% of ideal
Pulmonary hypertension—NYHA class III or IV, pulmonary artery pressure >55 mmHg, cardiac index <2 L/min	**Absolute**
Eisenmenger's syndrome—severe symptomatic impairment. The 2-year prognosis is not improved for these patients	HIV, hepatitis B, hepatitis C and liver disease, malignancy, other organ failure

DLCO = diffusion capacity for carbon monoxide; VC = vital capacity.

bronchiectasis). Note signs of infection—fever and areas of bronchial breathing or crackles. Look for sputum and assess the cough. Is the patient Cushingoid?

Management

The detection of complications and their management is likely to dominate the discussion.

1. *Rejection.* Early rejection episodes are common and treated with boost doses of prednisone. Symptoms of acute rejection include malaise, fever, dyspnoea and cough. Clinical assessment may reveal crackles, decreasing FEV_1, hypoxia and a raised white cell count. The chest X-ray may show infiltrates and pleural effusions. A transbronchial biopsy tends to be performed if there is any suspicion of rejection and allows an accurate diagnosis. In some places, routine biopsies are performed to detect asymptomatic rejection. It is not clear, however, whether these should be treated.
2. *Infection.* Most lung transplant patients develop infections requiring treatment. Infection is the most common cause of death. A combination of immunosuppression and local problems, such as impaired ciliary activity, seems to lie behind this. Infections with adenovirus, influenza A and paramyxovirus are common and associated with a significant mortality. Invasive fungal organisms, such as *Aspergillus*, result in an even worse prognosis. Patients now receive at least 3 months of routine prophylactic antibiotic, antiviral and antifungal treatment. This approach has improved the early postoperative prognosis.
3. *Immunosuppression.* The usual problems with immunosuppressive drugs occur in lung transplant patients. Renal impairment, hypertension and hyperlipidaemia are frequent problems. Osteoporosis and peripheral neuropathy are also possible problems. Five per cent of lung transplant patients develop post-transplant lymphoproliferative disorders.

4. *Bronchiolitis obliterans.* The gradual onset of small airways obstruction is a manifestation of chronic rejection. It does not usually begin until 2 or more years after transplant but is detectable in at least half of the transplant patients within 5 years. It may occur more often in those who have had more frequent acute rejection episodes and in those with a human leucocyte antigen (HLA) mismatch with the donor. There tends to be a very gradual onset of dyspnoea, fatigue and cough. Patients have a slowly decreasing FEV_1 but chest X-rays are often normal. CT scans may show a central mottling opacity. Biopsy will establish the diagnosis. The prognosis is not good. Sometimes an aggressive increase in immunosuppression may stabilise the condition but it cannot be reversed and often the patient deteriorates rapidly.

5. *Disease recurrence.* Sarcoidosis and some forms of idiopathic pulmonary fibrosis can recur in the transplanted lungs.

Gastrointestinal system

Peptic ulceration

This long case is usually a straightforward management problem.

It is now established that the most important causes of chronic peptic ulcer disease are *Helicobacter pylori* infection and traditional non-steroidal anti-inflammatory drugs (NSAIDs, including low-dose aspirin). The cyclo-oxygenase 2 (COX-2) specific NSAIDs have a lower incidence of peptic ulceration. Idiopathic ulcers (*H. pylori* negative, NSAID negative) are increasingly being reported. The Zollinger-Ellison syndrome (gastrinoma) is a very rare but important cause. As peptic ulcer disease affects 10% of the population, a history of this condition is not uncommon in the long case. Patients are usually admitted to hospital with peptic ulcer disease because of complications—typically haemorrhage, but more rarely perforation.

The history

1. Determine whether the patient currently has dyspepsia or a past history of dyspepsia (i.e. pain or discomfort centred in the upper abdomen). Typical ulcer symptoms include burning or sharp epigastric pain that may be related to meals, wakes the patient from sleep at night and is relieved by antacids or antisecretory drugs. However, many patients with these symptoms do *not* have peptic ulcer disease and ulcers are often associated with atypical symptoms. Duodenal and gastric ulcer cannot be distinguished from one another on the basis of symptoms. The differential diagnosis of dyspepsia includes gastro-oesophageal reflux disease (usually also causing heartburn or acid regurgitation), gastric cancer (especially in older patients with new onset of symptoms), biliary pain (which is usually severe, constant pain in the right upper quadrant or epigastrium that occurs episodically and lasts at least 20 minutes but usually hours), chronic pancreatitis, pancreatic cancer or intestinal angina (which causes severe postprandial pain such that the patient is afraid to eat and loses weight).

   Diabetes mellitus, thyroid dysfunction, hyperparathyroidism and connective tissue diseases can also cause dyspepsia. Ask about the course of the symptoms and, if intermittent, the number of recurrences and treatments given. Ask about alarm symptoms, such as weight loss (which suggests the possibility of malignancy) or recurrent vomiting (e.g. gastric outlet obstruction).

2. Ask patients about the types of investigations that they have had undertaken in the past. If an ulcer was apparently documented, determine whether this was by endoscopy (the most sensitive and specific test) or barium meal, or just by

symptoms alone (which is inadequate). Determine whether the patient knows whether *H. pylori* status was determined from gastric biopsies or by non-invasive tests, such as serology or urea breath testing.

3. A history of past ulcer surgery is important because of the associated complications (e.g. pain or bloating owing to bile reflux gastritis or an afferent loop syndrome, recurrent ulceration, early or late dumping, post-vagotomy diarrhoea, anaemia as a result of iron, vitamin B_{12} or folate deficiency, and osteomalacia or osteoporosis).

4. Inquire carefully about medication use—medications can induce dyspepsia, which can be confused with peptic ulcer (e.g. digoxin, potassium, iron, oral antibiotics). All NSAIDs are an important cause of dyspepsia with or without chronic ulceration. Alcohol can also induce acute dyspepsia (but not chronic ulcers). Patients with an ulcer history may be taking maintenance acid suppression. Treatment for *H. pylori* usually includes a proton pump inhibitor (PPI) plus two antibiotics for 7 days.

5. Determine why the patient is in hospital on this occasion. If the admission is because of acute gastrointestinal bleeding, then the treatment that was applied needs to be documented (e.g. blood transfusion, injection of a bleeding visible vessel in a peptic ulcer base with adrenaline, or surgical oversewing of an ulcer).

The examination

Physical examination in patients with suspected peptic ulcer disease is usually unhelpful. Epigastric tenderness is not a specific sign. An upper abdominal scar may indicate past ulcer surgery. Look for alarm signs, including evidence of anaemia (e.g. from bleeding), evidence of current bleeding (melaena, tachycardia, postural hypotension) or an abdominal mass (e.g. gastric or pancreatic carcinoma).

Investigations

1. *Endoscopy.* This is the standard test for determining that an active peptic ulcer is present. It is also the key test in a patient with upper gastrointestinal bleeding to determine whether the patient is at high risk of rebleeding and also to provide endoscopic therapy where required. Patients with active bleeding or a visible vessel at endoscopy need endoscopic therapy (e.g. injection with adrenaline followed by coagulation with a heater probe). Patients with a low risk of rebleeding (i.e. a clean ulcer base) can be discharged if stable. For patients with upper gastrointestinal tract bleeding, it is also important to exclude other causes, including variceal bleeding, erosions, angiodysplasia, a Mallory-Weiss tear or a Dieulafoy's lesion (rupture of a large submucosal artery). Where possible, biopsies should be obtained at the diagnostic endoscopy in ulcer patients to determine the *H. pylori* status.

2. *Abdominal imaging.* In the patient with unexplained dyspepsia where endoscopy is normal, ultrasound can be useful in certain clinical circumstances to investigate for biliary tract pathology. Computed tomography (CT) scanning is more sensitive for pancreatic disease.

3. *Atypical peptic ulcer.* Peptic ulceration in an unusual location, peptic ulcers resistant to therapy, an ulcer relapse after operation, or frequent or early ulcer recurrence can occur in the Zollinger-Ellison syndrome. This syndrome can also be associated with enlarged duodenal or gastric folds, or diarrhoea or steatorrhoea. The diagnosis is made by measuring the fasting serum gastrin level: a level of over 300 pg/mL is suggestive and over 1000 pg/mL almost diagnostic. Acid secretion can be confirmed by testing the pH of gastric juice obtained at endoscopy. The next diagnostic test of choice in uncertain cases is the secretin test, where a paradoxical increase in gastrin of over 200 pg/mL above basal levels is highly specific. Preoperative localisation of the tumour is then attempted by CT scanning and, if necessary, angiographic venous sampling. In patients with metastatic or multifocal

disease, surgery is avoided, but all other cases require surgical exploration. High-dose PPIs are used to control the disease medically.

Remember that hypergastrinaemia also occurs in hypochlorhydria (e.g. in type A atrophic gastritis and pernicious anaemia, following vagotomy or in renal failure). Other causes of hypergastrinaemia with acid hypersecretion include a retained gastric antrum after peptic ulcer surgery, massive small bowel resection, gastric outlet obstruction and thyrotoxicosis. If hypercalcaemia is present in patients with ulcer disease, this may suggest multiple endocrine neoplasia type I (MEN I, autosomal dominant) (with hyperplasia, adenoma or carcinoma of the parathyroid, pituitary and pancreatic islets; hyperparathyroidism and pituitary adenomas are most often associated with the Zollinger-Ellison syndrome in MEN I).

Management

There is now consensus that if peptic ulcer disease is documented and *H. pylori* is present, this infection should be treated. Almost all duodenal ulcers will be cured by this approach, as will most gastric ulcers, unless associated with NSAID use. Therapy with acid suppression alone for peptic ulcer disease is now obsolete unless no cause is identified. The optimal approach for curative treatment of *H. pylori* is currently three drugs (e.g. PPI plus amoxycillin plus clarithromycin), which give cure rates of approximately 80% if given for 1 week. Side-effects occur with such treatment in up to 20% of cases. PPIs cause an increase in gastrin secretion and may predispose the patient to the development of atrophic gastritis, particularly in the setting of *H. pylori* infection, but the risk is small.

Patients with gastric ulcers may be advised to have a repeat gastroscopy to confirm healing and exclude carcinoma. However, 98% of cancers will be detected at the initial gastroscopy and biopsy. Therefore, repeat endoscopy is usually only recommended if symptoms have not been relieved.

In peptic ulcer disease, confirm that *H. pylori* infection has been cured (e.g. by repeat endoscopic biopsy or urea breath testing at least 1 month after completing treatment). NSAID ulcers should initially be treated with a PPI, which is effective even if the NSAID is continued (although this does delay healing). PPIs are more effective than histamine H_2-receptor antagonists in promoting ulcer healing. NSAID use is an independent risk factor for peptic ulcer and therefore eradication of *H. pylori* in this situation may not prevent ulcer disease if NSAIDs are continued. Certain patients taking traditional NSAIDs have a higher risk of ulcer complications. These include elderly patients, those having their first 3 months of treatment, those on higher doses, those with a past history of peptic ulcer, those taking concomitant corticosteroid therapy or anticoagulants, and those with other serious medical illnesses. NSAID ulcers often present with complications without a history of dyspepsia because these drugs are analgesic agents that may mask symptoms. The prostaglandin E_1 analogue misoprostol and PPIs both substantially reduce the risk of NSAID-induced gastric and duodenal ulcers; histamine H_2-receptor antagonists in standard doses do not prevent NSAID-induced gastric ulcers. *H. pylori* eradication before treatment reduces, but does not eliminate, the risk of aspirin-induced ulcer development. *H. pylori* eradication alone provides insufficient protection from gastroduodenal complications arising from non-selective NSAID use in high-risk patients, who will still require a PPI.

Malabsorption

This is a difficult long case. It is usually a diagnostic problem. Coeliac disease (Table 6.27), chronic pancreatitis and previous gastric surgery account for 60% of cases of malabsorption.

Table 6.27   Coeliac disease
Diagnostic criteria for coeliac disease: 1. Evidence of malabsorption 2. Abnormal jejunal biopsy 3. Clinical, biochemical and histological improvement on a gluten-free diet (no wheat, rye or barley) 4. Relapse on reinstitution of gluten (rarely done today except in children)   *Note*: Splenomegaly in coeliac disease usually indicates that lymphoma has complicated the disease because otherwise splenic atrophy is characteristic and manifests with Howell-Jolly bodies in the peripheral blood smear.
Causes of lack of response to a gluten-free diet: 1. Incorrect diagnosis 2. Patient not adhering to the diet 3. Collagenous sprue 4. Intestinal lymphoma 5. Diffuse ulceration 6. Other intercurrent disease
Complications of coeliac disease: 1. T-cell lymphoma 2. Ulceration to the small bowel 3. Incidence of carcinoma of the gastrointestinal tract is generally slightly increased

The history

1. Ask about presenting symptoms:
   (a) pale, bulky, offensive stools (steatorrhoea)
   (b) weight loss
   (c) weakness (potassium deficiency)
   (d) anaemia (megaloblastic, iron deficiency etc.)
   (e) bone pain (osteomalacia)
   (f) glossitis and angular stomatitis (vitamin B group deficiency)
   (g) bruising (vitamin K deficiency)
   (h) oedema as a result of protein deficiency
   (i) peripheral neuropathy owing to vitamin B_{12} or B_1 deficiency
   (j) skin rash (eczema, dermatitis herpetiformis)
   (k) amenorrhoea owing to protein depletion.
2. Ask about time of onset of symptoms and their duration.
3. Ask aetiological questions:
   (a) gastrectomy, other bowel surgery
   (b) history of liver or pancreatic disease
   (c) drugs (e.g. alcohol, neomycin, cholestyramine)
   (d) history of Crohn's disease
   (e) previous radiotherapy
   (f) gluten-free diet treatment at any stage
   (g) history of diabetes mellitus
   (h) risk factors for HIV infection.

4. Ask about current treatment (e.g. diet, pancreatic supplements, vitamin supplements, cholestyramine, antibiotics).
5. Inquire about family history (e.g. coeliac disease, inflammatory bowel disease).
6. Ask about social problems related to the chronic illness.

The examination

Pay particular attention to the current weight and nutritional status (e.g. the body mass index [BMI]), the presence of abdominal scars, skin lesions (e.g. bruising, dermatitis herpetiformis, erythema nodosum, pyoderma gangrenosum, stomatitis, pigmentation, perianal lesions), signs of anaemia, signs of chronic liver disease, signs of peripheral neuropathy and lymphadenopathy.

Investigations (Table 6.28)

1. Demonstrate malabsorption:
   (a) faecal fat estimation over 3 days—more than 7 g per day is abnormal; note that patients with severe small bowel diarrhoea without fat malabsorption may lose up to 14 g a day
   (b) Schilling test for ileal disease if there is anything to suggest a vitamin B_{12} deficiency
   (c) xylose test for jejunal disease (of minor value); the glucose breath hydrogen test is of similar limited value.
2. Evaluate the consequences:
   (a) blood count with particular attention to red cell indices
   (b) serum iron and ferritin, serum and red cell folate, and vitamin B_{12} studies
   (c) serum albumin estimation
   (d) vitamin D assay, serum calcium, phosphate and alkaline phosphatase estimations
   (e) clotting profile—international normalised ratio (INR)
   (f) cholesterol and carotene.
3. Find the cause:
   (a) small bowel X-ray films for localised disease (e.g. Crohn's disease or anatomical causes of bacterial overgrowth such as diverticula or blind loops)
   (b) gastroscopy and small bowel biopsy (four biopsies) and duodenal aspirate for histology, parasites and bacterial overgrowth; look for multiple duodenal ulcers (e.g. as a result of Zollinger-Ellison syndrome, lymphoma, jejunoileitis).
      Subtotal villous atrophy may be present histologically in:
      (i) coeliac disease
      (ii) tropical sprue
      (iii) giardiasis
      (iv) lymphoma
      (v) hypogammaglobulinaemia
      (vi) Whipple's disease.
   Note that tissue transglutaminase and anti-endomysial antibodies are the most useful screening tests for sprue but they are not a substitute for small bowel biopsy, which remains the 'gold standard' test if coeliac disease is suspected.
   (c) Vitamin B_{12} absorption may be abnormal in ileal disease, bacterial overgrowth, pernicious anaemia and pancreatic disease.
   (d) The bile acid breath test (C14 glycocholate) can be used to detect bacterial overgrowth and ileal disease. The C14 xylose test is more sensitive and specific for the detection of bacterial overgrowth.
   (e) Greatly raised faecal fat levels (>40 g per day) strongly suggest pancreatic disease. This is investigated by plain abdominal X-ray films (for calcification), abdominal ultrasound and/or CT scan, magnetic resonance cholangiopancreatography (MRCP) and endoscopic retrograde cholangiopancreatography (ERCP). Pancreatic function testing is not performed routinely.

Table 6.28 Typical results of investigations in malabsorption

Investigation	Coeliac disease	Bacterial overgrowth	Whipple's disease	Terminal ileal disease	Chronic pancreatitis
Stool fat (or C14 triolein breath test)	High	High	High	High	Very high
D-Xylose*	Low	Low	Low	Normal	Normal
Schilling's test with or without IF†	Normal (rarely abnormal owing to ileal involvement)	Abnormal	Normal	Abnormal	Abnormal occasionally
Folate (serum)	Low (in >50%)	High to normal	Low	Normal	Normal
Small bowel biopsy (proximal)	Subtotal or total villous atrophy	Normal (>10⁵ organisms on quantitative jejunal fluid culture)	Clubbing and flattening of villi, PAS-positive macrophages	Normal	Normal
C14 glycocholate breath test	Normal	Abnormal (early peak)	Normal	Abnormal (late peak)	Normal

* This is a test of proximal small bowel function. Falsely low values occur in chronic renal failure, dehydration, ascites, hyperthyroidism and in the elderly.
† While pernicious anaemia corrects with intrinsic factor (IF), ileal disease does not correct. Bacterial overgrowth corrects with antibiotics and pancreatic insufficiency with pancreatic supplements. False-negative results occur with incomplete urinary collections, decreased extracellular volume and renal disease.

PAS = periodic acid-Schiff technique.

Treatment

Treatment depends on the cause and also involves the replacement of essential nutrients (Table 6.29).

Coeliac disease

The management of coeliac disease includes a gluten-free diet (exclusion of wheat, rye and barley; there is controversy about oats). Symptoms usually improve in weeks and the histology in months; anti-endomysial antibody also normalises in 3–6 months. A

Table 6.29   Causes and treatment of malabsorption

1. Lipolytic phase defects:

   Causes, e.g.
   (a) chronic pancreatitis
   (b) cystic fibrosis

   Treatment
   (a) reverse causes
   (b) pancreatic enzyme supplements
   (c) medium-chain triglycerides

2. Micellar phase defects:

   Causes, e.g.
   (a) extrahepatic biliary obstruction
   (b) chronic liver disease
   (c) bacterial overgrowth
   (d) terminal ileal disease (e.g. Crohn's disease or resection)

   Treatment
   (a) reverse causes (e.g. antibiotics for bacterial overgrowth)
   (b) cholestyramine if bile acid cathartic effect is important (e.g. <100 cm of ileum resected)
   (c) medium-chain triglycerides for steatorrhoea (e.g. >100 cm of ileum resected)
   (d) fat-soluble vitamin supplements

3. Mucosal and delivery phase defects:

   Causes, e.g.
   (a) coeliac disease (Table 6.27)
   (b) tropical sprue
   (c) lymphoma, intestinal lymphangiectasia
   (d) Whipple's disease
   (e) small bowel ischaemia, resection
   (f) amyloidosis
   (g) hypogammaglobulinaemia
   (h) HIV infection (Kaposi's sarcoma, idiopathic)

   Treatment
   (a) reverse causes—gluten-free diet (coeliac disease), antibiotics (Whipple's disease)
   (b) fat-soluble vitamin supplements

---

strict diet may reduce complications. It is reasonable to re-biopsy the duodenum in 3 months to confirm histological healing. Lack of response to a gluten-free diet may be caused by inadvertent gluten exposure, presence of another problem (e.g. lactose intolerance, pancreatic insufficiency, bacterial overgrowth), refractory sprue (which may respond to corticosteroids) or lymphoma (unresponsive to steroids).

Pneumococcal vaccine is recommended to these patients because of the hyposplenism of coeliac disease. Osteoporosis must be looked for and corrected. Latent coeliac disease can be diagnosed if the small bowel biopsy appears normal but there is a positive IgA anti-endomysial antibody test. For these patients, a gluten-free diet is not usually recommended but follow-up with repeat biopsy is indicated if the symptoms recur.

Inflammatory bowel disease

Both ulcerative colitis and Crohn's disease are common conditions in hospitals and in outpatient clinics. They present both diagnostic and treatment problems. Mutations in the *NOD2* gene (also called *CARD 15*) increases the risk of Crohn's disease (ileal and fibrostenosing). The patient will usually know the diagnosis but you may have to decide which type of inflammatory bowel disease is present.

The history

1. Ask about symptoms at presentation and, if relevant, current reason for admission. Ulcerative colitis typically presents in young adults with relapsing bloody diarrhoea, malaise, fever and weight loss. Crohn's disease has a variable presentation, including an insidious onset of pain, diarrhoea, weight loss, malabsorption, intestinal obstruction and 'appendicitis'.
2. Ask about local complications of the disease (Table 6.30).
3. Ask about extracolonic manifestations of the disease (Table 6.30).
4. Inquire about sexual preference (infective proctitis in homosexuals must be considered in the differential diagnosis).
5. Ask about medications—NSAIDs, gold, retinoic acid and possibly oral contraceptives can cause a similar picture.
6. Ask about investigations at the time of presentation and subsequently (and particularly whether infectious causes were considered).
7. Ask the number of hospital admissions.
8. Ask about whether regular follow-up colonoscopy has been performed in patients with longstanding ulcerative colitis.
9. Ask about treatment—medications, such as sulfasalazine, 5-aminosalicylic acid preparations (mesalazine, olsalazine), local or systemic steroids, budesonide, metronidazole, immunosuppressants (e.g. azathioprine), other antibiotics (consider pseudomembranous colitis), infliximab (tumour necrosis factor antibody), surgery.
10. Inquire about family history of inflammatory bowel disease or of bowel carcinoma.
11. Ask about smoking—a greater proportion than average of Crohn's disease patients are smokers and the risk of developing ulcerative colitis rises when people give up smoking.
12. Inquire about domestic arrangements and employment.

The examination

A thorough gastrointestinal system examination is important. Evaluate the general state of nutrition and hydration. Feel for any tenderness or abdominal masses and look for anal lesions externally. Always ask for the results of a rectal examination. Look for the signs of Cushing's syndrome if the patient is taking steroids. Search for the other extracolonic manifestations, being guided by the history (e.g. arthropathy, skin lesions, uveitis, anaemia, liver disease).

Investigations

It is important to exclude other causes of colitis (Table 6.31). For the investigation of inflammatory bowel disease, the following should be considered.

Table 6.30 Complications of inflammatory bowel disease (IBD)

Ulcerative colitis
Local:
1. Toxic megacolon (diameter of colon >6 cm on plain abdominal X-ray film)
2. Perforation
3. Massive haemorrhage
4. Strictures
5. Carcinoma of the colon—often multicentric and related to disease extent and duration

Extracolonic:
1. Liver disease
   (a) fatty liver
   (b) primary sclerosing cholangitis (large duct or small duct [pericholangitis])
   (c) cirrhosis
   (d) carcinoma of the bile duct
   (e) amyloidosis
2. Blood disorders
   (a) anaemia (owing to chronic disease, iron deficiency, ileal involvement, haemolysis from sulfasalazine or microangiopathy)
   (b) thromboembolism (as a result of antithrombin III deficiency, stasis, dehydration)
3. Arthropathy
   (a) peripheral (large joints)
   (b) ankylosing spondylitis
4. Skin and mucous membranes
   (a) erythema nodosum (coincides with active disease)
   (b) pyoderma gangrenosum
   (c) aphthous ulcers
5. Ocular—uveitis, conjunctivitis, episcleritis

Crohn's disease
Local:
1. Anorectal disease (including anal fissures or fistulas, pararectal abscess or rectovaginal fistula)
2. Obstruction (usually terminal ileum)
3. Fistula
4. Toxic megacolon and perforation (rare)
5. Carcinoma of the small and large bowel (incidence increased only slightly)

Extracolonic:
Similar to ulcerative colitis, except for the following:
1. Liver disease—primary sclerosing cholangitis is less common
2. Gallstones are more common (owing to decreased bile salt pool)
3. Renal disease includes urate and calcium oxalate stones, pyelonephritis (owing to fistulas), hydronephrosis (ureteric obstruction), amyloidosis
4. Malabsorption as a result of small bowel involvement
5. Osteomalacia

Table 6.31	Causes of colitis

1. Inflammatory bowel disease
2. Infections, including pseudomembranous colitis
3. Radiation
4. Ischaemic colitis
5. Diversion colitis (colonic loops excluded from the faecal stream)
6. Toxic exposure (e.g. peroxide or soapsud enemas, gold-induced colitis)
7. Microscopic or collagenous colitis
8. Lymphocytic colitis

1. Infection must be excluded. The causes include amoebiasis (diagnosed by rectal mucosal scraping or warm stool examination), *Shigella*, *Salmonella*, *Yersinia*, *Campylobacter*, *Escherichia coli* 0157:H7 and pseudomembranous colitis (*Clostridium difficile* toxin). Lymphogranuloma venereum (a chlamydial disease that is sexually transmitted), gonorrhoea and syphilis (particularly in homosexuals) and other infections in immunocompromised hosts (e.g. herpes, cytomegalovirus, cryptosporidium, *Isospora belli*) should be considered in patients at risk.
2. Sigmoidoscopy (and biopsy). Note decreased mucosal translucency, loss of vascular pattern, granular and friable mucosa, hyperaemia, ulceration and pseudopolyps.
3. Plain abdominal X-ray film. It is important to look for bowel wall thickening (oedema), gaseous distension and evidence of toxic megacolon in ulcerative colitis. In Crohn's disease also look for loops of matted bowel and small bowel obstruction.
4. Blood count. Check for anaemia (caused by chronic disease, blood loss, macrocytic anaemia in ileal disease, or haemolytic anaemia from an autoimmune process, microangiopathic disease or sulfasalazine). Check the white cell count (e.g. leukopenia from azathioprine). Look at the erythrocyte sedimentation rate (ESR) (or C-reactive protein [CRP]) for evidence of active disease.
5. Liver function tests and blood levels of electrolytes, urea and creatinine. These patients may develop liver disease. Crohn's disease may lead to renal stones, pyelonephritis, hydronephrosis or amyloidosis. Remember that hypoalbuminaemia is a sign of severe disease.
6. Barium enema is only uncommonly used to make a diagnosis. This is contraindicated in very active colitis and with toxic megacolon because of the risk of perforation. This investigation will help distinguish ulcerative colitis from Crohn's disease—in ulcerative colitis the rectum is nearly always involved and there are no skip lesions. Look for loss of haustrations, mucosal irregularity and ulceration, spasm, pseudopolyps and bowel shortening. Also look for evidence of strictures and carcinoma. In Crohn's colitis, look for thickening, 'cobblestoning', luminal narrowing, skip lesions, fistulas and transverse fissures (sinus tracts).
7. Colonoscopy is a very useful investigation to assess whether disease is patchy or not and its extent; the test is more sensitive than a barium enema. Mucosal biopsies may not differentiate ulcerative colitis from Crohn's disease. Mucus depletion and prominent crypt abscess formation are more suggestive of ulcerative colitis. Granulomas (in 25%) or focal inflammation are found in Crohn's colitis (but, note, granulomas also occur in biopsies from homosexual men with *Chlamydia trachomatis*, syphilitic proctitis, or in cases of tuberculosis). Patients with ulcerative colitis who have had pancolitis for more than 7 years or left-sided colitis for 15 years or more may have colonoscopic screening with biopsy offered every 1 or 2 years (although the benefits are contentious) to look for high-grade dysplasia and carcinoma. If high-grade

dysplasia is confirmed in the absence of severe inflammation, colectomy is indicated. If severe inflammation is present, assessment for dysplasia may be misleading.

8. Antibody testing: the presence of perinuclear antineutrophil cytoplasmic antibodies (p-ANCA) and anti-*Saccharomyces cerevisiae* antibodies (ASCA) does not make the diagnosis, but p-ANCA negative and ASCA positive patients are more likely to have Crohn's disease than ulcerative colitis (the test is specific but not sensitive).

Treatment

Ulcerative colitis

In ulcerative colitis, grade the severity of the disease:

1. mild—fewer than four motions per day, minimal bleeding, normal temperature and pulse
2. severe—more than six motions per day, profuse bleeding, temperature >37.5°C, pulse >90 beats/min, abdominal tenderness
3. fulminant—more than 10 motions per day, continuous bleeding, fever and tachycardia as above, abdominal tenderness and distension.

Other useful indices of severity are anaemia, hypoalbuminaemia and acute phase reactants (e.g. ESR, CRP).

In an acute attack, remember to correct hypokalaemia and avoid barium enema to prevent toxic megacolon or perforation. Do not prescribe opiates or anticholinergic agents for a similar reason. In severe colitis, intravenous broad-spectrum antibiotics (including metronidazole) are usually given. Intravenous steroids are the mainstay of treatment in moderate-to-severe disease. Cyclosporin may be given intravenously as a short-term alternative to colectomy for patients who do not respond to steroid treatment. Close cooperation with a surgeon who is interested in this field is important in severe disease.

In mild-to-moderate disease, sulfasalazine is useful; mesalazine is the active agent, while sulfapyridine is the cause of most intolerance (allergic reactions, e.g. skin rash—including Stevens-Johnson syndrome—Heinz body haemolytic anaemia; side-effects, e.g. nausea, headache, folate deficiency, reversible male infertility). The minimum dose is 4 g per day. Sulfasalazine decreases the relapse rate and administration should be continued indefinitely. Mesalazine is as effective as sulfasalazine but has fewer side-effects and higher doses may be given. Mesalazine is useful for patients with sulfasalazine intolerance. Note that the alternative, olsalazine, may cause diarrhoea in patients with active ulcerative colitis (because of ileal secretion)—as a result, it is normally used as maintenance treatment. Chronic steroid use does *not* reduce relapse rates. Remember to correct iron and folate deficiency if necessary.

If proctitis is the problem, first-line treatment is topical (steroid or mesalazine enemas twice daily) plus sulfasalazine or mesalazine orally for more active disease.

Azathioprine or 6-mercaptopurine is useful if there are repeated episodes. Side-effects include pancreatitis in 3% and reversible bone marrow suppression in <10% of patients. The use of methotrexate is controversial but there is some evidence of usefulness.

It is important to try to differentiate ulcerative colitis from Crohn's disease, from the clinical presentation, X-ray, endoscopic and histological findings. This is because ulcerative colitis that does not respond to medical management can be cured by colectomy, and because patients with extensive ulcerative colitis are at an increased risk of developing colorectal cancer. In up to 10% of patients, a specific distinction cannot be made.

Colectomy in ulcerative colitis is curative. Indications for surgery include chronic ill-health and severe disease, complications (e.g. perforation, massive bleeding) and severe disease not responding to optimal medical treatment in 7–10 days. Patients with a very high risk of carcinoma (confirmed high-grade dysplasia on biopsy or dysplasia in a lesion or mass) should be advised to undergo a colectomy. All manifestations of the disease are cured by colectomy, but ankylosing spondylitis, liver disease and occasionally pyoderma gangrenosum do *not* respond. While the standard Brooke ileostomy is the simplest procedure, the ileal pouch anal anastomosis is increasingly being used as it maintains intestinal continuity, although it does leave the patient with four to eight bowel movements daily and sometimes with minor incontinence (20%), and is often complicated by pouchitis (in up to 50% of patients). The latter usually responds to treatment with metronidazole.

Crohn's disease

For active disease, treatment is similar to ulcerative colitis. Sulfasalazine or mesalazine is more effective in colonic disease, while steroids are more effective in small bowel disease. Budenoside (a steroid derivative that acts locally and is 90% inactivated by the liver) is useful in ileocolonic disease. In quiescent disease mesalazine modestly reduces the frequency of relapse in the postoperative setting. Azathioprine (or 6-mercapto-purine) is useful for those who cannot cease steroids and to reduce relapse. Methotrexate is an alternative if azathioprine fails. Oral cyclosporin is largely ineffective. With extensive ileal disease, diarrhoea may respond to a bile salt sequestering drug (cholestyramine or colestipol).

Metronidazole is modestly useful for severe perianal disease and fistulae, which tend to recur once treatment is stopped; azathioprine may be tried in difficult severe cases. Infliximab (tumour necrosis factor alpha monoclonal antibody) heals fistulae and suppresses underlying inflammatory disease, but relapse is common after completion of the course of three infusions and maintenance treatment is now indicated. Infusion reactions, infection (including miliary tuberculosis), lymphoproliferative diseases and demyelination can occur on this drug. Infliximab is very expensive and not available everywhere but is becoming the standard of care for fistulas and refractory disease.

Surgery is reserved for the complications of Crohn's disease (e.g. internal fistula with abscess, intestinal obstruction not responding to medical management). The best operation is resection. Strictureplasty may allow relief of localised obstruction without the deleterious effects of multiple resections. When a total colectomy is needed, a standard ileostomy is the procedure of choice. The recurrence rate of the disease is unchanged by surgery.

Colon cancer

This is a particularly common tumour that usually develops in those 50 years of age or older, although patients at risk with hereditary syndromes will present at a younger age. As early disease is curable, there has been increased interest recently in colon cancer screening. Hence, a history of polyps or colon cancer is increasingly likely to be encountered in the examination.

The history

1. The patient may have been diagnosed recently as having a colon cancer. In this case, ascertain the reasons for diagnostic testing. A recent change in bowel habit, or bright red blood per rectum (from a rectal or left-sided colon cancer), symptoms of anaemia, new-onset abdominal pain or symptoms suggestive of small bowel obstruction (with a slow-growing caecal cancer) may be the presenting complaint. There may be symptoms from involvement of the bladder or female genital tract owing to local invasion. Sacral plexus pain is a very late manifestation.
2. If colon cancer was identified, determine the staging tests and treatment undertaken. If radiotherapy was given to the pelvis, inquire about any ongoing proctitis or cystitis.
3. Determine if the patient understands the prognosis and ascertain the social support network.

4. If there was a history of polyps, try to determine from the patient if this was an adenomatous polyp, its approximate size and the number present. Patients are often rather unclear about these issues and you may need to request, when discussing with the examiners, information from the medical record. Adenomatous polyps may be tubular or villous (or tubulovillous); invasive cancer is more likely in larger polyps (10% in those >2.5 cm). If polyps were detected, ask the patient whether surveillance colonoscopy has been conducted in the past, when this began, and how often. A frequency of approximately 3 years in those patients without previously documented colonic cancer who have a documented large (>1 cm) or multiple adenomatous polyps is generally recommended, although surveillance needs to be tailored to other risk factors, including the family history.

5. The family history needs to be carefully obtained in any patient with a history of polyps or colon cancer in the past. If the patient describes having had thousands of adenomatous polyps throughout the large bowel, then familial adenomatous polyposis (FAP) is the diagnosis (until proven otherwise). These polyps occur usually after puberty and most individuals are affected by the age of 25 years. If the colon is not removed, almost all will have colon cancer before the age of 40 years. In this type of clinical case, ask about the presence of any soft tissue or bony tumours (Gardiner's syndrome) or tumours in the central nervous system (Turkot's syndrome), which are variants of FAP. Most patients with FAP will have undergone a total colectomy with ileoanal anastomosis. Ask about continence and stool frequency if this operation has been performed. Screening for duodenal and periampullary cancers 1–3 yearly by endoscopy is generally recommended. Ask also if the offspring of a patient with this condition have been screened. Flexible sigmoidoscopy on an annual basis is recommended. DNA testing of peripheral blood mononuclear cells for the presence of the mutated *APC* gene at puberty is also useful (after first testing affected relatives to validate the *APC* mutation presence) in screening offspring.

    If there is a strong family history of colon cancer, consider the possibility of Lynch Syndrome (see below). There is a 70% lifetime risk of colon cancer in this autosomal dominant disease.

    There is often also a family history of either ovarian or endometrial carcinoma. Members of such families are typically screened by colonoscopy biennially beginning at the age of 25 years, as well as undergoing pelvic ultrasonography and endometrial biopsies.

6. Inquire about any history of documented inflammatory bowel disease. The risk of colorectal cancer in a patient with ulcerative colitis is small during the initial 7–10 years after pancolonic disease development, but then increases approximately 1% per year. You should inquire about whether colonoscopic surveillance has been undertaken or not. Patients with Crohn's disease may also be offered similar surveillance but there is less supporting data.

7. Inquire whether there has been any history of possible septicaemia. *Streptococcus bovis* bacteraemia indicates an underlying high risk of occult colon cancer as well as upper gastrointestinal tract cancer and requires aggressive investigation.

8. Haematomas of the gastrointestinal tract with mucocutaneous pigmentation (Peutz–Jeghers syndrome) increase the risk of both large and small bowel cancer, as well as breast, uterine and ovarian cancers. Affected patients should undergo surveillance by colonoscopy and gastroscopy three yearly from 18 years of age.

9. Determine if there is any history of a ureterosigmoidostomy for correction of congenital exstrophy of the bladder, which increases the risk of colon cancer 15–30 years later.

10. Diabetes mellitus and acromegaly may be associated with an increased risk.

The examination

Look for evidence of jaundice or anaemia. If the patient is currently undergoing fluorouracil-derived chemotherapy, look at the palms and soles for evidence of hand–foot syndrome. Carefully examine the abdomen, in particular looking for any evidence of malignant deposits in the liver, or other intraperitoneal masses or skin changes that are consistent with radiotherapy. Record any scars on the abdomen. Results of a rectal examination need to be obtained. Other lymph node groups should be examined and evidence of metastatic malignancy elsewhere (e.g. the lungs, bones or brain) should be sought. Look for the pigmentation of Peutz-Jeghers syndrome. Multiple skin lesions (e.g. sebaceous adenomas and carcinomas, basal cell and squamous cell carcinomas, keratoacanthomas) occur in a variant of hereditary non-polyposis colorectal cancer (Torres syndrome).

Investigations

1. *Screening.* If the patient has three or more relatives with a history of colon cancer, one of whom is a first-degree relative of the other two, or one or more cases of colorectal cancer diagnosed before the age of 50 in the family, or colorectal cancer involving at least two generations, consider the possibility of hereditary non-polyposis colon cancer (HNPCC or Lynch syndrome). In most kindreds with HNPCC, germ-line mutations have occurred in one of six DNA mismatch repair genes. Commercial testing is available for *hMSH2* and *hMLH1* mutations and these have a high sensitivity. 'Microsatellite instability' (MSI) is the expansion or contraction of short repeated DNA sequences. MSI has been observed in more than 90% of samples of tumour tissue from patients with HPNCC who fulfil the clinical (Amsterdam) criteria for this disease but also in up to 15% of tumours from patients with sporadic colorectal cancer. The presence of MSI may indicate a better prognosis and better response to adjuvant chemotherapy. Testing for the presence of MSI in a tumour or adenoma should be an initial screening test for patients suspected of having HPNCC and positive cases should undergo genetic screening.
2. *Symptomatic patients.* Most will have had the cancer identified by colonoscopy or barium enema examination. With the increasing introduction of screening measures in asymptomatic patients (e.g. faecal occult blood testing), earlier stage colon cancers will be detected by this means in average-risk patients. The prognosis depends on the stage of disease. Survival is decreased if the bowel wall is penetrated (Dukes's B2 stage) or with lymph node involvement (Dukes's C stage).

Treatment

For colon cancer, total tumour resection in local disease is the treatment of choice undertaken either endoscopically or surgically. Before surgery, patients should be evaluated for the possibility of metastatic disease, including a careful physical examination. Many physicians would also order a chest radiograph, liver function tests and measure the baseline carcinoembryonic antigen (CEA) level. If possible, a complete colonoscopy should be undertaken to look for evidence of synchronous cancers or polyps. If colonoscopy was not performed before the operation, it should be carried out as soon as practicable after the operation.

Following a resection, patients are often followed up for 5 years with annual physical examinations and surveillance colonoscopy 3 yearly. Measuring CEA levels 3 monthly for 2 years after surgery for Dukes's B or C stage disease, as a test for tumour recurrence, is often recommended but remains controversial.

If metastatic disease is present, resection of the primary colorectal tumour does not change prognosis and should be done only for symptomatic reasons. The exception is metastases to the liver only, where 25% may be cured by resection.

Determine if the patient has had radiation therapy to the pelvis, which may have been offered with a rectal cancer. Some patients may have received chemotherapy; in particular, patients with Dukes's stage C often have had adjuvant leucovorin modulated 5-fluorouracil for 6 months.

Chronic liver disease

Cirrhosis alone or in combination with other disease will often crop up, particularly in repatriation hospitals. (*Warning*: You may be exposed to prolonged war stories and discussions about shrapnel.) It is a pathological diagnosis. This discussion will be limited to aspects of cirrhosis and chronic hepatitis, which tend to be most frequent in the examination.

The history

Cirrhosis can present with jaundice, ascites, abdominal pain, acute bleeding or encephalopathy. Occasionally patients present with just weakness, lassitude or loss of libido. There may be no symptoms (incidental cirrhosis).

1. Ask about length of history of liver disease:
    (a) past history of hepatitis or jaundice, including contacts
    (b) alcohol intake (in men 80 g per day for more than 10 years is usually necessary; women need less exposure)
    (c) history of drug addiction (intravenous), sexual preference, transfusions, tattoos etc.
    (d) drug history (e.g. for chronic hepatitis: methyldopa, isoniazid, nitrofurantoin)
    (e) history of diabetes mellitus, cardiac failure or arthropathy (haemochromatosis)
    (f) overseas travel (e.g. acute hepatitis).
2. Ask about treatment (e.g. protein restriction, fluid restriction, alcohol abstinence, steroids, lactulose, neomycin).
3. Ask about complications, such as any history of encephalopathy, any history of portal hypertension (ascites or bleeding from varices), recent abdominal pain (gallstones—usually pigment stones, acute alcoholic hepatitis etc.).
4. Ask about investigations (e.g. liver biopsy).
5. Ask about operations (e.g. portacaval shunt).
6. Inquire about erectile dysfunction, loss of libido.
7. Inquire about social problems (e.g. employment, family).

The examination

Note the patient's racial origin. Hepatitis B and C viruses are endemic in South–East Asia, Italy and Egypt. Look for tattoos—tattoo needles are a source of infection. Examine carefully for the signs of chronic liver disease. Also note any hepatic encephalopathy, signs of portal hypertension, including splenomegaly, ascites, oedema and signs of bleeding (e.g. melaena).

Consider hepatocellular carcinoma (particularly in haemochromatosis and cirrhosis as a result of hepatitis B or C virus infection). In patients with decompensated cirrhosis, examine for a hard mass and liver bruit (hepatoma). Look for the signs of haemochromatosis. In young patients, consider Wilson's disease and look carefully for Kayser-Fleischer rings. If there is deep jaundice with scratch marks and xanthelasma, particularly in a woman, consider end-stage primary biliary cirrhosis. Exclude severe right heart failure, tricuspid regurgitation or constrictive pericarditis clinically in all patients. Other causes and sequelae are given in Tables 6.32 and 6.33.

Table 6.32   **Causes of cirrhosis in adults**

1. Alcohol
2. Postviral (hepatitis B, delta, C)
3. Non-alcoholic steatohepatitis (NASH)
4. Drugs (e.g. methyldopa, chlorpromazine, isoniazid, nitrofurantoin, propylthiouracil, methotrexate, amiodarone)
5. Autoimmune chronic hepatitis
6. Haemochromatosis
7. Wilson's disease
8. Primary sclerosing cholangitis
9. Primary biliary cirrhosis
10. Secondary biliary cirrhosis
11. Alpha$_1$-antitrypsin deficiency
12. Cystic fibrosis
13. Budd-Chiari syndrome
14. Cardiac failure, chronic constrictive pericarditis
15. Cryptogenic (idiopathic)

Table 6.33   **Sequelae of cirrhosis**

1. Portal hypertension and ascites
2. Portal vein thrombosis (rare)
3. Spontaneous bacterial peritonitis
4. Hepatic encephalopathy
5. Hepatorenal syndrome
6. Hepatocellular carcinoma

Investigations

Management of cirrhosis depends on aetiology, morphology and hepatic function. It is important to make a diagnosis and exclude potentially reversible causes of further liver deterioration.

1. Liver function tests. These should be used to confirm abnormalities, follow progress and give an idea of prognosis (particularly a low albumin level and prolonged INR). An aspartate aminotransferase (AST) to alanine aminotransferase (ALT) ratio of >2.0 suggests alcoholic liver disease.
2. Full blood count. This is helpful as anaemia may be caused by chronic disease, blood loss, folate deficiency, bone marrow depression, hypersplenism, haemolysis or sideroblastic anaemia. Round macrocytes are common in alcoholics. Remember that leukopenia and thrombocytopenia occur in hypersplenism.
3. Renal function tests are important to exclude the hepatorenal syndrome. Hyponatraemia is common in cirrhosis.
4. Ascitic tap (Tables 6.34 and 6.35).
5. Ultrasound. This may help exclude biliary obstruction and infiltration. The texture of the liver may suggest infiltration (e.g. fat) or nodularity (cirrhosis).
6. In the setting of dyspnoea, consider hepatopulmonary syndrome. Platypnoea (dyspnoea that is worse when the patient sits up and is relieved by lying down)

Table 6.34 Causes of ascites and interpretation of ascitic fluid studies

Causes
1. Related to portal hypertension (serum-to-ascites albumin gradient (SAAG) ≥11 g/L):
   (a) cirrhosis
   (b) alcoholic hepatitis
   (c) cardiac ascites
   (d) fulminant hepatic failure
   (e) veno-occlusive disease
   (f) Budd-Chiari syndrome (hepatic vein thrombosis) or inferior vena caval obstruction (Table 6.35)
   (g) myxoedema
2. Not related to portal hypertension (SAAG <11 g/L):
   (a) peritoneal carcinomatosis
   (b) peritoneal tuberculosis
   (c) pancreatitis
   (d) nephrotic syndrome (Table 6.71)

Examination of ascitic fluid following a diagnostic paracentesis
1. SAAG—≥11 g/L in portal hypertension (e.g. cirrhosis)
2. Blood—suggests malignancy or a recent invasive test
3. Turbid or white fluid—suggests infection or chylous ascites
4. Cell count (0–300 × 10^6/L mononuclear cells is normal: >500 cells or >250 polymorphs × 10^6/L suggests spontaneous bacterial peritonitis)
5. Lactate—increased in spontaneous bacterial peritonitis
6. Amylase—elevated in pancreatic ascites
7. Cytology—for malignant cells
8. Culture—for spontaneous bacterial peritonitis

---

and orthodexia (arterial desaturation when upright) is strongly suggestive; intrapulmonary vascular dilatation diagnosis may be possible by contrast echocardiography.

7. Liver biopsy. This is a definitive test and probably should be done if the diagnosis is uncertain, unless there are specific contraindications (e.g. coagulopathy).

Always assess for possible causative factors (see Table 6.32). Hepatitis B and C serology should be obtained. Screen for antimitochondrial antibody (AMA) if primary biliary cirrhosis is suspected. Test for antinuclear antibody (ANA), smooth muscle antibody, and anti-liver and kidney microsomes type 1 (anti-LKM1) antibody in suspected chronic hepatitis (e.g. young woman with raised globulins). In type I autoimmune chronic hepatitis there is marked hyperglobulinaemia, and ANA and anti-smooth muscle antibody (ASMSA) are present. In type IIa, ANA is negative but anti-LKM1 is present in high titre and responds to interferon treatment (this antibody also occurs in low titre in hepatitis C). In the rare overlap syndromes, the only serological abnormality may be AMA, but the histology shows autoimmune hepatitis, or the patient is ANA or ASMA (but not AMA) positive and has primary biliary cirrhosis (autoimmune cholangiopathy) on histology.

Iron studies and, in a young patient, caeruloplasmin levels should be ordered. Alpha$_1$-antitrypsin deficiency should be considered; absence of the alpha$_1$ fraction on a protein electrophoresis is a useful clue. Evaluate for evidence of inflammatory bowel

Table 6.35 **Budd-Chiari syndrome**

Typically young adults who have pain (owing to hepatic congestion), hepatomegaly and ascites

Causes
1. Idiopathic—thrombosis or fibrous obliteration of hepatic vein
2. Myeloproliferative disease, especially polycythaemia rubra vera
3. Malignant disease (e.g. renal, pancreatic, hepatoma, adrenal, testicular, thyroid)
4. Oral contraceptives or pregnancy
5. Paroxysmal nocturnal haemoglobinuria (PNH)
6. Drugs (e.g. azathioprine, adriamycin)
7. Fibrous membrane, trauma, schistosomiasis, amoebiasis

Diagnosis
1. Liver function tests—non-specific, but serum alkaline phosphatase level may be high
2. Ascitic tap
3. Ultrasonography with Doppler flow studies—less sensitive than angiography but diagnostic in >85% of cases
4. Technetium sulfur colloid liver scan (increased caudate lobe uptake)—less useful
5. Liver biopsy (highly suggestive—'nutmeg' liver)
6. Angiography and venography (most important)

disease if there are colonic symptoms. Perinuclear antineutrophil cytoplasmic antibodies (p-ANCA) occur in up to 80% of patients with ulcerative colitis and are a marker for primary sclerosing cholangitis (60% of cases).

Screening for hepatocellular carcinoma (HCC) is often undertaken despite a lack of definite evidence of its usefulness. It should certainly be performed in patients with Child's A cirrhosis who would be suitable for a partial hepatectomy if carcinoma were discovered. It should also be carried out for patients being assessed for transplant. Screening is by 6 monthly measurement of alpha-fetoprotein and liver ultrasound. It is expensive.

Finally, assess the hepatic functional reserve of patients with known or suspected cirrhosis (Table 6.36).

Treatment

Decide whether the patient has acute or acute-on-chronic disease, and decide whether the disease is compensated or decompensated. Management includes treating hepatocellular failure (synthetic function) and portal hypertension (plumbing). Cirrhosis is irreversible. However, removing causative factors, such as alcohol, iron overload and drugs, or treating viral infection is of value.

Hepatocellular failure

Acute hepatic encephalopathy is precipitated by bleeding into the gastrointestinal tract or electrolyte disturbances (alkalosis increases the ammonia crossing the blood–brain barrier, whereas hypokalaemia increases renal ammonia production). Hypokalaemia may be caused by recent diuretic use. Infection (e.g. spontaneous bacterial peritonitis), drugs (e.g. sedatives), a high-protein diet, constipation, deteriorating liver function (e.g.

Table 6.36   Child's classification of patients with cirrhosis in terms of hepatic functional reserve

	A	B	C
Degree of impairment	Minimal	Moderate	Severe
Serum bilirubin (mmol/L)	<35	35–50	>50
Serum albumin (g/L) (μmol/L)	>35 (>507)	30–35 (435–507)	<30 (<435)
Ascites	None	Easily controlled	Poorly controlled
Encephalopathy	None	Minimal	Advanced; 'coma'
Nutrition	Excellent	Good	Poor; 'wasting'

alcoholic binge, hepatoma) and rarely metabolic disturbances (e.g. hypoglycaemia, hypoxia) may also precipitate encephalopathy.

Management consists of removing the precipitating factors. This means removing blood from the gut (e.g. enemas), giving a low-protein diet, treating infection, correcting electrolyte disturbances, avoiding sedatives and attacking the urea-splitting organisms with lactulose or lactitol (lactulose causes more diarrhoea), or neomycin, or both.

Chronic hepatocellular failure should be managed by treating the cause where possible and manipulating the protein diet as required. Control encephalopathy and ascites. Watch for gastrointestinal bleeding and renal failure. In cases of autoimmune chronic hepatitis, steroids are helpful in patients without viral markers.

Portal hypertension

Clinical features include splenomegaly, the presence of collaterals, ascites and fetor hepaticus.

Investigations include endoscopy for oesophageal varices, ascitic tap and abdominal ultrasound with Doppler arterial and venous flow studies. An attempt should be made to assess the bleeding risk for a patient with varices. High-risk patients (75% risk of haemorrhage over 1 year) are those with Child's class C cirrhosis, gross ascites and large varices. All high-risk patients should be recommended prophylactic treatment—usually with beta-blockers.

Bleeding varices should be managed acutely by replacing blood and correcting coagulation abnormalities. Intravenous octreotide (or vasopressin combined with glyceryl trinitrate) is first-line therapy but is only a temporary measure. Oesophageal variceal banding therapy is effective (and superior to sclerotherapy) in stopping acute bleeding. Balloon tamponade at the gastro-oesophageal junction with the gastric balloon is now uncommonly required; oesophageal balloon tamponade may worsen the prognosis. To prevent recurrent variceal bleeding, elective endoscopic banding to obliterate varices may be effective. Beta-blockers (propranolol) can reduce portal pressure and may be useful in patients with good liver function. Portosystemic shunting is controversial—it probably does not reduce mortality in the long term. TIPS is preferable to shunt surgery. Mortality is high for 'crash' shunts.

Treatment of ascites consists of gentle diuresis (maximum weight loss of 500 g per day). Begin with bed rest, salt restriction and spironolactone but increase the dose slowly. If the urinary sodium to potassium ratio is >1, a dose of 150 mg/day is usually adequate; if the ratio is less than 1, higher doses are needed. Frusemide is given if necessary. A combination of frusemide 40 mg daily and spironolactone 25 mg daily may be the most helpful, although there is evidence that spironolactone alone may be as effective. Therapeutic paracentesis is a safe alternative in patients with tense ascites, especially when there is also peripheral oedema. Intravenous salt-poor albumin is given to replace the protein lost in ascitic fluid, and 5–10 L can be removed; the procedure can be repeated if necessary. Therapeutic paracentesis is contraindicated in renal failure or severe coagulopathy.

In resistant ascites, alternatives include transjugular intrahepatic portosystemic shunts (TIPS) or surgical shunts. Le Veen shunts do not improve the prognosis. Complications of Le Veen shunting include disseminated intravascular coagulation, infection, cardiac failure, pulmonary oedema and variceal bleeding; shunt failure is common.

Liver transplantation is the definitive treatment in suitable patients (in the absence of hepatorenal syndrome).

Hepatitis B

Hepatitis B virus (HBV) may be transmitted parenterally (intravenous drug users, infected blood products etc.) or sexually. Most infected individuals seroconvert and develop immunity; however, a small proportion become chronic carriers or progress to chronic hepatitis and ultimately cirrhosis. The risk of developing hepatocellular carcinoma (HCC) in the latter group is high.

The diagnosis of hepatitis B is made by positive serology (HBsAg-positive) and active disease is usually associated with the HBeAg-positive state as well as elevated serum transaminase levels, particularly the serum ALT level. Measuring for HBV-DNA provides a more accurate assessment of viral load. Precore mutants of HBV are usually diagnosed in patients who are HBeAg-negative and HBeAb-positive, but have elevated transaminase and HBV-DNA levels. The most accurate method of staging the disease is by means of a liver biopsy. The liver biopsy is important to assess the extent of the inflammation and fibrosis in those with chronic hepatitis.

The aim of antiviral therapy is to stop viral replication (i.e. seroconversion from positive HBeAg to negative HBeAg and HBV-DNA levels), as well as normalising ALT levels and histology. Treatment is with subcutaneous interferon, most commonly 5 million units thrice weekly for 2–6 months, or lamivudine at 100 mg or adefovir 10 mg daily for as long as necessary. Interferon produces a response rate of approximately 30% with loss of HBeAg status. Nevertheless, the drug has many debilitating side-effects. Lamivudine has minimal side-effects, with a seroconversion rate after 2 years of about 30%. Lamivudine is an orally active nucleoside analogue that interferes with HBV replication. Long-term use of lamivudine may be associated with the development of a *YMDD* mutant form of HBV. To date these variants have not been shown to cause any additional liver damage. Patients should be maintained on lamivudine despite the presence of the variant. This is because re-emergence of wild-type virus may have a worse outcome. Adefovir is active against lamivudine-resistant HBV; entecavir is an alternative.

Liver transplantation can be considered in patients with decompensated HBV liver disease but without proper preparation HBV infection recurs in the transplanted liver and may cause very aggressive liver disease. Fortunately, new strategies are becoming available to overcome this problem. Currently, antiviral drugs are used prior to transplantation to lower HBV-DNA levels, and then large doses of hepatitis B immunoglobulin are used in the peritransplantation period. This strategy is extremely effective in preventing recurrence after liver transplantation.

Hepatitis C

Hepatitis C virus (HCV) is predominantly parenterally transmitted and is particularly common in intravenous drug users. The virus is also commonly found in migrants from endemic regions, including South-East Asia, Egypt and Italy. The majority of patients are incidentally found to be infected and are usually asymptomatic, although fatigue is a common symptom. Extrahepatic manifestations are listed in Table 6.37. The disease process is insidious in onset. Approximately 80% of infected individuals go on to develop chronic hepatitis over a 20-year period. It is estimated that 20–30% of patients with chronic hepatitis C develop cirrhosis, but the process is generally slow and insidious. Once cirrhosis develops, symptoms are more common and the signs of end-stage liver disease can appear with jaundice, weakness, wasting and gastrointestinal bleeding. After 25 years of infection about 4% of patients with cirrhosis develop HCC.

Table 6.37   **Extrahepatic manifestations of hepatitis C**

Mixed cryoglobulinaemia
Porphyria cutanea tarda
Cutaneous necrotising vasculitis
Membranoproliferative glomerulonephritis
Lichen planus
Hashimoto's thyroiditis
B-cell lymphoma
Polyarthralgias and polyarthritis

Diagnosis is usually based on a positive HCV antibody ELISA test. If there is any doubt, HCV-polymerase chain reaction (PCR) testing is useful as a confirmatory test. Quantitative HCV-PCR is useful in monitoring the response to treatment.

A liver biopsy is necessary to stage the disease and estimate the extent of fibrosis. Patients with cirrhosis respond poorly to antiviral therapy and are also at risk of development of HCC.

Current therapy is based on a combination of oral ribavirin and pegylated interferon for 12 months. Sustained response rates of approximately 40% can be achieved. Vaccination against hepatitis A and B is recommended for patients who are not already immune.

Patients who develop end-stage liver disease may be transplant candidates. Hepatitis C-related liver disease is the commonest reason for liver transplantation today.

Haemochromatosis

This is an autosomal recessive disease marked by progressive iron loading of parenchymal cells of the liver, pancreas, heart and other organs. The diagnosis is now often made before symptoms develop (the result of routine iron studies). Symptomatic patients usually present with hepatomegaly and abdominal pain. HCC occurs in up to 30% of patients with cirrhosis. Diabetes mellitus is common, as is skin pigmentation, dilated cardiomyopathy, arthropathy and impotence (owing to iron pigmentation in the pituitary gland). Hereditary haemochromatosis is a common genetic disorder in Caucasians, with a prevalence of at least 1 in 250.

Diagnosis is suggested by an increased transferrin saturation (>62% men, >50% women) and a raised ferritin level (>300 μg/L in men and >200 μg/L in women is suggestive). The serum ferritin level is an acute-phase reactant and may be elevated in other chronic inflammatory conditions, notably those involving the liver, including NASH, alcoholic liver disease and chronic viral hepatitis. Liver biopsy is useful to measure the amount of iron overload and the extent of liver disease (fibrosis, cirrhosis, etc.). There are specific features on biopsy; a Perl's Prussian blue stain visually demonstrates the extent of iron overload. It is important to determine the hepatic iron concentration and index (usually >1.9) on liver biopsy specimens.

The genetic defect has been localised to the short arm of chromosome 6. The gene has been termed *HFE*. Two mutations have been described—*C282Y* and *H63D*. Better identification of family members is now able to be undertaken based on documenting the presence of these two mutations. Patients with phenotypic haemochromatosis are usually homozygous for the *C282Y* mutation; a few are compound heterozygotes (*C282Y* and *H63D* mutation). Homozygotes for *H63D* may not be at risk; 5% of those with haemochromatosis have none of these mutations. Genetic testing is recommended for all first-degree relatives of the proband. In those cases homozygous for *C282Y*, there is a 1 in 4 chance of the siblings being homozygous. The children's chance of developing haemochromatosis depends on the spouse (homozygous normal indicates no risk).

Treatment is through regular venesection (weekly) for approximately 2 years and then once every 3 months. The optimal regimen is not established but the aim is to reduce iron stores as quickly as possible. Fifty units of blood contains 12.5 g of iron. Patients with iron overload as a result of mutations of the iron export protein ferroportin may not tolerate this rate of removal. The avoidance of alcohol is important. Arthropathy and endocrine changes do not respond to treatment. Hepatocellular carcinoma is not prevented by venesection in patients with established cirrhosis but life-expectancy is normal in those without end-organ damage whose iron stores are reduced.

Non-alcoholic steatohepatitis

NASH is defined by histological features, resembling those of alcoholic hepatitis, that are present in patients who have not consumed excessive quantities of alcohol. The majority of patients present because they are inadvertently found to have abnormal liver function tests or steatosis detected on imaging. Even though clinical findings are uncommon, hepatomegaly is the most frequent sign detected. The typical liver function abnormalities are a two- to threefold elevation of the serum aminotransferase levels, with the serum ALT greater than the serum AST level (the opposite of alcoholic liver disease). The serum gamma-glutamyl transferase (GGT) levels are also similarly elevated. Viral markers are absent.

NASH is more common in women and the most frequently associated underlying clinical conditions are obesity, type 2 diabetes mellitus and hyperlipidaemia, particularly hypertriglyceridaemia. Nevertheless, studies have documented lean men with NASH. While the peak age of presentation is the fifth and sixth decades of life, NASH is now the commonest cause of liver disease in adolescents.

The definitive diagnostic test is a liver biopsy. The histopathological features should be evaluated in conjunction with a detailed history of alcohol and drug intake (e.g. methotrexate). Where relevant, other liver disease must be excluded (e.g. haemochromatosis, chronic viral hepatitis) (Table 6.38). The typical histological features are macrovesicular steatosis with an associated necroinflammatory infiltrate (usually mononuclear) and a variable degree of fibrosis.

Another group of patients has fatty liver disease without inflammation and with normal transaminase levels—non-alcoholic fatty liver disease (NAFLD).

A proportion of patients will progress to more chronic liver disease with fibrosis and ultimately cirrhosis. NASH may explain many cases previously labelled as cryptogenic. Studies have documented elevations in both cardiovascular and hepatic mortality. Management options are limited to treating the underlying clinical condition, with slow weight loss recommended for obese patients, and strict control of hyperlipidaemia and hyperglycaemia. Drug trials evaluating the role of urodeoxycholic acid,

Table 6.38 Causes of hepatic steatosis	
Metabolic disorders	**Drugs and toxins**
Obesity	Alcohol
Diabetes mellitus	Methotrexate
Hyperlipidaemia	Organic solvents
Jejunoileal bypass	Amiodarone
Total parenteral nutrition	

lipid-lowering agents and hypoglycaemic drugs are currently being pursued. Vitamin E may be of some benefit.

Liver transplantation

Liver transplantation is now an important therapeutic option in the patient with irreversible, progressive liver disease for which there is no acceptable alternative therapy and no absolute contraindication. The 1-year survival rate overall is now 75%. In the examination setting, a patient will either have chronic liver disease and be a candidate for transplantation or be a transplant recipient who has a problem.

The history

1. Obtain details of the patient's liver disease, including diagnosis and duration. Candidates for liver transplantation include patients with cirrhosis, primary sclerosing cholangitis, autoimmune chronic hepatitis, chronic portal-systemic encephalopathy, Budd-Chiari syndrome, inherited metabolic diseases (e.g. Wilson's disease, alpha$_1$-antitrypsin deficiency) and acute or subacute hepatic failure.
2. The timing of the transplantation is crucial. This should be considered when the patient is invalided but before complications have occurred that may preclude proceeding (e.g. preterminal variceal bleeding, irreversible hepatorenal syndrome, development of a catabolic state, irreversible coagulopathy, vascular instability with ascites or incapacitating osteopenic bone disease). Those with end-stage liver disease who have had a life-threatening episode of decompensation or whose quality of life has become unbearably reduced are potential candidates. Accepted criteria include a Child-Pugh score >6, an episode of variceal bleeding or spontaneous bacterial peritonitis or stage II encephalopathy in acute liver failure. A model for end-stage liver disease (MELD), which has been developed at the Mayo Clinic and based on three parameters (serum bilirubin, INR and creatinine), helps predict survival and is widely used.
3. If the patient may be a candidate for liver transplantation, inquire about potential contraindications. Relative contraindications include active sepsis outside the liver, metastatic malignancy, cholangiocarcinoma, continuing alcohol consumption, the acquired immunodeficiency syndrome (AIDS), diffuse portal vein thrombosis and advanced cardiopulmonary or renal disease, a prior portacaval shunt, intrahepatic or biliary infection, localised portal vein thrombosis, prior complex hepatobiliary surgery, severe hypoxaemia as a result of intrapulmonary shunting (patients with the hepatopulmonary syndrome and hypoxia can benefit, but a PaO_2 of <50 mmHg is a relative contraindication), and renal impairment.
4. Ask about tests that have been done in preparation for transplant. These typically include cardiac and pulmonary (electrocardiogram [ECG], echocardiogram, stress

test, chest X-ray, pulmonary function tests), renal (24-hour urine protein and creatine and glomerular filtration rate estimation), and liver (imaging to exclude a hepatoma and to define the vascular anatomy).

5. Inquire about complications of the patient's liver disease (e.g. previous haemorrhages, ascites, pre-coma, hypoxaemia caused by hepatopulmonary syndrome, etc.).

6. If the patient has had a transplant, inquire about the postoperative course, including whether further surgery was carried out (e.g. drainage of abscesses, reconstruction of the biliary tract, for control of bleeding, retransplantation for graft failure, for hepatic arterial thrombosis). Also inquire about postoperative infections.

7. Ask about complications of liver transplantation. Early on (in the first 5 days), primary graft failure, technical problems (e.g. bleeding, hepatic arterial thrombosis, bile leaks, portal vein thrombosis), renal failure and pulmonary complications (atelectasis, pleural effusion, infection) may occur. Major problems after discharge from hospital include rejection, infection, biliary complications, hypotension, recurrent disease, bone disease, nutrition and de-novo cancer. Infections occur in most patients largely related to immunosuppression; chronic opportunistic infections usually occur from 4 weeks after transplantation. Biliary strictures may also occur from 4 weeks after transplantation. Acute liver rejection is rarely seen after the initial 6 months. Chronic rejection usually occurs 6 weeks to 9 months after transplantation; there is progressive cholestasis, and diagnosis is best made by liver biopsy. Bone disease and ectopic calcification may occur some months after transplantation.

8. Ask about current medications and related complications with their use. Cyclosporin may induce cholestasis (dose-dependent), hypertension, nephrotoxicity, gum hypertrophy, seizures (controlled by phenytoin, which itself induces cyclosporin metabolism), and central nervous system effects, including tremor and central pontine myelinolysis. Patients with a low serum cholesterol level are at increased risk of central nervous system toxicity. Steroids in high doses may induce a number of problems, including aseptic necrosis of long bones, cataracts and psychosis. Inquire about drug compliance.

9. Ask about the specific complications of immunosuppression. Systemic and local infection are frequent problems and can be rapidly fatal if not treated aggressively. Opportunistic infections include *Pneumocystis carinii* and *Candida albicans*. Cytomegalovirus infection remains a major problem. Try to find out tactfully whether there has been any problem with malignancy. The incidence of skin cancers and lymphomas (especially in the central nervous system) is increased with immunosuppression.

The examination

The pretransplant patient should be examined for signs of chronic liver disease and complications of liver disease.

The post-transplant patient should be examined for liver tenderness (e.g. acute rejection) and jaundice (e.g. vanishing bile ducts in chronic rejection, biliary stricture). Examine the chest for infection and the mouth for candidiasis. The temperature must be taken (Table 6.39). Examine the central nervous system (e.g. cyclosporin toxicity or cerebral infarction from perioperative hypotension or air embolism). Tap the spine for tenderness (e.g. vertebral collapse). Take the blood pressure (hypertension may occur at any time after transplantation; it is often caused by cyclosporin).

Investigations and treatment

Pretransplant patients need tests to confirm the diagnosis, determine current liver synthetic function (e.g. serum albumin, prothrombin time) and rule out contraindications. Ultrasound and CT scanning are routine. In patients with possible or definite

Table 6.39	Causes of fever in the outpatient with a liver transplant

Biliary tract (stricture and cholangitis)
Pneumonia (e.g. *Pneumocystis*, bacterial, fungal)
Urinary tract sepsis
Hepatitis (acute or recurrent)
Central nervous system infection (especially fungal)
Viral infection (e.g. cytomegalovirus, herpes, varicella-zoster)

malignancy, metastases must be sought. The hepatic arterial tree, portal vein and inferior vena cava need to be visualised by angiography. The bile ducts should be visualised (e.g. by endoscopic retrograde cholangiopancreatography [ERCP] or percutaneous cholangiography if ERCP fails). Assess bone density; osteopenia is common in liver disease and increases following transplant. Psychiatric evaluation is important.

Routine outpatient monitoring after transplantation should include a full blood count, electrolyte levels, renal and liver profile, and trough cyclosporin levels. Remember drug interactions with cyclosporin. Diabetes mellitus may supervene as a result of treatment with tacrolinus or steroids. Hypertension should be treated. Diseases that can recur in the graft include hepatitis B and C, Budd–Chiari syndrome and primary biliary cirrhosis.

Haematological system

Haemolytic anaemia

This is an uncommon but important long case. It is usually a diagnostic problem. Coombs' positive haemolytic anaemia is most often encountered in the examination.

The history

1. Presenting symptoms. Ask about the symptoms of anaemia (e.g. fatigue, shortness of breath on exertion) and whether the patient has noticed or been told about jaundice.
2. Determine whether there is a history of known haemolytic episodes. Onset at an early age or a family history suggests an intrinsic red cell defect (e.g. hereditary spherocytosis or elliptocytosis [both autosomal dominant], sickle cell anaemia).
3. Ask about symptoms of connective tissue disease. Joint pain or swelling may also occur in acute sickle cell crisis and especially affect the knees and elbows. Refractory leg ulcers occur in hereditary spherocytosis and sickle cell syndromes. Systemic lupus erythematosus (SLE) and other connective tissue disorders may be associated with warm antibody immunohaemolytic anaemia. Lymphoma is associated with both warm and cold antibodies and anaemia.
4. A history of pain in the abdomen, back and elsewhere suggests sickle cell anaemia or paroxysmal nocturnal haemoglobinuria. Congenital haemolytic anaemias can result in pigment gallstones that can cause symptomatic cholelithiasis and even acute cholecystitis; these episodes can be confused with acute crises.
5. Ask about neurological problems. Spinal cord lesions can occur with hereditary spherocytosis. Paraspinal masses (extramedullary haemopoiesis) may be seen in any hereditary haemolytic anaemia or lymphoma. Acute sickle cell crisis can also result in neurological impairment, particularly stroke. In thrombotic thrombocytopenic

purpura there are often fluctuating neurological abnormalities. Tertiary syphilis may cause paroxysmal cold haemoglobinuria.

6. List all drugs that have been taken; for example, methyldopa, penicillin and quinidine can cause warm antibody immunohaemolytic anaemia, and antimalarials, sulfonamides and nitrofurantoin cause haemolysis in subjects deficient in glucose-6-phosphate dehydrogenase (G6PD). *Note*: Between 10% and 20% of people taking methyldopa have a positive direct Coombs' test. Only a small minority of these develop haemolysis. The drug alters Rh antigens so that antibodies are produced against them, which then cross-react with normal Rh antigens. The indirect Coombs' test is therefore positive, even when the drug is not added to the test. The other drugs produce an indirect Coombs' test result only when the drug is added to the mixture because here the antibodies are directed against a combination of drug and cell membrane. Fludarabine, which is increasingly used as second-line treatment of chronic lymphatic leukaemia and non-Hodgkin's lymphoma, may cause exacerbation of warm autoimmune haemolytic anaemia.

7. Inquire about any operations, particularly mechanical heart valve replacement (10% of those with aortic valve prostheses have significant haemolysis; this percentage is lower with mitral valve prostheses unless a paravalvular leak is present, as the pressure gradient is lower). Severe haemolysis in these patients suggests a paravalvular leak. Consider the other occasional cause of haemolysis within the circulation—external trauma, such as occurs in joggers who wear thin-soled shoes, and the traditional group, bongo drummers.

8. Determine the patient's ethnic background (e.g. Greeks or Italians may inherit the beta-thalassaemia trait, while black men may have G6PD deficiency).

9. The patient may have an underlying medical problem associated with the risk of developing microvascular fragmentation of red cells. These conditions include: disseminated intravascular coagulation (DIC), which is usually caused by vessel wall changes related to an underlying disease, such as disseminated malignancy, renal graft rejection or malignant hypertension; thrombotic thrombocytopenic purpura (TTP), which is of unknown aetiology; and haemolytic uraemic syndrome, which can follow gastroenteritis caused by *E. coli* infection.

The examination

A careful haematopoietic system examination is required. The characteristic 'chipmunk' facies in a young person with thalassaemia is caused by maxillary marrow hyperplasia and frontal bossing. Look for pallor and icterus. Examine the heart for a valve prosthesis or severe aortic stenosis (traumatic haemolysis). Profound anaemia may be associated with high-output cardiac failure. An iron overload state in thalassaemia major from repeated transfusions may cause skin pigmentation, cardiac failure and hepatomegaly.

Carefully palpate for the spleen; splenomegaly from any cause (see Table 8.19) may result in haemolysis. Lymphadenopathy may indicate lymphoma (associated with warm or cold antibody haemolysis), or chronic lymphocytic leukaemia, or glandular fever (cold agglutinin haemolysis). Signs of chronic liver disease should be noted—in severe cirrhosis spur-cell (acanthocyte) anaemia is occasionally observed. Examine for focal neurological signs. Look in the fundi—retinal detachment, retinal infarcts and vitreous haemorrhages can be manifestations of sickle cell anaemia, while Kayser-Fleischer rings may be present in the cornea when haemolysis is caused by Wilson's disease.

Joint swelling and tenderness, and occasionally aseptic necrosis of bone (e.g. neck of femur), also occur in sickle cell anaemia; bony infarcts may become infected (e.g. *Salmonella* osteomyelitis). Look for leg ulceration. Note any signs of connective tissue disease. Test the urine—urobilinogen may be present with haemolysis, it may be dark from haemoglobin in intravascular haemolysis, and the sediment may be abnormal (e.g. thrombotic thrombocytopenic purpura). Fever may occur with septicaemia or malaria-associated haemolysis, with acute crises in sickle cell anaemia and in TTP.

Investigations

It is important to confirm that haemolysis is present, exclude intravascular haemolysis and perform tests to determine the aetiology. Ask for the results of a blood count, reticulocyte count, serum bilirubin and lactate dehydrogenase. Haemolysis is likely to be present if there is a normochromic normocytic anaemia with an increased reticulocyte count (but reticulocytosis also occurs with blood loss or partially treated anaemia) and release of red blood cell components (increased unconjugated bilirubin and, more variably, lactate dehydrogenase). In thalassaemia, the anaemia is often hypochromic and microcytic.

If in doubt, the definitive test for haemolysis is a red cell survival study (using chromium-51 tagged red cells). Intravascular haemolysis is documented by the presence of methaemalbumin in the plasma (Schuum's test) and less often of haemoglobin in the urine; usually serum haptoglobin is absent, and haemosiderin is present in the urine. The presence of fragmented red cells (schistocytes) suggests valve haemolysis, DIC, TTP or haemolytic uraemic syndrome. TTP is very likely when fragmented red cells occur in association with thrombocytopenia, normal coagulation studies and renal impairment.

The history and physical examination may have provided hints about the likely aetiology. The blood film usually shows polychromasia; it may show other red cell changes (Tables 6.40 and 6.41). If a congenital intracorpuscular defect seems unlikely, ask for a Coombs' test next to determine whether the anaemia is immunohaemolytic. The polyspecific direct Coombs' test measures the ability of anti-IgG and anti-C3 to agglutinate the patient's red blood cells. 'Warm' antibodies react at body temperature and may occur with lymphoma (usually non-Hodgkin's), chronic lymphocytic leukaemia, SLE and drugs, or be idiopathic. 'Cold' reactive antibodies are precipitated by exposure to cold—cold agglutinin disease (IgM antibodies) may occur acutely with glandular fever, mycoplasma infection or hepatitis C, and chronically may be caused by lymphoma or be idiopathic; paroxysmal cold haemoglobinuria (IgG antibodies) is rare.

If the haemoglobinuria occurs usually at night and there is pancytopenia and venous thrombosis, paroxysmal nocturnal haemoglobinuria (PNH) should be strongly suspected. The disease may also complicate recovery from aplastic anaemia. Here the neutrophil alkaline phosphatase score is low (but this test is now rarely performed). The sucrose lysis and acid haemolysis (Ham's) test are usually positive. The most reliable test now is analysis by flow cytometry for glycosylphosphatidylinositol-(GPI) linked proteins (e.g. decay accelerating factors [DAF]) on the red cell surface. PNH, which is an acquired clonal disease, is a result of a mutation that causes faulty or absent production of the GPI anchor molecule. Various linked proteins are missing from the red cell surface and, as a result, the cells are not protected from lysis by complement. Tests for haemolysis owing to other causes are presented in Table 6.41.

Treatment

This depends on the underlying disease process, which should be reversed if possible (e.g. drug withdrawal, treatment of transplant rejection, adoption of another musical instrument) (Table 6.41). Steroids are useful in immunohaemolytic anaemia caused by warm-reactive antibodies. The usual approach is to commence at a starting dose of 1 mg/kg/day of prednisolone. The haemoglobin level will usually rise within the first week. Concurrent use of folate is often recommended. Once a normal haemoglobin level has been achieved the steroid dose must be tapered slowly. Recently, subtotal splenectomy has been advocated but remains of unclear efficacy. Immunosuppressive

Table 6.40 Full blood count and liver function tests from a female patient with autoimmune haemolytic anaemia

Parameter	Value	Normal range
Haemoglobin	63 g/L	115–165 g/L (female)
Mean corpuscular volume (MCV)	100 fL	80–100 fL
White cell count (WCC)	15.0×10^9/L	$4.5–13.5 \times 10^9$/L
Platelet count	350×10^9/L	$150–400 \times 10^9$/L
Erythrocyte sedimentation rate (ESR)	58 mm/h	3–19 mm/h (female < 50 years)
Reticulocyte count	18%	0.2–2.0% of red cell count
Bilirubin (total)	45 mmol/L	<20 mmol/L
Aspartate aminotransferase (AST)	30 U/L	<45 U/L
Alanine aminotransferase (ALT)	40 U/L	<40 U/L
Lactate dehydrogenase (LDH)	451 U/L	110–230 U/L
Protein (total)	72 g/L	62–80 g/L
Albumin	42 g/L	32–45 g/L
Haptoglobin	< 0.2 g/L	0.3–2.0 g/L

• Blood film: moderate anisocytosis, numerous spherocytes, prominent polychromasia. Nucleated red cells, neutrophilia and band forms.
• Direct Coomb's test positive: reaction grade 8–12

Comment
The patient has a severe normochromic anaemia with marked reticulocytosis. The very high reticulocyte count suggests haemolysis rather than blood loss. The polychromasia, nucleated red cells and reticulocytosis are signs of increased marrow erythroid activity. The raised bilirubin and reduced haptoglobin levels are consistent with haemolysis. The classical triad suggesting haemolysis is a raised LDH level, reduced haptoglobin level and unconjugated hyperbilirubinaemia. The presence of spherocytes suggests hereditary spherocytosis or immune haemolysis. If there were fragmented red cells, mechanical haemolysis or microangiopathic haemolysis would be likely. Normal red cell morphology would suggest hypersplenism or paroxysmal nocturnal haemoglobinuria. The presence of 'bite' cells would suggest G6PD deficiency.

In this case the candidate should ask for a Coomb's test to distinguish autoimmune haemolytic anaemia from hereditary spherocytosis.

Table 6.41   Haemolytic anaemia

Classification	Peripheral blood morphology	Diagnostic test	Treatment
Extracorpuscular			
1. Immune haemolysis			
(a) 'Warm' antibody	Spherocytes	Coombs' (antiglobulin) test; differential Coombs' test (IgG, complement)	Clinically significant haemolysis—steroids; if steroids not tolerated or do not control disease—splenectomy; if still refractory—azathioprine, cyclophosphamide or danazol
(i) autoimmune (lymphoma, connective tissue disease, idiopathic)			
(ii) drug-induced			Discontinue drugs
(b) 'Cold' antibody	Red cell agglutination in cold	Cold agglutinins Coombs' test—C3 on red cell surface Anti-I (e.g. mycoplasma) or anti-i (e.g. glandular fever)	Maintain warm environment; immunosuppressives only if severe disease
(i) cold agglutinin (post-infection, lymphoma, idiopathic)			
2. Mechanical haemolysis			
(a) Microangiopathic (DIC, TTP, vasculitis etc.)	Schizocytes, microspherocytes	Evidence of intravascular haemolysis, evidence of underlying disease state	Microangiopathic TTP: plasma-pheresis
(b) Heart valve			Correct iron deficiency; replace valve if indicated
(c) March haemoglobinuria (e.g. marathon runners)			Avoid marathons
3. Infection			
(a) Septicaemia	Spherocytes, fragments, intraerythrocyte parasites	Blood cultures, thin and thick smears	Treat infection
(b) Parasitic (e.g. malaria)			
4. Acquired membrane abnormalities			
(a) Cirrhosis	Spur-cells (acanthocytes)	Liver function tests etc.	Splenectomy if severe haemolysis
(b) Uraemia	Burr cells (echinocytes)	Renal function tests	Treat renal failure Correct iron deficiency

(c) Paroxysmal nocturnal haemoglobinuria	Spherocytes, microcytes	Acid serum lysis test, sucrose lysis test, decreased red cell acetylcholinesterase, deficiency of DAF in red cell membrane	Steroid or androgen therapy may reduce haemolysis; transfuse with washed red cells
Intracorpuscular 1. Haemoglobinopathies (a) Amino acid substitutions (e.g. sickle cell)	Sickle forms, hypochromic	Sickle preparation, Hb electrophoresis	Detect infection early and treat, maintain adequate folic acid levels, acute crises— analgesia, oxygen if hypoxic
(b) Thalassaemias— beta-thalassaemia alpha-thalassaemia	Microcytic, target cells, tear drops	HbA_2 and HbF levels, globin synthesis study, gene mapping, family study of HbS	Beta-thalassaemia major—supportive: transfusion, iron chelating therapy
(c) HbH disease: inherited or acquired (myeloproliferative, myelodysplastic)	Heinz bodies on incubation	Hb electrophoresis, brilliant cresyl blue preparation	Folic acid, avoid oxidant drugs, treat underlying disease, bone marrow transplant
2. Inherited membrane abnormalities (e.g. spherocytosis)	Spherocytes	Osmotic fragility (increased), red cell membrane protein study	Splenectomy corrects the anaemia
3. Metabolic abnormalities (e.g. G6PD deficiency)	'Bite' cells, spherocytes	G6PD assay, G6PD electrophoresis	Prevent haemolytic episodes (avoid oxidant drugs, fava beans)

DAF = decay accelerating factors; DIC = disseminated intravascular coagulation; G6PD = glucose-6-phosphate dehydrogenase; Hb = haemoglobin; HbH = haemoglobin H; TTP = thrombotic thrombocytopenic purpura.

treatment is reserved for those who do not respond to steroids and splenectomy. Azathioprine and cyclophosphamide have each been used with some benefit. Normal human immunoglobulin may also be of use. Transfusion is not usually indicated unless there is symptomatic anaemia with a haemoglobin level <90 g/L; it may exacerbate haemolysis. The antibody in immunohaemolytic anaemia is likely to react with all normal donor cells so that standard cross-matching is not possible. When cold-reactive antibodies are responsible, steroid treatment is less effective. Avoidance of cold can be helpful. The disease tends to progress unless the underlying malignancy can be treated. The chimeric antibody, rituximab, which attaches to the CD20 binding site on B lymphocytes and induces their destruction, may be useful in severe cases.

The acute haemolytic episodes of patients with G6PD deficiency are self-limiting (only older red blood cells are affected) and require no specific treatment. Hydration should be maintained to protect renal function. Patients should be warned to avoid precipitating factors (e.g. fava beans, antimalarials and sulfonamides).

Valve haemolysis may be improved by iron supplements and an increase in haemo-globin (reduced cardiac output). Paravalvular leaks often need to be repaired and occa-sionally the prosthetic valve may have to be replaced with a larger one.

TTP is now treated with plasmapheresis, which improves the mortality rate from almost 100% to 10%. Twice-daily treatment is combined at first with high-dose steroids. Even severe neurological deficit, including coma, may be reversible. Antiplatelet drugs are of uncertain benefit. Cyclophosphamide and vincristine are used when plasmapheresis has been unsuccessful. Relapse (10%) can usually be treated successfully. Platelet transfusions must be avoided. The preferred replacement solution is cryosupernatent or fresh frozen plasma.

Splenectomy is virtually curative for patients with hereditary spherocytosis and elliptocytosis (only 10% have severe haemolysis) and may be useful in selected patients with massive splenomegaly, immunohaemolytic anaemia, certain haemoglobinopathies and enzymopathies. All patients undergoing splenectomy should receive pneumo-coccal vaccine preoperatively if possible. Sometimes, prophylactic treatment with peni-cillin is recommended for 2 years following splenectomy. Failure of splenectomy to control haemolysis may be caused by an accessory spleen (which can be detected by a liver–spleen scan).

PNH can be treated with washed red cell transfusions. Heparin and warfarin should be used for thrombotic episodes. Bone marrow transplant may be curative.

Thrombophilia

The discovery of new thrombophilic factors has made the patient with recurrent or even a single thrombotic episode a very suitable long case. Suspect this possibility if the patient is under 50 or has a history of recurrent thromboses. (Table 6.42).

Table 6.42	Occurrence and risk associated with the thrombophilic factors			
	Deep venous thrombosis	Normal population	Relative risk	Arterial thrombosis
APC resistance	50%	4%	8 times	–
Antiphospholipid antibodies	Common	Sometimes— at low titre	8 times	+
AT III, C & S deficiency	10%	1%	20 times	–
Prothrombin gene mutation	15%	3%	4 times	–
High homocysteine	15%	5%	3 times	+
Factor V Leiden	20%	3–7%	5–10 times	–
APC = activated protein C; AT = antithrombin.				

The history

1. Ask about the reason for the patient's current admission. There may have been a recent episode of venous or arterial thrombosis or the patient may have been admitted to hospital for a procedure that has a high risk of thrombosis.
2. Ask about the nature of thrombotic episodes. These may have been arterial, venous or both. Find out how often the problem has occurred and what part of the body was involved.
3. Ask whether a thrombotic tendency has been identified and how this was done (the patient may know).
4. Ask what anticoagulation therapy is currently being used. The possibilities include intravenous unfractionated heparin, fractionated heparin given subcutaneously, warfarin, aspirin or (less likely) clopidogrel or dipyridamole.
5. If the patient is or has been on treatment with warfarin, find out how much he or she understands about the drug, including the importance and necessary frequency of international normalised ratio (INR) testing and the target INR. The patient should probably know the most recent INR result and have some understanding of food and drug interactions with warfarin. For a patient on warfarin, ask about the usual frequency of blood tests and whether practical difficulties have been encountered in getting to the pathology laboratory. Ask who usually relays INR results and dose changes to the patient, and whether the patient has ever used a home INR tester.
6. Inquire about a family history of thrombosis and whether the patient's own problem has led to the testing of other members of the family. In general, 50% of first-degree relatives will inherit the mutation if there is an identified autosomal dominant hereditary factor (e.g. protein C, protein S and antithrombin deficiency).
7. Ask about other factors that may increase thrombotic risk, including smoking, oestrogen-containing oral contraceptives, pregnancy, malignancy, recent surgery and immobility; long-aeroplane flights are controversial as a risk factor but are receiving extensive discussion in the popular press.
8. If the event has followed a surgical operation, ask about what prophylaxis was used to try to prevent thrombosis.
9. In women, ask about previous unexplained miscarriages. This can be associated with the presence of antiphospholipid antibodies, which are autoantibodies against various platelet surface molecules, including phospholipids.
10. Specifically ask about previous myocardial infarction. The occurrence of myocardial infarction in young women with normal coronary arteries has been associated with factor V Leiden deficiency.
11. Ask whether there have been chronic venous problems in the legs. Damage to the venous system can cause chronic oedema and ulceration that can be quite disabling. If there have been chronic problems, detailed questions about their effect on the patient's life are essential.
12. Ask about the congenital abnormality, homocysteinuria, which is associated with a Marfanoid habitus and premature strokes and coronary artery disease. Homocysteine is a thrombophilic agent.
13. Ask about PNH—recurrent episodes of dark urine, anaemia and pancytopenia.

The examination

Note the presence or absence of an intravenous heparin infusion. If one is present, look at the infusion rate. Note the presence of obesity, and look for signs of venous insufficiency from previous venous thromboses. Examine the legs for oedema, venous ulceration and venous valvular insufficiency. Check the peripheral pulses for evidence of arterial obstruction. Note the presence of abdominal wall bruising from subcutaneous low-molecular-weight heparin injections.

There may be evidence of a myeloproliferative disorder, SLE or a malignancy.

Investigations

There is a case now for testing anyone with a significant arterial or venous thrombosis for thrombophilic factors (Table 6.42), especially those with a family history of thromboembolic disease. Certainly, unusual or repeated thromboses should be investigated, as set out below. The currently available routine screening tests are listed in Table 6.43.

Table 6.43 Tests for thrombophilia

Full blood count and ESR (and tests for myeloproliferative disorders and possibly malignancy)
Factor V Leiden (APC resistance)
Antiphospholipid antibodies, including lupus anticoagulant
Antithrombin III
Protein C and S (off warfarin for 2 weeks)
Prothrombin gene mutation
Plasma homocysteine

APC = activated protein C; ESR = erythrocyte sedimentation rate.

---

1. *Factor V Leiden* is an abnormal factor V molecule. The abnormality is caused by a point mutation that affects the cleavage site on the activated molecule. The abnormal factor V is resistant to neutralisation by activated protein C (APC), which forms part of the natural anticoagulation pathway. The condition is also called APC resistance. The mutation occurs in 4% of the general population in Australia and in up to 50% of people with a family history of recurrent venous thrombosis. The condition is autosomal dominant. The heterozygous state is associated with an eightfold increase in venous thrombotic risk. The homozygous state also occurs and these people have 100 times the average risk.

    The thrombotic risk is higher for women with this condition because of their additional risk associated with pregnancy and the use of oral contraceptives containing oestrogen. Use of these drugs causes a 35 times increased risk of a thrombotic event (approximately a 3% risk over 10 years). The mechanism is probably that of lowering antithrombin III levels.

2. *Antithrombin III deficiency* is present in a mild form in about 1 in 2000 of the population. The thrombotic risk is somewhat unpredictable, but the occurrence of a first thrombotic event in these patients is a relative indication for lifelong anticoagulation therapy with warfarin.

3. *Proteins C and S* are natural anticoagulants. Their deficiency is associated with recurrent venous thrombosis and pulmonary embolism, but the level of increased risk is less clear than that for the abnormalities above. There is overlap between the serum levels in people with, and apparently without, an increased risk of thrombosis. Testing must occur after at least 2 weeks without warfarin treatment. In homozygotes with protein C deficiency, warfarin may induce skin necrosis.

4. *Prothrombin gene mutation* is present in about 3% of the Australian population. This point mutation leads to an increased plasma level of prothrombin. Its detection

requires DNA polymerase chain reaction (PCR) analysis. It is an autosomal dominant trait, and leads to a fourfold increase in the risk of venous thrombosis.

5. *Homocysteine* levels are increased in patients with venous thrombosis and are also an independent risk factor for coronary artery disease. The test is now widely available.

6. *Combined thrombophilic abnormalities* are relatively common and further increase thrombotic risk.

7. *Antiphospholipid antibodies* are of two main types, although the exact nature of the antibodies is very variable, even in the same person. *Anticardiolipin* antibodies and *lupus anticoagulant (IgG or IgM antiphospholipid)* antibodies are associated with an increased risk of venous thrombus and arterial embolus. In most cases, both are abnormal. The transient presence of these antibodies at low titres is common, is often associated with infection, and is probably not of clinical significance. They may be present as part of SLE or occur alone (primary antiphospholipid syndrome).

8. Consider investigations for other illnesses that are 'prothrombotic'. These include malignancy, cardiac failure and haematological conditions, such as PNH, polycythaemia rubra vera and thrombocythaemia.

Management

Try to identify transient and continuing risk factors.

In general, an initial episode of thrombosis is treated in the usual way, with intravenous non-fractionated heparin or subcutaneous fractionated heparin. This should be followed by at least 6 months of treatment with warfarin, for idiopathic above-knee deep venous thromboses (DVTs) or for pulmonary embolism. Patients with antithrombin III deficiency will still respond to treatment with heparin because of the presence of small amounts of antithrombin III. Tests for the vitamin K-dependent proteins C and S should be performed before the patient is begun on warfarin.

Patients with protein C and S deficiency or heterozygous APC resistance do not need long-term anticoagulation until after their second thrombotic event. Homozygous APC deficiency is an indication for long-term warfarin treatment. All these patients and their affected asymptomatic relatives need aggressive prophylaxis before surgery or during periods of immobilisation, such as long aeroplane flights. Surgical prophylactic treatment should include heparin, compressive stockings and foot pumps, and early mobilisation. Long aeroplane flights may be an indication for prophylactic subcutaneous fractionated heparin. Aspirin is of unproven benefit for the prevention of venous thrombosis. Pregnant women with a history of DVT require prophylaxis (with heparin) throughout pregnancy and until the puerperium.

The detection of antiphospholipid antibodies in women with miscarriages is an indication for treatment with low-molecular-weight heparin with or without low-dose aspirin during pregnancy. They should be advised strongly against smoking and avoid oestrogen contraceptives. Progesterone-only preparations appear to be safe.

There is still controversy about the long-term treatment of these patients and their relatives, but thrombosis may be an indication for long-term anticoagulation with warfarin maintaining a high INR (3.5). Relatives should be tested for the appropriate defect and offered prophylaxis, if affected.

Polycythaemia

The myeloproliferative disorders (Table 6.44) often occur in the clinical examination. They present a diagnostic and management problem. Polycythaemia rubra vera (erythraemia) is the commonest myeloproliferative disease encountered. This disease occurs in later middle life and is slightly more common in males. No specific gene

---

Table 6.44   Myeloproliferative disorders

1. Polycythaemia rubra vera
2. Myelofibrosis
3. Essential thrombocythaemia
4. Chronic myeloid leukaemia

---

defect has been isolated but the condition is a clonal disease. Secondary causes of polycythaemia (erythrocytosis) must be excluded.

The history

The patient will probably know the diagnosis. If you suspect polycythaemia, ask about:

1. symptoms of polycythaemia or polycythaemia rubra vera:
   (a) vascular problems, such as transient ischaemic episodes, angina, peripheral vascular disease (thrombosis and digital ischaemia); intra–abdominal venous thrombosis, including the Budd-Chiari syndrome
   (b) bleeding from the nose
   (c) symptoms of peptic ulceration (increased four to five times in polycythaemia rubra vera)
   (d) abdominal pain or discomfort from gross splenomegaly or urate stones
   (e) pruritus after showering ('aquagenic pruritis')
   (f) gout
2. symptoms owing to disease causing secondary polycythaemia (Table 6.45), such as chronic respiratory diseases, chronic cardiac or congenital heart diseases, renal diseases (especially polycystic kidneys, hydronephrosis or carcinoma); ask about the use of coal tar derivatives, which can cause the production of abnormal haemoglobin, such as methaemoglobin, as secondary polycythaemia may occur as a result
3. investigations performed and how the diagnosis was made (e.g. blood counts, red cell mass measurement, abdominal imaging, and renal, pulmonary and cardiac investigations); the patient may know if the erythropoietin level has been measured
4. the treatment initiated (e.g. phlebotomy [how often and for how long], radioactive phosphorus, treatment of renal, pulmonary or cardiac disease)
5. resolution of symptoms with treatment
6. social problems related to chronic disease.

The examination

Look at the patient. Note plethora, the state of hydration, cyanosis and any Cushingoid features.

Examine the hands for nicotine stains, clubbing and signs of peripheral vascular disease. Note any gouty tophi. Look for scratch marks and bruising on the arms, and take the blood pressure (systolic hypertension accompanies an increased red cell mass, and phaeochromocytoma is associated with increased erythropoietin).

Look at the eyes for injected conjunctivae and examine the fundi for hyperviscosity changes. Examine the tongue for central cyanosis.

Examine the cardiovascular system for signs of cyanotic congenital heart disease if appropriate, and the respiratory system for signs of chronic lung disease.

Table 6.45   Causes of polycythaemia

Absolute polycythaemia (increased red cell mass)
1. Primary—polycythaemia rubra vera
2. Secondary polycythaemia
   (a) increased erythropoietin:
       (i) renal disease (e.g. polycystic disease, hydronephrosis, tumour)
       (ii) hepatoma
       (iii) cerebellar haemangioma
       (iv) uterine myoma
       (v) virilising syndromes (see Table 8.38)
       (vi) Cushing's syndrome
       (vii) phaeochromocytoma
       (viii) self-injection of erythropoietin (e.g. athletes)
   (b) Hypoxic states (erythropoietin secondarily increased):
       (i) chronic lung disease
       (ii) hereditary haemorrhagic telangiectasia (because of pulmonary arteriovenous malformations)
       (iii) sleep apnoea
       (iv) cyanotic congenital heart disease
       (v) abnormal haemoglobins (high-affinity variants)
       (vi) carbon monoxide poisoning

Relative polycythaemia (decreased plasma volume)
1. Dehydration
2. Smokers' polycythaemia—carboxyhaemoglobinaemia (erythrocyte mass also increased)
3. Stress polycythaemia—Gaisbock's disease (? a distinct entity)

Examine the abdomen for hepatomegaly (hepatoma must be excluded) and splenomegaly, which occurs in 80% of cases of polycythaemia rubra vera, but not in secondary polycythaemia. Palpate for renal masses (polycystic kidneys, hydronephrosis, carcinoma). Rarely, uterine fibromas may be found, or very rarely virilisation may be noted.

Look at the legs for scratch marks (pruritus may be secondary to elevated plasma histamine levels), gout and evidence of peripheral vascular disease. Auscultate over the cerebellar regions for a bruit (cerebellar haemangioblastoma). Note any upper motor neurone signs (cerebrovascular disease owing to thrombosis or the hyperviscosity syndrome).

Check the urine for evidence of renal disease.

Investigations

Confirm the presence of polycythaemia and establish whether this is primary or secondary. Remember that erythrocytosis is an increase in the absolute red cell mass, which occurs as a result of some stimulus (usually hypoxia) and erythraemia (polycythaemia vera) is an increase in red cell mass of unknown aetiology (Table 6.46).

1. **Full blood count.** In polycythaemia rubra vera the following are increased: haemoglobin value, haematocrit value, red cell count, white cell count (including the absolute basophil count), platelet count, and more variably the neutrophil alkaline

---

Table 6.46 Criteria for a diagnosis of polycythaemia rubra vera

1. Elevated red cell mass
2. Splenomegaly
3. Normal Pao_2
4. Splenomegaly, or leucocytosis and thrombocytosis
5. Reduced plasma erythropoietin level

---

phosphatase (NAP) score. Check the mean corpuscular volume and red cell distribution width (RDW). Microcytic erythrocytosis can only be caused by polycythaemia rubra vera or hypoxic erythrocytosis (RDW usually elevated), or beta-thalassaemia (RDW normal). The erythrocyte sedimentation rate (ESR) is very low in both primary and secondary polycythaemia.

2. Confirm that absolute polycythaemia is present with an elevated red blood cell mass (chromium-51-labelled red cells) and usually a normal or sometimes increased plasma volume (isotope-labelled albumin).
3. Assess for splenomegaly (and renal disease) with an abdominal ultrasound or computed tomography (CT) scan.
4. Check the arterial blood gases (in polycythaemia rubra vera, 80% of patients have an arterial oxygen saturation >92% and in almost all it is >88%).
5. Serum erythropoietin level is usually substantially reduced or absent in polycythaemia rubra vera and elevated in secondary polycythaemia. Remember, however, that certain tumours (haemangioblastoma, renal cell carcinoma, renal sarcoma and carcinoma of the liver) cause polycythaemia by excreting erythropoietin.
6. Vitamin B_{12} binding capacity. The total vitamin B_{12} level is elevated in 75% of cases of polycythaemia rubra vera. The vitamin B_{12} level is raised owing to increased transcobalamin I and III, made by the neutrophils, which have an increased turnover.
7. Rule out renal disease with abdominal ultrasound and CT scanning, if indicated.
8. Bone marrow. In polycythaemia rubra vera there is significant panhyperplasia and iron stores are often reduced, but in secondary polycythaemia the bone marrow is usually normal. There are no consistent cytogenetic markers. Bone marrow biopsy is not essential for the diagnosis. It is only necessary if another myeloproliferative disorder is suspected. Fibrosis may be seen in the advanced stages of polycythaemia rubra vera.

Treatment

The aim is to lower the haematocrit value to 0.42–0.45 (haemoglobin <140 g/L for men and <120 g/L for women) and maintain it at this level. Patients may die of thrombosis, which seems related entirely to the elevated red cell mass. The presence of thrombocytosis does not increase the risk of thrombotic events and antiplatelet treatment and anticoagulation are not indicated. Untreated cases have a median survival of 2 years because of the thrombotic risk. This is extended to over 10 years with phlebotomy alone.

Polycythaemia rubra vera should be treated by phlebotomy. Frequent venesection is required until a state of iron deficiency has been produced. This will then limit red cell production and the frequency may be reduced to about 3 monthly.

Radioactive phosphorus (phosphorus-32) irradiates the bone marrow and is easy to use and effective, but it increases the incidence of acute myeloid leukaemia and should be avoided in patients under the age of 70 years (and perhaps in all patients). Alkylating agents (e.g. busulphan) must be monitored closely for the same reason and should not be given routinely. Hydroxyurea is a much safer drug in these circumstances. Pruritus may not respond to antihistamines and interferon alpha or PUVA therapy (combination drugs and ultraviolet light) may be required, and hyperuricaemia should be treated with allopurinol. Low-dose aspirin is recommended to prevent thrombosis without excessive gastrointestinal bleeding (avoid high doses).

Secondary polycythaemia is treated by removal of the cause, and phlebotomy if the haematocrit exceeds 0.55.

Idiopathic myelofibrosis

This is a rare form of chronic myeloproliferative disorder. Patients are often asymptomatic at the time of diagnosis. The condition is often diagnosed following a routine full blood count or the discovery of splenomegaly.

Occasionally there may be signs of aggressive extramedullary haematopoiesis: bowel or urethral obstruction, ascites, pericardial effusion, skin masses or spinal cord compression. Rapid splenic enlargement can cause splenic infarction (with the sudden onset of left upper quadrant pain and tenderness). The typical patient is over 50 years of age and has marked splenomegaly (>10 cm) and mild-to-moderate hepatomegaly. The white cell counts may be normal, increased or decreased. The blood film will show teardrop poikilocytes and a leukoerythroblastic picture (presence of myelocytes, metamyelocytes and nucleated red blood cells). Median survival is 4–5 years, but patients with severe anaemia (<100 g/L) have a worse prognosis (median survival about 2 years).

Bone marrow biopsy (aspiration is usually impossible) may reveal karyotypic abnormalities on cytogenetic examination. This finding is associated with a worse prognosis.

The condition must be distinguished from myelofibrosis secondary to other conditions, such as lymphoma, leukaemia, myeloma, polycythaemia, chronic myeloid leukaemia (CML) and SLE. These may be amenable to specific treatment.

Treatment with hydroxyurea is helpful for symptomatic patients with organomegaly or marked thrombocytosis. Folate and vitamin B_{12} may help if they are deficient; erythropoietin has not been particularly effective. Allopurinol is used when there is hyperuricaemia. Most patients are treated with repeated blood transfusions. Splenectomy may be indicated if massive splenomegaly has occurred. Alkylating agents are contraindicated. Cure is possible only with bone marrow transplantation for the few patients who are young enough and for whom a suitable donor can be found. Leukaemic transformation may occur in 10% of patients.

Essential thrombocythaemia

This is a relatively common form of chronic myeloproliferative disorder. Patients usually present with symptoms related to a high platelet count (>800 × 10^9/L)—poor memory, erythromelalgia (painful red extremities) and thromboembolism. Up to 50% of patients have haemorrhagic problems, especially from the gut and easy bruising. A prolonged bleeding time and abnormal platelet aggregation may be present. There are, however, no consistent platelet abnormalities. Modest splenomegaly (<5 cm) is seen in 50% of patients. Many patients are asymptomatic and the diagnosis has been made on a routine platelet count.

A definitive diagnosis requires exclusion of reactive thrombocytosis secondary to infection, polycythaemia, malignancy, inflammation, bleeding, recent surgery or an asplenic state. Cytogenetic studies may be necessary to exclude CML.

Asymptomatic patients, even if they have a platelet count of over one million, may need no treatment. Unexpectedly, bleeding tends to be more of a problem when the platelet count is over a million and thrombosis when it is less than a million. Neurological symptoms should first be treated with aspirin. Failure of response is an indication to reduce platelet numbers, usually with hydroxyurea. Bleeding problems may be improved with tranexamic acid; this may be useful if given before surgery. Transformation to acute leukaemia is uncommon (<10%) and often the result of prior alkylating chemotherapy. Anagrelide is a more specific anti-megakaryocyte agent that can be useful for symptomatic patients.

The condition usually runs an indolent and benign course and the temptation to treat asymptomatic patients should be strongly resisted.

Chronic myeloid leukaemia

The typical patient has moderate splenomegaly (6–8 cm) and a white cell count >50 $\times$ 10^9/L. The white cell differential count will show two peaks, one at the neutrophil stage and the other at the myelocyte stage. Basophilia is common. A low NAP score is another typical laboratory feature, as is the Philadelphia (Ph) chromosome (in the absence of Ph chromosome, 50% have hybrid gene *BCR/ABL* rearrangement). The platelet count is usually elevated and there is mild normochromic anaemia.

The disease will eventually undergo blastic transformation. While in its chronic phase, it can be controlled with hydroxyurea or busulphan, but a cure can be achieved only with bone marrow transplantation from a compatible donor. Interferon alpha therapy is sometimes helpful in the chronic phase. It may induce differentiation of the immature cells. The tyrosine kinase inhibitor, imatinib, has revolutionised treatment of CML and is now available in Australia. It is now first-line treatment for younger patients without a suitable donor and for older patients (>65 years). Its use can be associated with hepatotoxicity, myalgia and fluid retention.

Median survival is 22 months. The current recommendations are that for patients under the age of 65, interferon alpha should be given for the first year and should be followed by bone marrow transplant. This should be from a related donor (sibling) with full human leucocyte antigen (HLA) compatibility or single HLA mismatch. Autologous transplant has been performed successfully.

Lymphomas

These diseases provide complicated diagnostic and management problems. Treatment in expert units is important, as many patients can be cured. Cure should be possible in over 85% of patients with Hodgkin's disease and in up to 40% of those with non-Hodgkin's lymphomas. Remember that the cell lineage is uncertain for Hodgkin's disease (although probably mostly B cell) but 80% of non-Hodgkin's lymphomas are of B cell origin. There are a number of slightly different classification systems. Some are based on the cell type, some are clinical (staging) and others histopathological (Tables 6.47–6.49).

Hodgkin's disease (Table 6.48) presents either with discrete, rubbery, painless nodes or with generalised symptoms (fever, night sweats, weight loss and sometimes pruritus). Mediastinal adenopathy usually occurs in young people with nodular sclerosing disease. Older people with generalised symptoms, in whom the only enlarged nodes may be in the abdomen, often have lymphocyte-depleted Hodgkin's disease.

The majority of cases of non-Hodgkin's lymphomas (Table 6.48) present with painless enlargement of peripheral lymph nodes (a lymph node of more than 1 cm diameter and present for 6 weeks or more for no obvious reason should be biopsied). Localised or generalised painless adenopathy with or without hepatosplenomegaly may also occur. It may present with just an abdominal mass. Presentation with mediastinal adenopathy is much less common than in patients with Hodgkin's disease. In some patients the disease may arise at an extranodal site (e.g. the gastrointestinal

Table 6.47   World Health Organization (WHO) classification of lymphomas (lymphoid malignancies)—more common types

B cell	T cell	Hodgkin's disease
Precursor B cell neoplasm	**Precursor T cell neoplasm**	Nodular lymphocyte predominant
Precursor B cell lymphoblastic leukaemia/lymphoma	Precursor T cell lymphoblastic lymphoma/leukaemia	**Classic Hodgkin's disease**
Mature (peripheral) B cell neoplasms	**Mature (peripheral) T cell neoplasms**	Nodular sclerosis Hodgkin's disease
B cell chronic lymphocytic leukaemia/small lymphocytic lymphoma	Adult T cell lymphoma/leukaemia	Lymphocyte-rich Hodgkin's disease
Plasma cell myeloma/plasmacytoma	Mycosis fungoides	Mixed cellularity Hodgkin's disease
MALT lymphoma, mantle cell lymphoma	Peripheral T cell lymphoma	Lymphocyte-depleted Hodgkin's disease
Follicular lymphoma	Angioimmunoblastic T cell lymphoma	
Diffuse large B cell lymphoma	Anaplastic large cell lymphoma	
Burkitt's lymphoma		

Note: There is an overlap of cell types between leukaemias and lymphomas. Leukaemia is diagnosed when the malignant cells are primarily found in the blood and bone marrow, and lymphoma when there are solid tumours of the immune system.

tract—5%). These patients may present with abdominal pain, obstruction or haemorrhage. Most non-Hodgkin's lymphomas are diffuse and aggressive. Waldeyer's ring, mesenteric and epitrochlear node involvement are more common in non-Hodgkin's than in Hodgkin's disease. Systemic symptoms are less common in non-Hodgkin's lymphoma. In low-grade non-Hodgkin's lymphoma, lymphadenopathy has often been present for a long time. Other uncommon presentations include skin infiltration and direct renal infiltration. Primary neurological infiltration is also uncommon. Low-grade gastro-intestinal lymphomas (e.g. MALT [mucosa-associated lymphoid tissue] lymphomas) are less common.

The history

1. Presenting symptoms and causes of symptoms, such as palpable nodes, cough as a result of mediastinal node involvement, systemic symptoms, bone pain owing to

Table 6.48   Histopathological classification of lymphoma

Hodgkin's disease
1. Lymphocyte predominant
2. Nodular sclerosing
3. Mixed cellularity
4. Lymphocyte-depleted

Non-Hodgkin's lymphoma

The Rappaport classification has largely been replaced. There are a number of new classifications, including the International Working Formulation.
   International Working Formulation (this classification translates into the clinical setting better than the others)
I   Low-grade lymphoma
   1. Small lymphocytic cell
   2. Follicular, mixed cleaved cell
   3. Follicular, mixed small cleaved and large cell
II   Intermediate-grade lymphoma
   1. Follicular large cell
   2. Diffuse small cleaved cell
   3. Diffuse mixed small cleaved cell
   4. Diffuse large cell
III   High-grade lymphoma
   1. Large cell immunoblastic
   2. Lymphoblastic cell
   3. Small non-cleaved cell (Burkitt and non-Burkitt)

Table 6.49   Staging of lymphoma—Ann Arbor classification

Stage I   Disease confined to a single lymph node region or a single extralymphatic site (Ie)
Stage II   Disease confined to two or more lymph node regions on the same side of the diaphragm, plus or minus splenic involvement
Stage III   Disease confined to lymph node regions on both sides of the diaphragm (III$_1$ = upper abdomen; III$_2$ = lower abdomen), with or without localised involvement of the spleen (IIIs), other extralymphatic organ or site (IIIe), or both
Stage IV   Diffuse disease of one or more extralymphatic organs (with or without lymph node disease)

For any stage:
   A. No symptoms
   B. Fever, weight loss >10% in 6 months or night sweats

marrow infiltration or pathological fractures, spinal cord compression, splenic pain, alcohol-induced pain (rare).
2. History of infection (as a result of decreased cell-mediated immunity in Hodgkin's disease or depressed humoral immunity from chemotherapy or radiotherapy).

3. History of a predisposing condition, such as Klinefelter's syndrome, HIV infection, congenital or acquired immune deficiency, use of immunosuppressive drugs, autoimmune disease, or use of phenytoin (pseudo-lymphoma).

4. Investigations performed—particularly lymph node biopsy, CT and gallium scans, and bilateral bone marrow aspirations. Magnetic resonance imaging (MRI) scanning may have been used for suspected spinal cord, brain or bone marrow involvement. Lymphangiography and staging laparotomy are rarely indicated now. Lumbar puncture is important in high-grade lymphoma investigation if central nervous system involvement is suspected.

5. Treatment undertaken—an indication of the stage and type of disease. Ask about the side-effects of any treatment (e.g. mantle radiation can result in pneumonitis, hypothyroidism, pericarditis, myocardial fibrosis and spinal cord injury). Ask if the patient been informed about possible long-term complications of treatment.

6. The prognosis given and what the patient's understanding of this seems to be.

7. The social situation—dependent family members, social support, ability to work, reactions to disease (e.g. depression, coping mechanisms), etc.

The examination

Examine the haemopoietic system thoroughly. Attempt to stage the disease clinically (Table 6.49). Remember that staging is much less relevant for non-Hodgkin's lymphomas because spread is haematogenous and not contiguous. Fewer than 10% of even nodular non-Hodgkin's lymphomas are localised and suitable for local irradiation at the time of presentation. Note any radiotherapy marks (and the field covered). Look for evidence of infection (e.g. herpes zoster).

Investigations

Investigations are aimed at determining the grade and stage of the disease. The first step is to obtain histological confirmation of disease. Ask to see the pathology report if excision lymph node biopsies have already been performed. Fine-needle biopsy is not good enough to define lymph node architecture. Reed-Sternberg cells are *not* pathognomonic of Hodgkin's disease, but may occur in cases of glandular fever, other viral diseases and with other malignancies.

The next step is to stage the disease further. Ask for a full blood count and ESR, a bilateral bone marrow aspirate and trephine, liver function tests, chest X-ray film and abdominal, pelvic and chest imaging (usually CT scan). In Hodgkin's disease, agranulocytosis (sometimes with marked eosinophilia or a leukaemoid reaction), an elevated ESR, reversed CD4/CD8 ratio, skin test anergy and a mildly elevated alkaline phosphatase level are often present but may *not* indicate widespread disease. The ESR remains the best indicator of disease activity. Lymphangiography is less often done these days, especially if the CT, single-photon emission CT (SPECT) and gallium scans are normal. Positron emission tomography (PET) scanning may be more sensitive than gallium scanning in staging the disease at diagnosis and in monitoring residual disease. Staging laparotomies are now only rarely performed but previously treated patients may bear the scar. Staging in this invasive way is less relevant now that systemic treatment is more often used for all patients.

Treatment

Hodgkin's disease (85% of patients are curable)
Treatment depends on the stage of the disease (see Table 6.49). Histological type is less important here.

- Stages IA, IIA and IIIsA—radiotherapy or abbreviated course of chemotherapy followed by radiotherapy.

- Stage IIIA (with para-aortic node involvement with or without radiotherapy to involved sites), IIIB and IV—combined chemotherapy (e.g. ABVD [adriamycin, bleomycin, vinblastine and dacarbazine]).

Salvage treatment

Relapse less than 1 year after initial treatment or failure to achieve complete remission is an indication for second-line therapy. For relapse after more than 1 year retreatment can be given using the original regimen. Further radiotherapy can be used for relapse outside the radiation field if the patient has early stage disease.

Prognosis

This depends on the stage. In general, in:

- stage I, expect 85–95% 10 years' disease-free survival
- stage II, expect 80–90% 10 years' disease-free survival
- stage III and IV, expect 60% 10 years' disease-free survival.

Complications of treatment

The improvement in survival achieved with current treatment means that complications of treatment are more likely to cause death than the disease. Secondary malignancies, including leukaemia and carcinomas, are associated with the use of alkylating agents. Breast cancer risk is associated with chest irradiation. Chest radiotherapy also increases the risk of coronary artery disease after 10 years or more, and of hypothyroidism. Infertility can occur in men and women treated with chemotherapy. The chance of recovery of fertility is much greater for young patients.

Non-Hodgkin's lymphoma

Prognosis and treatment depend mainly on the histological type (particularly whether it is nodular or diffuse and based on the International Working Formulation—Table 6.48); most cases of low-grade lymphomas are stage III or IV at presentation. The International Prognostic Index (Table 6.50) has proved an accurate way of assessing the patient's likely course. More recently, treatment decisions have been based on the WHO classification (see Table 6.47).

Table 6.50 International Prognostic Index—clinical risk factors for a poor outcome

Age >60
Lactate dehydrogenase level elevated
Ann Arbor stage III or IV
>1 extranodal site
Physical performance e.g. Karnosky score >70 (self-caring, mobile, etc.)

0–1 risk factors	= low risk
2 risk factors	= low-to-intermediate risk
3 risk factors	= intermediate-to-high risk
4 or 5 risk factors	= high risk

Treatment protocols: International Working Formulation classification

1. *Low-grade lymphoma.* Follicular mixed cleaved cell low-grade lymphoma has a good prognosis for survival but is not generally curable. Commonly it presents as stage IVA.

(a) For asymptomatic low-grade lymphoma no treatment is indicated.

(b) For symptomatic low-grade lymphoma, chlorambucil with or without prednisone, or CVP (cyclophosphamide, vincristine and prednisone), is the usual initial treatment.

For stages I and II low-grade lymphoma (uncommon), extended field radiation may be used in younger patients with curative intent but they must be very carefully staged first. More aggressive regimens (as for intermediate-grade) may produce more complete remissions but have not been shown to increase survival. Maintenance single-agent chemotherapy has not reduced the relapse rate.

2. *Intermediate and high-grade lymphoma.* These have a poor prognosis if untreated. Diffuse large cell lymphoma and high-grade lymphomas are potentially curable with treatment.

(a) Stage I and some stage II: aggressive treatment to try for cure is essential but careful staging must be carried out first.

(b) Stages II, III and IV:

   (i) diffuse large cell lymphoma—combination chemotherapy, such as CHOP (cyclophosphamide, adriamycin, vincristine and prednisone); high-dose methotrexate and intrathecal methotrexate may be added if indicated

   (ii) diffuse well-differentiated lymphocytic lymphoma—this is the most indolent type and prognosis is indistinguishable from that for chronic lymphocytic leukaemia; no treatment is required unless symptomatic

   (iii) other diffuse types: combination chemotherapy

   (iv) salvage chemotherapy—failure of remission or relapse is an indication of a poor prognosis; salvage treatment is usually attempted with drugs such as cisplatin or cytosine arabinoside, but remission rates are only 20–30%.

(c) AIDS-related lymphomas: these tumours tend to be of the large B cell or Burkitt's type and very aggressive. Results of combination chemotherapy, so far, have been poor. The best regimens, using central nervous system prophylaxis, granulocyte-macrophage colony stimulating factor (GM-CSF) (to limit neutropenia) and a modified chemotherapeutic combination have produced 50% complete response rates. There is a high mortality from associated infection in these immunodeficient patients.

Treatment Protocols—WHO classification

1. *Precursor B cell neoplasms.* Precursor B cell lymphoblastic leukaemia/lymphoma is usually the childhood malignancy acute lymphocytic leukaemia (ALL). The lymphoma is rare in adults and rapidly progresses to become leukaemia. Combination chemotherapy is used to induce remission and continuing treatment to attempt cure. The cure rate in adults is about 50%.

2. *Mature B cell neoplasms.* B cell chronic lymphoid leukaemia/small lymphocytic lymphoma is the most common lymphoid leukaemia and represents about 75% of non-Hodgkin's lymphomas. Patients with only bone marrow involvement and lymphocytosis are not usually treated. They have a median survival of over 10 years. Once liver and splenic involvement have occurred, treatment is likely to be required at some stage but may not be recommended until bone marrow failure is present. Oral chlorambucil or the more potent intravenous drug, fludarabine, are most often recommended. Young patients may benefit from bone marrow transplant.

3. *MALT-type lymphoma* (extranodal marginal zone B cell lymphoma—8%). These gastric mucosal lymphomas are curable when localised. MALT is associated with *Helicobacter pylori* infection. Eradication of the infection will usually induce remission (75%). Otherwise chlorambucil is the drug of choice. Endoscopic follow-up is important.

4. *Mantle cell lymphoma* (6%). The majority of these present as a systemic disease. Treatment is not very successful. The usual approach is combination chemotherapy followed by radiotherapy. Chemotherapy may be used with rituximab (the anti-CD20 antibody). Bone marrow transplant is offered to younger patients.

5. *Follicular lymphoma* (22%). Asymptomatic patients may require no treatment. Chlorambucil alone or combination treatment (CVP or CHOP) can achieve a 75% remission rate. Interferon alpha seems to prolong survival once remission has been achieved and rituximab can be helpful for patients who have relapsed.

6. *Diffuse large B cell lymphoma* (30%). Treatment is usually begun with combination chemotherapy (often CHOP). This may be followed by radiotherapy if there is bulky stage I or II disease. Six cycles of treatment will produce a cure in up to 70% of patients. Bone marrow transplant is more effective than further chemotherapy for patients who relapse. It can achieve up to 40% long-term disease-free survival.

7. *Burkitt's lymphoma*. This is a rare disease in Australia but more common in Africa. Intensive combination chemotherapy with attention to the central nervous system will produce a cure in about 70% of patients.

Bone marrow transplant

Disease resistant to standard-dose chemotherapy can be treated with bone marrow ablation using chemotherapy or radiotherapy or both. Bone marrow transplant is then performed with autologous stem cells or, less often, from a compatible donor. The mortality rate associated with this procedure (now <5%) and the success of engraftment have improved with the use of haematopoietic growth factors. Long-term outcomes are uncertain, as are the indications for the use of this treatment in patients with less aggressive disease.

Multiple myeloma (myeloma)

This is a disseminated malignant disease of plasma cells. It can present as a diagnostic or a management problem. Myeloma occurs more commonly in the elderly—the median age is 60 years—and more often in men. It is more common in people whose occupations involve exposure to petroleum and in people exposed to nuclear radiation. Chronic antigenic stimulation may play a role in B cell clonal transformation. A number of chromosomal deletions and translocations have been identified in myeloma patients. The most important of these is 13q. Its presence has prognostic significance. Some myeloma begin as monoclonal gammopathies of uncertain significance (MGUS). These evolve to myeloma at a rate of 10% a year—'smouldering myeloma'.

The history

1. Ask about presenting symptoms:
   (a) bone pain or pain with movement affects nearly three-quarters of patients, occurs particularly in the ribs or axial skeleton, and may cause pathological fractures; the association with movement may distinguish it from the bone pain of metastatic malignancy, which can be worse at night (persistent pain suggests a pathological fracture)
   (b) bacterial infection is the presenting problem in one-quarter of patients—particularly pneumonia and urinary tract infections (the level of normal functional immunoglobulins is reduced as a result of reduced production and increased destruction; in advanced marrow disease there is white cell depletion); the most common organisms are *Streptococcus pneumoniae*, *Staphylococcus aureus* and *Klebsiella pneumoniae* in the lungs and *Escherichia coli* in the urinary tract

    (c) symptoms of anaemia (normochromic and normocytic)—as a result of bone marrow depression from infiltration, chronic disease, renal failure or treatment

    (d) bleeding tendency—caused by paraprotein inactivation of plasma procoagulants and reduced platelet function (coating of platelets with antibodies) and thrombocytopenia as a result of bone marrow suppression

    (e) renal disease symptoms (owing to stone formation secondary to hypercalcaemia, hyperuricaemia, tubular damage by light chains, therapy, urinary tract infection, contrast studies, plasma cell infiltration or amyloid); renal failure affects one-quarter of patients and half develop renal impairment; renal impairment at the time of diagnosis means a poor prognosis

    (f) hypercalcaemic symptoms owing to bone lysis

    (g) hyperviscosity symptoms once plasma viscosity exceeds 5 (normal is about 1.8)

    (h) spinal cord compression or, rarely, diffuse sensorimotor neuropathy

    (i) skin changes, such as pruritus, purpura, yellow skin, hypertrichosis (rare), erythema annulare (rare)

    (j) systemic amyloid deposition (10–15%).

2. Ask about how the diagnosis was made.
3. Ask about treatment—ask about drugs (e.g. bisphosphonates, thalidomide) and their side-effects, radiotherapy and bone marrow transplant (actual or planned).
4. Inquire about the social history, including dependants, work, activities of daily living (ADLs), etc.
5. Inquire about the patient's understanding of this life-threatening condition and its prognosis—how much information he or she has about possible further problems and treatment.

The examination

Inspect the patient for signs of weight loss, anaemia, chest infection and general debility.

    Examine the haemopoietic system. Pay particular attention to a search for bony tenderness. Kyphosis may be caused by compression fractures. Note signs of anaemia and purpura. Look for skin rash. Check carefully for any signs of spinal cord compression. Check the urine analysis and temperature chart. Look for signs of infection (e.g. pulmonary consolidation).

Investigations

Once the diagnosis is suspected, check the full blood count (and film) for anaemia (and plasma cells) and a raised ESR. Obtain a protein electrophoretogram (EPG) of serum and urine, and an immunoelectrophoretogram (IEPG). An M component (monoclonal globulin peak) is found in 95% of cases. In the urine, light chains are present in 50–75% of patients (Bence-Jones proteinuria cannot be detected by dipstick urine analysis). The bone marrow must be examined for plasma cells. Check the beta$_2$-microglobulin level (see below).

    Look at X-ray films of the skull, chest, pelvis and proximal long bones for fractures, osteoporosis and lytic lesions. The latter is a result of the secretion of osteoclast activating factors by the tumour cells. Since there is little osteoblastic activity, bone scans are less sensitive than plain X-rays. Also check the serum calcium and urate levels, and the renal function.

    The three major diagnostic features of multiple myeloma, in order of importance, are:

1. plasma cells in the bone marrow (>10% involvement is consistent with the diagnosis)
2. production of serum paraprotein (50% are IgG, 33% IgA, 5% IgM, 10% only light chains, 2% nil)
3. bone destruction (lytic lesions).

The disease can be staged according to certain criteria:

- stage I—(i) haemoglobin near normal (>100 g/L); (ii) calcium not elevated; (iii) low M component; (iv) up to one lytic bone lesion
- stage II—intermediate between stages I and III
- stage III—poor prognostic features include anaemia (haemoglobin <85 g/L), hypercalcaemia (>3 mmol/L), advanced lytic bone lesions, high M component production rates.

In addition, subclassification is made on the basis of serum creatinine levels: (A) creatinine <200 mmol/L; (B) creatinine >200 mmol/L.

On this basis, median survival can be estimated as follows:

- stage IA—61 months
- stage IIA or B—55 months
- stage IIIA—30 months
- stage IIIB—15 months.

An elevated serum beta$_2$-microglobulin level (which reflects the myeloma cell burden and renal functional impairment) indicates a median survival of 12 months.

Other poor prognostic features include advanced age, increased interleukin-6 (IL-6; correlates with C-reactive protein) and cytogenetic abnormalities (e.g. any translocation, deletion chromosome 13).

Treatment

Irradiation is helpful for localised bone pain and spinal cord compression. Patients with a single bone plasmacytoma will often get prolonged disease-free survival after treatment with local radiotherapy. Pamidronate or one of the other bisphosphonates should be given to patients with more than stage I disease. Bisphosphonates reduce bone pain, fracture rates and episodes of hypercalcaemia. There is evidence that they improve the prognosis. For those with more diffuse disease, general measures, such as adequate hydration and use of bicarbonate for Bence-Jones proteinuria, are important to prevent renal failure. Intravenous contrast material must be used cautiously and only with excellent hydration. Allopurinol may protect renal function from urate nephropathy related to treatment. Treat hypercalcaemia and bacterial infection. Avoid live vaccines. Erythropoietin may improve the anaemia.

Chemotherapy is indicated for patients with stage II or III disease and for those with stage I disease if they are symptomatic or have rising myeloma protein levels or progressive lytic bone lesions. Melphalan and prednisone are standard treatments but other alkylating agents (e.g. cyclophosphamide) are probably equally effective. Resistance to one alkylating agent is often but not always associated with resistance to the others. Typically treatment is given intermittently. A week's course is repeated 4 weeks later for up to 2 years. The patient's progress must be monitored with regular protein EPG studies. Interferon alpha may be used as maintenance therapy after induction, or in light-chain or IgA disease. It probably does not prolong survival.

Secondary acute leukaemia is being seen increasingly, related to alkylating agent therapy. Autologous bone marrow transplantation is the treatment of choice for these patients if they are less than 60 years old. The mortality rate is about 15% a year. Causes of death include infection, renal failure, leukaemia, concomitant illnesses and progressive myeloma.

Differential diagnosis

Monoclonal gammopathy of undetermined significance (MGUS)

A smaller IgG or IgA peak (<30 g/L), less than 10% plasma cells in the bone marrow and absence of lytic bone lesions suggest this diagnosis.

Waldenström's macroglobulinaemia

The EPG has a peak consisting of monoclonal IgM. These patients are generally older than those with myeloma. The hyperviscosity syndrome is often present; symptoms and signs include lassitude, confusion, bleeding, anaemia, infection, lymphadenopathy and splenomegaly, dilated retinal veins and perivenous haemorrhages, and (rarely) renal failure. Lymphadenopathy and splenomegaly do not usually occur in patients with myeloma. Lytic bone destruction is rare. Ten per cent of the macroglobulins are cryoglobulins. An underlying lymphoproliferative disorder may be present. Treatment with plasmapheresis is effective in removing IgM paraprotein. Prednisone and chlorambucil are useful. Median survival is 4 years.

Localised myeloma

Only one plasma cell tumour is present. Solitary plasmacytomas often occur in the nasopharynx or paranasal sinuses. The major complications of myeloma are absent. Only 50% of cases show a monoclonal peak. Local radiotherapy is the usual treatment.

POEMS syndrome

This is an atypical form of myeloma. The features include *p*olyneuropathy, *o*rganomegaly, *e*ndocrinopathy, *m*onoclonal gammopathy (osteosclerotic myeloma, or IgA or IgG M proteins with lambda light chains) and *s*kin changes. There is a progressive sensorimotor polyneuropathy associated with myeloma-like bone lesions. Unlike multiple myeloma, over half the patients have hepatomegaly and lymphadenopathy, and some have splenomegaly. Male impotence and gynaecomastia, and female amenorrhoea, occur as a result of hyperprolactinaemia. A few patients have hypothyroidism and a third have type 2 diabetes. Skin changes include clubbing, hypertrichosis, thickening and increased pigmentation.

There are often high levels of the cytokines, IL-1, IL-6 and tumour necrosis factor (TNF).

Treatment of the myeloma component in the usual way often helps the other manifestations. Local bone lesions often respond to radiotherapy.

Bone marrow transplantation

Bone marrow transplantation is being performed for an increasing number of indications. Patients are chronically ill and often available for examinations. Two groups of patients are treated in this way: those with a malignant condition (Table 6.51), who have their bone marrow destroyed by irradiation or chemotherapy given in marrow-toxic doses to treat a malignancy; and those with a defective bone marrow that is destroyed

Table 6.51 Malignant indications for bone marrow transplant

Condition	Autologous	Allogenic
Acute leukaemia	Yes	Yes
Chronic myeloid leukaemia	Yes	Yes
Lymphoma	Yes	Yes
Hodgkin's disease	Yes	Yes
Carcinoma of the breast	Yes	No
Carcinoma of the testis	Yes	No
Multiple myeloma	Yes	Yes
Wilm's tumour	Yes	No

and then replaced (Table 6.52). Autologous transplants (when the patient's own marrow or stem cells are stored and then reinfused) are now more common than allogenic transplants (when another person is used as the donor of marrow or stem cells).

Table 6.52 Non-malignant indications for bone marrow transplant		
Condition	Autologous	Allogenic
Aplastic anaemia	No	Yes
Sickle cell disease	No	Yes
Thalassaemia	No	Yes
Gaucher's disease	No	Yes
Severe combined immunodeficiency	No	Yes
Fanconi's anaemia	No	Yes

The history

1. What was the indication for the bone marrow transplant?
2. Has there been a problem leading to the current admission to hospital (if the patient is an inpatient)?
3. Has other treatment been tried unsuccessfully? (For example, bone marrow transplant is often the treatment of choice for relapse after treatment for leukaemia or lymphoma.)
4. Was the bone marrow transplant autologous or allogenic? How was the marrow ablated before transplant (radiotherapy, chemotherapy or both) and, if the transplant was autologous, how were the stem cells harvested (from peripheral blood or by bone marrow aspiration)?
5. If the transplant was allogenic, does the patient know the donor? Only about 30% of people have an HLA-compatible relative. HLA antigens are inherited together and rarely cross over. The patient may know how close the match was.
6. How long was the patient in hospital after transplantation? (Engraftment is usually quicker and complications fewer after autologous transplant.) Ask specifically about problems with infection in the early period and how complications were managed.
7. Find out what effects this complicated illness and treatment have had on the patient's life and ability to work. Ask about family and financial problems. Young patients are likely to have been made sterile by the treatment. Total body irradiation and the use of alkylating agents are more likely to cause permanent sterility than other treatments. Women more often regain fertility than men. Ask tactfully whether the patient is aware of this.
8. How effective has the treatment been? Does the patient feel better or worse than before, and what medium- and long-term prognosis has he or she been given?
9. Have there been specific transplant-associated problems? Ask specifically about the symptoms and signs of graft versus host disease (GVHD) and the other complications of allogenic transplantation (Table 6.53).
10. What are the patient's current medications?

The examination

Examine for persisting or recurrent signs of the condition for which the bone marrow transplant was performed.

Table 6.53 Complications of allogenic bone marrow transplant

Early complications	Late complications

Induction-related
• Mucositis
• Cystitis
• Interstitial pneumonitis
  (usually CMV infection)
• Renal impairment
Graft failure
Infection
Immunodeficiency
Acute GVHD
Veno-occlusive disease of the liver
  (hepatomegaly, ascites, jaundice)
	Treatment-related
	• Gonadal toxicity
	• Cataracts
	• Neurological
	
	Chronic GVHD
	Infection
	Relapse of treated condition
	Second malignancy
	Immunodeficiency

CMV = cytomegalovirus; GVHD = graft versus host disease.

Examine for signs of GVHD. These include skin changes similar to those of scleroderma, dry eyes and mouth (sicca syndrome), alopecia and bronchiolitis obliterans (signs of airflow obstruction).

Examine for hepatic enlargement and ascites (veno-occlusive disease of the liver). Feel all the lymph node groups (e.g. enlarged as a result of a second malignancy, such as ALL, melanoma) and examine the eyes (e.g. secondary glioblastoma). Look for signs of infection in the lungs and for herpes zoster. Examine the hips (aseptic osteonecrosis).

Patients who have had radiotherapy may show evidence of hypothyroidism.

Management

Detailed discussion about methods of transplantation is unlikely to be required.

Management after transplant begins with supportive treatment to prevent infection and bleeding before engraftment occurs. Platelet and blood transfusions may be required and the patient is usually kept isolated. Transfused products are irradiated to prevent GVHD from transfused lymphocytes. Most patients receive colony-stimulating factors to speed recovery. Platelet recovery is usually the slowest and tends to determine the time of discharge from hospital.

Patients who have had an allogenic transplant are at risk of GVHD. This risk is reduced if the HLA match is a good one (only one locus is mismatched). Prophylaxis against GVHD with some combination of prednisone, methotrexate and cyclosporin is usual. The donor marrow may be treated to remove T cells to reduce the incidence of GVHD, but this increases the risk of graft rejection. The risk of GVHD is also increased by previous exposure to blood products and by previous pregnancy.

Acute GVHD can occur even when the major HLA antigens match. It occurs by definition in the first 3 months after transplant and is characterised by diarrhoea, skin rash and liver function test changes. Severe acute GVHD (generalised erythroderma or desquamation) reduces survival and requires aggressive treatment. It is usually treated with high doses of prednisone, antithymocyte globulin and monoclonal antibodies to T cells. Some centres use prophylactic treatment after transplant with methotrexate and tacrolimus or cyclosporin. Remember that the presence of some GVHD reduces the risk of tumour recurrence as a result of graft versus tumour activity.

Chronic GVHD develops after 3 months and affects up to half of transplant recipients. Patients develop an autoimmune-like illness with sicca syndrome, arthritis, cholestasis and bronchiolitis obliterans. It is treated with immunosuppression. It is rare for it to persist for more than 3 years.

Infection can be a problem at various times after transplant. Bacterial infection is most common during the early period before the neutrophil count reaches normal levels. It is treated with isolation and appropriate antibiotics. Fungal infection can become a problem within a week of transplant but usually resolves once engraftment has occurred. *Pneumocystis carinii* infection and cytomegalovirus (CMV) infection can occur within a week of transplant but are uncommon after 3 months. Interstitial pneumonitis occurs in up to 10% of patients. This is usually the result of CMV infection and is treated with supporting measures and ganciclovir. CMV-negative recipients should receive only CMV-negative blood products and CMV-positive patients should receive prophylactic ganciclovir.

Prophylactic treatment with fluconazole, cotrimoxazole and ganciclovir is often used to prevent these problems.

Graft rejection is usually a result of the activity of functional host lymphocytes and is most common in patients who have not had their marrow ablated (e.g. those with aplastic anaemia).

Recurrence of leukaemia may be treated with infusion of more donor T cells, although this increases GVHD. Veno-occlusive disease of the liver occurs in up to 50% of patients. Most recover but in severe cases treatment with tissue plasminogen activator may be indicated.

In general, autologous bone marrow transplant is associated with similar but less severe complications. GVHD, however, does not occur.

The prognosis for these patients varies with the indication for the treatment (Table 6.54). In general, malignant conditions have a better prognosis when treated with bone marrow transplant as a primary or secondary therapy than when it is used only after all else has failed. Patients with non-malignant conditions can often be very successfully treated with bone marrow transplant. For example, aplastic anaemia patients can expect up to 90% disease-free survival. Opinions differ about the use of bone marrow transplant as initial treatment for these patients.

Remember that, as with any complicated and life-threatening illness, pay great attention to the patient's ability to cope and the availability of support at home; these are important issues you must be able to discuss.

Table 6.54 Survival of bone marrow transplant patients	
Condition	**Five-year survival rate**
Acute myeloid leukaemia	50%
Acute lymphatic leukaemia	50%
Chronic myeloid leukaemia (CML), chronic phase	70%
CML accelerated	40%
CML blast crisis	15%
Chronic lymphocytic leukaemia (CLL)	50%
Hodgkin's disease	50%
Non-Hodgkin's lymphoma	40%
Aplastic anaemia	90%
Severe combined immunodeficiency	90%
Thalassaemia	90%

Rheumatology

Rheumatoid arthritis

This is a very common long case in which the diagnosis is usually straightforward and the patient has many physical signs. The peak incidence of the onset of rheumatoid arthritis is in the fourth decade, and it is three times as common in women as in men. There is a familial incidence (human leucocyte antigen [HLA]-DR4 in 70% of patients).

The history

1. Ask about when the diagnosis was made—the onset of rheumatoid arthritis in patients over the age of 60 is associated with a worse prognosis for those who are rheumatoid factor positive.
2. Ask about the presenting features—most patients present with vague generalised symptoms, such as fatigue, anorexia and non-specific musculoskeletal pains, a minority present with obvious oligoarticular arthritis and a few with severe constitutional symptoms and acute arthritis. Morning stiffness lasting for more than an hour is very characteristic of inflammatory arthritis but not of osteoarthritis.
3. Ask about the initial treatment.
4. Ask about the disease progression and what joints have been involved. The lumbar spine is never involved and the distal interphalangeal joints are only rarely affected.
5. Inquire about the alterations in treatment over time and any complications encountered.
6. Ask about the non-articular features of the disease:
   (a) skin—Raynaud's phenomenon, leg ulcers
   (b) lungs—dyspnoea owing to diffuse interstitial fibrosis or pleural effusion, pain as a result of pleuritis
   (c) eyes—dry eyes and mouth (Sjögren's syndrome), scleritis, episcleritis or scleromalacia perforans, cataracts (caused by steroids)
   (d) nervous system—peripheral neuropathy, mononeuritis multiplex, cord compression (owing to cervical spine involvement or rheumatoid nodules), entrapment neuropathy (particularly carpal tunnel syndrome)
   (e) blood—anaemic symptoms owing to chronic disease, iron deficiency (from blood loss), folate deficiency (diet), Felty's syndrome (rheumatoid arthritis with leukopenia and splenomegaly)
   (f) heart—chest pain owing to pericarditis
   (g) renal—infection, analgesic use, amyloid.
7. Ask about drug complications:
   (a) aspirin (e.g. pain or nausea, gastric erosions or ulcers causing bleeding, tinnitus)
   (b) non-steroidal anti-inflammatory drugs (NSAIDs) (e.g. ulceration, renal impairment)
   (c) methotrexate is often used and has a number of side-effects that need to be monitored, including hepatic and pulmonary toxicity, low white cell count and thrombocytopenia; the patient should know not to drink alcohol while taking methotrexate
   (d) penicillamine (e.g. nephrotic syndrome, thrombocytopenia, rashes, mouth ulcers, alteration in taste and, rarely, systemic lupus erythematosus [SLE], polymyositis, myasthenia gravis, Goodpasture's syndrome, or pulmonary infiltration)
   (e) cyclosporin—monitor renal function and blood pressure
   (f) hydroxychloroquine (e.g. nausea, pigmentation, regular ophthalmological review)

(g) gold (e.g. proteinuria, thrombocytopenia, rash, mouth ulcers or, rarely, enterocolitis or hepatitis)

(h) sulfasalazine (e.g. rash, nausea, haematological abnormalities, abnormal liver function tests)

(i) steroids; anti-tumour necrosis factor (TNF) monoclonal antibody (e.g. increased risk of infections).

8. Ask about the major current problem—decreasing hand power, paraesthesiae.
9. Ask about current activity of the disease. This can be assessed historically by asking about the number of joints that have recently been involved with active synovitis, the severity and duration of early morning stiffness (very important), functional ability, changes in weight and the degree of systemic ill-health.
10. Inquire about past medical history, especially of peptic ulceration, drug reactions or renal disease.
11. Inquire about social background—ability to cope at home, ability to climb steps, independence in daily activities, ability to perform fine activities, the work environment, availability of support services.
12. Ask about family history.

The examination (Fig 6.15)

Figure 6.15   Rheumatoid arthritis.

1. GENERAL INSPECTION
   Cushingoid appearance
   Weight

2. HANDS

3. ARMS
   Entrapment neuropathy (e.g. carpal tunnel)
   Subcutaneous nodules
   Elbow joint
   Shoulder joint
   Axillary nodes

4. FACE
   Eyes—dry eyes (Sjögren's)—scleritis, episcleritis
   Scleromalacia perforans—anaemia
   Cataract (steroids, chloroquine)
   Fundi—hyperviscosity
   Face—parotids (Sjögren's)
   Mouth—dryness, ulcers, dental caries, temporomandibular joint (crepitus)

5. NECK
   Cervical spine
   Cervical nodes

6. CHEST
   Heart—pericarditis, valve lesions
   Lungs—effusion, fibrosis, infarction, infection, nodules (and Caplan's syndrome)
   Tuberculosis (steroids)

7. ABDOMEN
   Splenomegaly (e.g. Felty's syndrome)
   Epigastric tenderness (drugs)
   Inguinal nodes

8. HIPS

9. KNEES

10. LOWER LIMBS
    Ulceration (vasculitis)
    Calf swelling (ruptured synovial cyst)
    Peripheral neuropathy
    Mononeuritis multiplex
    Cord compression

11. FEET

12. OTHER
    Urine: protein, blood (drugs, vasculitis, infection, amyloidosis)
    Rectal examination (blood)

A thorough general examination is important. In addition to assessing for synovitis in *every* joint, look particularly for the following.

1. General appearance—steroid complications, weight. Remember that the pain arises mostly from the joint capsule and that acutely inflamed joints are held in the flexed position to increase the volume of the capsule and reduce pain.
2. The hands—including vasculitis and hand function. The wrist joints are almost always affected.
3. Arms—the elbow and shoulder joints, rheumatoid nodules and axillary node enlargement.
4. The face. The eyes for Sjögren's syndrome, scleritis, episcleritis, scleromalacia perforans, cataracts, anaemia and signs of hyperviscosity in the fundi. Enlarged parotid glands (Sjögren's syndrome). Assess the mouth (dryness, dental caries, ulcers), listen for a hoarse voice and palpate the temporomandibular joints (crepitus). *Note*: Rheumatoid arthritis does not cause iritis.
5. The neck—for signs of cervical spine involvement.
6. The chest. Examine the heart (for pericarditis, conduction defects, aortic and mitral regurgitation) and the lungs (for pleural effusion, fibrosis, nodules, infarction, Caplan's syndrome).
7. The abdomen—for splenomegaly and epigastric tenderness.
8. The hips and knees.
9. The lower legs—for ulcers, calf swelling (ruptured Baker's cyst), neuropathy, mononeuritis multiplex and signs of cord compression.
10. The feet.
11. The peripheral nervous system for peripheral neuropathy or mononeuritis multiplex (caused by vasculitis).
12. The skin, for cutaneous vasculitis (ischaemic ulcers on the legs or brown discoloured areas in the nail beds).
13. Urine analysis for protein and blood, and rectal examination for blood (if there is a history suggestive of NSAID complications).

Differential diagnosis

Consider the differential diagnosis of a deforming symmetrical chronic polyarthropathy:

1. rheumatoid arthritis
2. psoriatic arthropathy and other seronegative spondyloarthropathies
3. chronic tophaceous gout (rarely symmetrical)
4. primary generalised osteoarthritis.

Remember that the causes of arthritis plus nodules include:

1. rheumatoid arthritis (seropositive)
2. SLE—rare
3. rheumatic fever (Jaccoud's arthritis)—very rare
4. amyloid arthropathy (most usually in association with multiple myeloma).

Note: Gouty tophi and xanthoma may sometimes cause confusion.

Investigations

To support the diagnosis (remembering that this is primarily a clinical diagnosis, see Table 6.55), investigations include:

1. serological tests
    (a) rheumatoid factor—70% of patients are seropositive; patients may at first be seronegative and seroconvert later (*Note*: Most patients are rheumatoid factor positive if they have nodules or associated vasculitis; remember that over 10%

Table 6.55 Criteria for the diagnosis of rheumatoid arthritis*
1. Morning stiffness ≥1 hour for ≥6 weeks 2. Arthritis of three or more joint areas (soft-tissue swelling or fluid for ≥6 weeks of PIP, MCP, wrist, elbow, knee, ankle, MTP joints) 3. Arthritis of hand joints ≥6 weeks (*not* DIP joint) 4. Symmetrical arthritis ≥6 weeks (for joints defined in 2) 5. Rheumatoid nodules 6. Serum rheumatoid factor 7. X-ray changes of rheumatoid arthritis
* >4 of 7 criteria is diagnostic. DIP = distal interphalangeal; MCP = metacarpophalangeal; MTP = metatarsophalangeal; PIP = proximal interphalangeal.

of well people over the age of 65 have rheumatoid factor and that it is commonly found in association with infections and other inflammatory conditions, in relatives of patients with rheumatoid arthritis and transiently after some vaccinations)

(b) antinuclear antibody (ANA)—positive results in about 20% of cases.

2. X-ray films of involved joints—changes to look for are:
    (a) soft-tissue swelling
    (b) joint space narrowing
    (c) juxta-articular osteoporosis
    (d) joint erosions.

To assess the activity of the disease, investigations include:

1. erythrocyte sedimentation rate (ESR) or C-reactive protein (CRP)—remember that the differential diagnosis of a raised ESR in rheumatoid arthritis includes:
    (a) active disease
    (b) amyloidosis
    (c) infection
    (d) Sjögren's syndrome
2. anaemia—the severity of normochromic anaemia usually correlates with activity
3. rheumatoid factor titre—the higher the titre the more likely the patient is to have extra-articular features; it does *not* correlate with the activity of the arthritis
4. progressive erosions on serial X-ray films.

Treatment

Remember that treatment is palliative rather than curative and the limitations and problems of treatment should be made clear to the patient from the start. The principles of treatment include:

1. education
2. physiotherapy, including exercise and splinting of the joints to prevent deformity
3. occupational therapy
4. drug treatment aimed at reducing pain and inflammation (with NSAIDs or cyclo-oxygenase 2 [COX-2] inhibitors) and at preventing progression of the disease—the gastrointestinal toxicity of the traditional NSAIDs (i.e. peptic ulceration) is

reduced by the COX-2 inhibitors; however, all can cause dyspepsia and renal disease (e.g. acute interstitial nephritis); COX-2 inhibitors are associated with an increased risk of myocardial infarction.

The use of slow-acting, or disease-modifying, antirheumatic drugs (DMARDs) is now recommended early on for patients with active progressive disease, especially if there is evidence of joint destruction. These drugs include methotrexate, sulfasalazine, hydroxychloroquine, cyclosporin, leflunomide, azathioprine, penicillamine and gold (oral or injected). These medications have a slow onset of action (weeks for methotrexate to months for gold). There is evidence that they can lead to healing of bone erosions. It is not clear that any one is more effective than the others but failure of one does not mean another will not be effective. Monitoring should include full blood count, urine testing for proteinuria and specific tests for certain drugs, such as liver function tests for methotrexate or ophthalmological examination and assessment of visual fields for hydroxychloroquine.

Methotrexate can be given orally or intramuscularly, usually 10–25 mg weekly, but starting with a low dose. It is usually better tolerated than the other DMARDs and is often the drug of first choice and given early in the course of the disease to decrease inflammation and sometimes the development of synovitis. Methotrexate may sometimes cause an increase in the number of rheumatoid nodules. It can be given alone or in combination with hydroxychloroquine and sulfasalazine. This triple therapy has been shown to be more effective in leading to remission. To decrease the risk of side-effects of methotrexate, especially mouth ulcers, folic acid is given daily. Safety monitoring includes full blood count and liver function tests. Adverse reactions include rash, abnormal liver function tests (transaminases), leukopenia, thrombocytopenia and interstitial pulmonary fibrosis. It should not be given to patients with glucose-6-phosphate dehydrogenase deficiency.

Newer regimens include the use of cyclosporin in combination with methotrexate when other agents have failed. Other agents in use include leflunomide (a pyrimidine antagonist that inhibits activated T cells) and cytokine-targeted monoclonal antibodies (anti-TNF, interleukin [IL]-1-receptor antagonists).

Anti-TNF antibodies have been shown to be effective treatment when used in combination with methotrexate. These agents may be directed against TNF (infliximab, adalimumab) or against the TNF receptor (etanercept). They are given as subcutaneous injections or as an infusion (infliximab). The antibodies are either chimeric (infliximab) or completely humanised (adalimumab). Anti-TNF is effective in controlling symptoms but has not yet been shown to reduce erosions. It increases susceptibility to serious infections.

Parenteral gold therapy is also disease-modifying; it should always be given with a test dose first (5–10 mg), then 50 mg weekly until 1000 mg is reached, then decrease the frequency of the injections over several months to 50 mg once a month. It is now used less often, having been superseded by the above regimens. Oral gold may be less effective. Monitor regularly for proteinuria (0.500 mg/24 hours) and bone marrow depression (leukopenia or thrombocytopenia), which are indicators for the cessation of therapy. D-penicillamine use is restricted by complications of renal toxicity and bone marrow depression; it is not often used now.

Local steroid injections are helpful for acute involvement of a joint and may give prolonged relief from pain and swelling and improve function.

Low-dose steroid treatment may retard joint damage. The main indications for steroid use are:

1. vasculitic complications of rheumatoid arthritis (where high doses are needed)
2. severe progressive disease, until suppressive treatment with another slow-acting antirheumatic drug becomes effective
3. chronic low-dose treatment, which may be justifiable in the elderly.

Surgery may be very effective treatment for severely diseased joints. Hip, shoulder and knee replacements are the most successful operations. Arthroplasty and relief of contractures can be of value, especially in the hands.

The prognosis of this chronic but often intermittent disease varies. Only a small minority have no permanent joint problems 10 years after diagnosis. Half have a disability that interferes with work by this time. The greater the number of involved joints at the outset, and the more abnormal the inflammatory markers, the worse the prognosis. Life-expectancy has been reduced by up to 7 years, partly as a result of the increased risk of gastrointestinal bleeding and partly because of an increased risk of infection. There is now evidence to suggest an increased risk of atherosclerosis in patients with these chronic inflammatory conditions.

Systemic lupus erythematosus

This multisystem disorder occurs usually in patients between 20 and 40 years of age. Women are more often affected than men (8:1) and there is an increased incidence in families (monozygotic twins have a 50% concordance). There are associations with HLA-DR2, HLA-DR3 and with homozygous deficiencies of the early components of complement. It presents diagnostic as well as long-term management problems.

The history

1. Ask about presenting symptoms (Table 6.56):
    (a) general symptoms—malaise (100%), weight loss (60%), nausea and vomiting (50%), thrombosis of veins or arteries (15%)
    (b) musculoskeletal symptoms (95%)—arthralgia and arthritis, myalgia and myositis
    (c) dermatological symptoms (85%)—skin rash, alopecia
    (d) fever (77%)
    (e) neuropsychiatric symptoms (60%)—delirium, dementia, convulsions, chorea, neuropathy, loss of vision (optic neuritis), headache, symptoms resembling multiple sclerosis, anxiety and depression
    (f) renal tract symptoms (50%)—haematuria, oedema, renal failure
    (g) respiratory tract symptoms (45%)—pleurisy
    (h) cardiovascular symptoms (40%)—pericarditis
    (i) haematological symptoms (50%)—lymphadenopathy, anaemia
    (j) gastrointestinal symptoms (30%)—nausea, diarrhoea, pseudo bowel obstruction, perforation
    (j) thrombophlebitis, recurrent abortions or fetal death in utero (suggests antiphospholipid syndrome [p 173])
    (k) sicca symptoms (secondary to Sjögren's syndrome)
    (l) reduced activities of daily living and ability to work as a result of the effect of this chronic and relapsing disease on the patient's life.
2. Ask about any drug history (e.g. procainamide, hydralazine) (Table 6.57). Newer antiarrhythmic and antihypertensive drugs have made drug-induced lupus less common and typically the symptoms resolve rapidly with cessation of the drug. Autoantibody levels diminish slowly.
3. Ask about any treatment given and any complications of treatment.
4. Ask about problems during pregnancy and use of contraception.
5. Inquire about the family history.
6. Inquire about the patient's understanding of the implications of this chronic and incurable disease and its prognosis.

Table 6.56 The American Rheumatism Association criteria for systemic lupus erythematosus (revised)

Clinical features
1. Malar rash (flat or raised erythema)
2. Discoid lupus (patches raised and red with scaling)
3. Photosensitivity
4. Oral ulcers (usually painless)
5. Arthritis (non-erosive, involving ≥2 peripheral joints)
6. Pericarditis or pleuritis
7. Seizures or psychosis or an organic mental syndrome or neuropathy (e.g. cranial nerve) or ocular field defects, hemiparesis, aphasia or movement disorder, tremor

Laboratory features
8. Proteinuria (>0.5 g/day) or cellular casts
9. Haemolytic anaemia or leukopenia (<4 × 10^9/L) or lymphopenia (<1.5 × 10^9/L) or thrombocytopenia (<100 × 10^9/L)
10. Positive ANA in the absence of drugs associated with lupus
11. Antibody to double-stranded DNA (dsDNA) or Smith antigen (Sm) (relatively specific) or antiphospholipid antibodies or false-positive results in serological tests for syphilis
12. Presence of anticardiolipin antibodies

Note: Four or more manifestations of the 12 must be present serially or simultaneously (but are *not* diagnostic).

Table 6.57 Drugs inducing systemic lupus erythematosus (SLE)

1. Procainamide (most patients are ANA-positive within 1 year; 15–20% develop SLE)
2. Hydralazine (most patients are ANA-positive within 1 year; 5–10% develop SLE)
3. Isoniazid*
4. Methyldopa*
5. Penicillamine*
6. Chlorpromazine*
7. Anticonvulsants,* particularly phenytoin (not sodium valproate)

Note: There is an increased incidence of drug-induced lupus in slow acetylators who will develop a positive ANA and clinical manifestations sooner than rapid acetylators. Drug-induced lupus is more common in the elderly because of the more frequent use of drugs in this group. There is usually no renal or nervous system disease, no antibody to dsDNA, and improvement *may* occur if the drug is withdrawn.

*Rarely cause overt SLE, but ANA is commonly positive.

The examination (Fig 6.16)

Figure 6.16 Systemic lupus erythematosus (SLE).

1. **GENERAL INSPECTION**
   Cushingoid
   Weight
   Mental state

2. **HANDS**
   Vasculitis
   Rash
   Arthropathy

3. **ARMS**
   Livedo reticularis
   Purpura
   Proximal myopathy (SLE, steroids)

4. **HEAD**
   Alopecia, lupus hairs
   Eyes—scleritis, cytoid lesions etc.
   Mouth—ulcers, infection
   Rash (e.g. butterfly)
   Cranial nerve lesions
   Cervical adenopathy

5. **CHEST**
   Cardiovascular system—
      endocarditis

   Respiratory system—pleural
      effusion, pleurisy, pulmonary
      fibrosis, collapse or infection

6. **ABDOMEN**
   Hepatosplenomegaly
   Tenderness

7. **HIPS**
   Aseptic necrosis

8. **LEGS**
   Feet—small joint synovitis
   Rash
   Proximal myopathy
   Cerebellar ataxia
   Neuropathy (uncommon)
   Hemiplegia
   Mononeuritis multiplex

9. **OTHER**
   Urine analysis (proteinuria)
   Blood pressure (hypertension)
   Temperature chart

Inspect the patient for weight loss, Cushingoid appearance (because of steroid treatment) and assess the general mental state.

Examine all the skin. Remember that discoid lupus erythematosus (DLE) occurs in 20% of SLE patients. This disfiguring skin disease leads to permanent hair loss with telangiectasia scaling, circular erythematous lesions and follicular plugging. There is often destruction of skin appendages. DLE can occur without other features of SLE.

Look at the hands for vasculitis, which can produce nail-fold infarcts and ischaemia or gangrene, and rash (e.g. photosensitivity, diffuse maculopapular rash). Also look for Raynaud's phenomenon and arthropathy (fusiform swelling of the PIP joints or synovitis, possibly in a rheumatoid arthritis distribution—10% develop swan neck deformity and ulnar deviation of the fingers).

Look at the forearms for livedo reticularis and purpura as a result of vasculitis or thrombocytopenia. Test for proximal myopathy caused by actual disease or secondary to steroid treatment.

Inspect the head. Look for alopecia. Lupus hairs are characteristic: they occur above the forehead and are short, broken hairs that grow back quickly after hair loss (except in patients with DLE). Look at the eyes for keratoconjunctivitis sicca and for pale conjunctivae owing to anaemia, and look at the fundi for cytoid lesions (hard exudates secondary to vasculitis). Look in the mouth for ulcers and infection. Note any facial rash (butterfly photosensitivity rash, discoid lupus or diffuse maculopapular rashes). Feel the cervical and axillary nodes.

Examine the chest. In the cardiovascular system, note signs of pericarditis or murmurs (Libman-Sacks endocarditis is very uncommon). In the respiratory system, note signs of pleural effusion, pleuritis, pulmonary fibrosis or atelectasis.

Examine the abdomen for splenomegaly (usually mild) and hepatomegaly. Feel for abdominal tenderness.

Examine the hips for signs of aseptic necrosis and examine for proximal weakness in the legs, cerebellar ataxia, hemiplegia and transverse myelitis.

Also examine for neuropathy (mainly sensory) and mononeuritis multiplex, as well as thrombophlebitis and leg ulceration.

Look at the urine analysis (for evidence of renal disease—haematuria and proteinuria) and take the blood pressure (may be elevated in renal disease). Also look at the temperature chart (for fever indicating active disease or secondary infection).

Investigations

Diagnosis depends on a combination of the symptoms, signs and laboratory test results (Tables 6.56–6.59).

Patients who do not fit the criteria may have another connective tissue disease.

Mixed connective tissue disease (MCTD) is suggested by the overlapping clinical features of scleroderma, polymyositis and SLE and the presence of characteristic antibodies to nuclear ribonucleoprotein (nRNP), which is one of the extractable nuclear antigens. Anti-nRNP is present in high titre and produces a speckled pattern on fluorescent antibody testing in patients with MCTD. When these patients are followed for many years, they may start to resemble patients with progressive systemic sclerosis or SLE, or may continue with a relatively undifferentiated connective tissue disease.

The important laboratory tests in SLE are haematological and serological. Magnetic resonance imaging (MRI) scans and lumbar puncture (increased protein and mononuclear cells) may be indicated if central nervous system lupus is suspected. Central nervous system symptoms often correlate poorly with serological measures of the activity of the disease.

Haematological tests

Anaemia—normochromic, normocytic and related to the chronic inflammatory processes—is very common. Immune haemolytic anaemia is less common and the Coombs' test then gives a positive result.

Leukopenia (especially lymphopenia) occurs in over half the patients and may be caused by antibody directed against leukocytes.

Table 6.58   **Antinuclear antibody (ANA) patterns**

1. Rim or shaggy pattern—antibody to dsDNA = SLE (50–60%). These antibodies are quite specific and high titres suggest disease activity and nephritis
2. Homogeneous pattern—antibody to deoxyribonucleoprotein = connective tissue disease, including SLE
3. Speckled pattern—antibody to extractable nuclear antigen = SLE or scleroderma or mixed connective tissue disease
4. Nucleolar pattern—antibody to RNA found especially in scleroderma, myositis

SLE = systemic lupus erythematosus. ANA present in 99%.

Table 6.59   Antibodies associated with connective tissue diseases

Disease	Antibodies associated
Systemic lupus erythematosus (SLE)	Anti-single-stranded DNA (not specific) Anti-dsDNA (50–60%) Antibody to extractable nuclear antigen Anti-Sm (30%)—specific for lupus Anti-RNP (30% in low titre)—high titre in MCTD Anti-Ro-SS-A (30%)—associated with primary Sjögren's syndrome, congenital heart block, can cause nephritis Anti-SS-B (15%)—associated with Sjögren's syndrome Antihistone (drug-induced SLE: 95%) Antiphospholipid (50%)—include anticardiolipin and lupus anticoagulant Antierythrocyte (60%)—occasionally causes anaemia Antiplatelet Antilymphocyte (70%)—possible leukopenia
Scleroderma and CREST	Anticentromere (CREST: 70%; scleroderma: 10%) Antinucleolar, anti-Scl-70 (scleroderma 40%) Anti-RNP, anti-SS-A (scleroderma occasionally in low titre) Antinuclear antigen (90%)
Sjögren's syndrome	Anti-SS-A (70%), anti-SS-B (60%)
Mixed connective tissue disease (MCTD)	Anti-RNP (100%) Anti-SS-A (occasionally in low titre)
Polymyositis and dermatomyositis	Anti-PM1 (polymyositis: 50%; dermatomyositis: 10%)

CREST = calcinosis cutis; Raynaud's phenomenon; (o)esophageal involvement; sclerodactyly; telangiectasia; RNP = ribonucleoprotein.

The lupus anticoagulant and anticardiolipin antibodies, or both, are found in about 10% of cases. Characteristically, there is a prolonged partial thromboplastin time with kaolin (PTTK), which is not corrected by the addition of normal plasma. It is associated with thrombosis rather than bleeding.

Thrombocytopenia occurs in 15% of cases and is associated with antiplatelet antibodies.

Immunological tests

The characteristic abnormalities are the presence of autoantibodies (Tables 6.58, 6.59). Antibodies to ANA are present in 99% of cases. The antigens involved include single- and double-stranded DNA, SS-A and SS-B and Sm antigen (an acidic nuclear protein). Many antibodies persist even when the disease is quiescent. Antibodies to dsDNA and Sm are the most specific for SLE and are therefore the most useful diagnostically. The latter, however, is not very sensitive.

Complement abnormalities are usual during exacerbations of the disease, with a reduction in total haemolytic complement (CH50) and in the components of the classical pathway (C3 and C4). The combination of a low CH50 and normal C3 suggests an inherited deficiency of complement components and is strongly associated with SLE. The finding of high levels of anti-dsDNA and lower complement levels is usually associated with active disease and especially renal involvement.

Positive rheumatoid factor occurs in 10% of cases at low titre. Skin biopsy in SLE can be helpful; positive immunofluorescence of the basement membrane in involved skin occurs in 95% of patients.

Treatment

Current work suggests that appropriate treatment to suppress exacerbations of SLE will prolong life. Many patients have mild disease without life-threatening complications.

Arthralgias, myalgia and fever respond to rest and NSAIDs. Exposure to sunlight should be avoided and sunscreen used. Hydroxychloroquine is useful in the management of arthritis and skin rash. Annual retinal and visual field examinations must be performed in patients on these drugs because of the cumulative risk of retinal toxicity. Raynaud's phenomenon may respond to calcium channel antagonists. Steroids are indicated for central nervous system involvement, pericarditis, myocarditis, pleurisy, severe haemolytic anaemia and thrombocytopenia. Use of high initial doses with gradual reduction once improvement occurs is the proper method of treatment. Hypercoagulability may be treated by anticoagulants—warfarin treatment with a target international normalised ratio (INR) of 2.5–3 is effective.

Management of renal disease is difficult. Renal biopsy usually shows abnormalities but often only mild changes. Renal biopsy is indicated early if there is any clinical or biochemical evidence of renal disease or if the urine sediment is abnormal. Four groups of biopsy abnormalities can be identified: mesangial proliferation, focal glomerulonephritis, diffuse proliferation and membranous proliferation. Mesangial proliferation has the best prognosis—disease is unlikely to progress. Diffuse proliferative glomerulonephritis has the worst prognosis and aggressive treatment (e.g. high-dose pulse steroids plus cyclophosphamide) is recommended. Membranous proliferation has a low rate of response to treatment. SLE is not a contraindication to dialysis or renal transplant in those patients who develop renal failure but there is a higher than average risk of graft failure. Calcium and vitamin D supplements should be offered to protect against osteoporosis. Calcitonin and bisphosphonates should be considered if long-term steroid treatment is likely.

Azathioprine is indicated as a steroid-sparing agent. Cyclophosphamide is a more toxic alternative. Intermittent pulses of cyclophosphamide may be helpful. These agents are particularly indicated in active glomerulonephritis. Plasmapheresis is sometimes used in severe disease but is not of established benefit. Autologous stem cell transplant is experimental treatment.

The prognosis of SLE is generally good. There is a 75% 10-year survival rate; the major causes of death are infections and renal failure.

Remember that postpartum exacerbations of lupus may occur. Spontaneous abortions are common in women with antiphospholipid antibodies. Treatment with anticoagulation may be effective in reducing the risk of abortion. Steroids may be used in pregnancy as, except for dexamethasone, these do not cross the placenta. Women with the anti-Ro antibody may have babies with permanent complete heart block and transient erythematous rashes.

Systemic vasculitis

Patients with a systemic vasculitic illness will often be used for the long-case examination because of the complex nature of these illnesses and the frequent need for hospitalisation. The fact that the illness tends to affect multiple body systems across numerous specialties is ideal to test the candidates' general approach to internal medicine. The majority of cases seen in the examination will have a vasculitis such as Wegener's granulomatosis, giant cell arteritis or polyarteritis nodosa. Occasionally, less common adult vasculitides, such as Churg-Strauss syndrome or microscopic polyarteritis, will be encountered.

The long-case examination for the patient with systemic vasculitis will require the candidate to take a careful history and examine the patient in a thorough general sense, as well as look for specific abnormalities in each disease. Candidates will be expected to have a good knowledge of the various investigative tools available to diagnose vasculitis. The course of treatment will invariably be discussed in this type of case, particularly the side-effects of long-term medications and likely prognosis.

The history

In most cases, the onset of a systemic vasculitic illness is subacute rather than acute. The patient has often seen several practitioners before a diagnosis is made.

The history will be critical in determining the diagnosis if the patient has a systemic vasculitis and presents a diagnostic problem, or indeed if there are significant management issues. First, ask about the systemic features that would suggest a vasculitic illness: fatigue, malaise, fever, myalgia and arthralgia will be very frequent in these patients. Ask about vasculitic skin rash, which would normally be in the form of palpable purpura. Ask about the pattern of joint involvement.

In Wegener's granulomatosis, frequent symptoms are nasal congestion, rhinorrhoea and bloody nasal discharge, cough (which is initially a dry cough but may evolve into haemoptysis), and breathlessness. The upper and lower respiratory tract are almost invariably involved in Wegener's granulomatosis. Next ask about a history of renal disease, particularly hypertension or renal failure, and any gastrointestinal symptoms.

In giant cell arteritis, the patient is generally in the sixth, seventh or eighth decades of life, but it can occasionally occur in younger people. The usual specific symptoms for giant cell arteritis are severe bitemporal headache and, less commonly, visual disturbance or visual loss, and jaw claudication. Other focal neurological systems can also occur.

In polyarteritis nodosa, the specific symptoms will depend on which arteries are involved. Remember that these are usually medium-sized arteries and so the disease tends to cause ischaemic problems in the territory of the coronary arteries, mesenteric arteries and renal arteries. Ask about risk factors for hepatitis B.

In Churg-Strauss vasculitis, the patients almost invariably have a previous history of allergic rhinitis, asthma and possibly eczema. They then develop problems with cough and breathlessness and subsequently peripheral nervous system disease either in the form of symmetrical peripheral neuropathy or mononeuritis multiplex. Skin rash may occur with Churg-Strauss syndrome.

In microscopic polyarteritis, the major problem is usually with renal impairment, which may not have any specific symptoms. Systemic symptoms of vasculitis are generally very prominent.

The examination

The patient with systemic vasculitis usually looks quite unwell. Check for fever, sinus tachycardia, pallor and signs of recent weight loss. Other physical signs will be more specific to the actual underlying illness. In Wegener's granulomatosis, there may be evidence of tachypnoea and crackles throughout the lung field. Fluid overload may occur in the setting of worsening renal failure. In giant cell arteritis, tender and indurated temporal arteries will often be present. There may be abnormal eye signs if there is retinal involvement. Focal neurological signs should be sought.

In Churg-Strauss syndrome, look for signs of allergic disease, such as swollen nasal turbinates, nasal polyps, and evidence of bronchospasm. Examine the peripheral nervous system carefully, looking for single nerve lesions or symmetrical peripheral neuropathy generally affecting the lower limbs. In polyarteritis nodosa, there may be evidence of painful skin nodules in rare cases. In microscopic polyarteritis, urinalysis is the key, looking for any evidence of proteinuria or haematuria.

Investigations

Investigations will be critical in determining the diagnosis in systemic vasculitis. In most cases a biopsy of affected tissue is the most reliable way of making the diagnosis; other investigations will raise the suspicion that vasculitis is the problem and direct the clinician to a suitable biopsy site.

It will often be necessary to exclude systemic infection, malignancy or generalised autoimmune disease. In vasculitis, the ESR is invariably raised, often at levels of >70 mm/h. There is frequently a normochromic normocytic anaemia and there may be neutrophilia. The platelet count may be elevated. Renal function will often be impaired in Wegener's granulomatosis, polyarteritis nodosa and microscopic polyarteritis. Abnormal liver function tests, particularly elevated transaminase levels, may be found in Wegener's granulomatosis and in polyarteritis nodosa. Liver function abnormalities are also reported in giant cell arteritis. Urine abnormalities will often be found in the form of urinary casts and the presence of dysmorphic red blood cells in the urine, particularly in Wegener's granulomatosis, microscopic polyarteritis and polyarteritis nodosa. The chest X-ray will often show a bilateral diffuse interstitial abnormality in Wegener's granulomatosis and a peripheral fluffy, patchy infiltrative pattern in Churg-Strauss syndrome.

The critical investigation in Wegener's granulomatosis is the cytoplasmic (c) antineutrophil cytoplasmic antibody (c-ANCA). This will be present in a vast majority of cases of Wegener's granulomatosis. Further testing of this antibody will reveal the presence of anti-pr3 antibodies. The presence of a typical clinical syndrome with a positive c-ANCA and pr3 antibodies is virtually diagnostic of Wegener's granulomatosis. The need for a tissue biopsy may be avoided if these tests are positive. Occasionally, patients with upper airways disease only will not have a positive c-ANCA test.

Diagnosis of giant cell arteritis depends on a positive tissue sample. Temporal artery biopsy should reveal the diagnosis as long as a generous biopsy is taken by the surgeon.

In polyarteritis nodosa, tissue samples are often not available. Many organs may be involved (Table 6.60). Angiography is sometimes helpful in this illness, particularly of the mesenteric arteries but possibly also of the coronary arteries. Bead-like aneurysmal dilation of the arteries is suggestive of polyarteritis.

Fifty per cent of patients who have Churg-Strauss syndrome will have a positive perinuclear (p) ANCA test. The other important diagnostic tool is the tissue biopsy, which will reveal intense eosinophilia. Sural nerve biopsy will sometimes be required in the setting of neuropathy and this will show vasculitis.

Microscopic polyarteritis is characterised by a positive p-ANCA result. This antibody is directed against myeloperoxidase. Renal biopsy is usually necessary to establish the diagnosis. p-ANCA and c-ANCA are rare in other inflammatory diseases

Table 6.60   Clinical findings in patients with polyarteritis nodosa

Site	Clinical problem	Incidence
Muscles and joints	Myalgia, arthritis	65%
Kidneys	Hypertension, renal impairment	60%
Gut	Nausea, vomiting, abdominal pain, bowel, liver or pancreatic infarcts	45%
Peripheral nervous system	Mononeuritis multiplex, peripheral neuropathy	50%
Central nervous system	Strokes and seizures	25%
Skin	Purpura, infarcts, Raynaud's phenomenon	40%
Heart	Cardiac failure, infarction, pericarditis	35%
Genitourinary	Ovarian, testicular pain or infarction	20%

but common in patients with vasculitis. ANCA titres do not correspond with the clinical severity of the patient's illness and they may only be markers of disease.

Treatment

Systemic vasculitis will generally require aggressive immunosuppressive medication. Failure to suppress the vasculitis aggressively can result in permanent injury, progressive deterioration and death. Once the diagnosis of Wegener's granulomatosis is established, high-dose corticosteroids and daily oral cyclophosphamide should be instituted. Antibiotics are adjunctive therapy. In giant cell arteritis, high-dose oral corticosteroids are required. In polyarteritis nodosa, the untreated 5-year survival rate is less than 20%. A combination of high-dose prednisone and cyclophosphamide will usually be very effective treatment (90% long-term remission). Treatment may often be discontinued after remission is obtained and the long-term prognosis is very good. Interferon alpha, or the antiviral drug vidarabine, may help to induce remission if there is associated hepatitis B infection. The eosinophilic vasculitis of the Churg-Strauss syndrome is generally very steroid responsive but occasionally other cytotoxic agents need to be used. Steroids alone have been shown to increase the 5-year survival rate from 25% to 50%. Corticosteroids combined with immunosuppressive agents are usually required for microscopic polyarteritis with renal support in patients who develop renal failure.

The duration of treatment for all of these vasculitic illnesses needs to be individualised. Patients with giant cell arteritis can come off treatment after about 2 years but some have disease for several years. Most of the other diseases will require maintenance therapy. Patients often suffer the effects of long-term steroid therapy and immuno-suppression, such as osteoporosis, hypertension, diabetes and accelerated vascular disease. Infection is common in this group and can be serious or fatal. Patients on cyclophosphamide need careful monitoring of their blood count and careful counselling to ensure adequate fluid intake and avoid haemorrhagic cystitis.

Antiphospholipid syndrome

Antiphospholipid syndrome is a disease which not infrequently requires patients to be admitted to hospital for its various complications. It therefore may crop up as a long case in the examination. The disease can be either primary or secondary. The secondary form is usually a complication of other autoimmune conditions. The most common of these is SLE. The main antibody in this disease is directed against the phospholipid–beta$_2$-glycoprotein 1 complex, on which it exerts a procoagulant effect. It has also been described in HIV infection.

The history

Patients with antiphospholipid syndrome commonly suffer thrombosis.

1. Ask about venous thromboses. The most common site is the deep lower limb or pelvic veins, but the axillary veins can be involved.
2. Ask about arterial thromboses. Stroke and myocardial infarction are the most common arterial complications.
3. Inquire about a history of recurrent first-trimester abortion. Antiphospholipid syndrome is far more common in females and otherwise unexplained first trimester abortions are very characteristic of this disease. Other obstetric complications include intrauterine growth retardation and an increased tendency for hypertension in pregnancy.
4. Ask about bleeding problems associated with thrombocytopenia, livedo reticularis, central nervous system complications, such as migraine and chorea, and rarely the HELLP syndrome (*h*aemolysis, *e*levated *l*iver enzymes and *l*ow *p*latelets).
5. Ask about features of the underlying disorder, such as SLE, which suggest the patient has a secondary form of antiphospholipid syndrome.

The examination

Unless the patient has an active thrombosis there are unlikely to be any abnormal physical signs. Look for:
1. the signs of any associated autoimmune diseases, particularly skin rashes and joint abnormalities in lupus, and dry eyes and mouth in Sjögren's syndrome
2. the typical features of scleroderma
3. the livedo reticularis rash on the lower limbs.

Investigations

The detection of IgG anticardiolipin antibodies is diagnostic for the antiphospholipid syndrome if the antibodies are in high titre and found in the correct clinical context. IgM anticardiolipin antibodies may be detected, although these are less specific. The lupus inhibitor is a related antibody (both are antibodies to phospholipid) which confers an even greater risk of thrombosis and pregnancy complications. The lupus inhibitor is also associated with a prolonged activated partial thromboplastin time (APPT). In any patient with antiphospholipid syndrome, it is worth checking the ANA and other autoimmune serology as indicated. The platelet count should also be measured.

Treatment

Any patient with thrombotic complications of the antiphospholipid syndrome should be treated with anticoagulants for life. The patient with anticardiolipin antibodies but no clinical abnormalities presents a difficult clinical situation. There are no data to support routine anticoagulation in this situation but clearly there is a risk of arterial thrombosis. The patient who has had obstetric problems in the past but no history of thrombosis also presents a dilemma for clinicians. The literature supports the use of anticoagulation therapy only in those with anticardiolipin antibodies or lupus inhibitor in whom a thrombotic complication has previously occurred.

Women who have suffered recurrent abortion will require treatment during pregnancy. Low-molecular-weight heparin would normally be used throughout the pregnancy, possibly with the addition of aspirin. There is no good evidence that corticosteroids improve survival of the fetus.

Systemic sclerosis (scleroderma)

This is a progressive disease of multiple organs. Although a rare disease, it crops up commonly in examinations. It is more common in women (3:1).

The history

1. Ask about symptoms:
    (a) dermatological symptoms—Raynaud's phenomenon (commonly the first symptom), tight skin, disability from sclerodactyly
    (b) arthritis—arthropathy in a rheumatoid distribution, carpal tunnel symptoms
    (c) gastrointestinal symptoms—dysphagia, heartburn (oesophagitis), diarrhoea (malabsorption), jaundice (primary liver cancer), pruritis (rare)
    (d) renal tract symptoms—hypertension, renal failure
    (e) respiratory symptoms—symptoms of pulmonary fibrosis, pleurisy, known diagnosis of pulmonary hypertension
    (f) cardiac symptoms—symptoms of pericarditis, palpitations (arrhythmias), symptoms of cardiac failure (dilated cardiomyopathy)
    (g) other symptoms—impotence, hypothyroidism, history of non-melanoma skin cancer.
2. Ask about a history of exposure to polyvinyl chloride (PVC), L-tryptophan (eosinophilic myalgia syndrome), drugs (e.g. bleomycin, pentazocine). Also ask about drugs likely to aggravate Raynaud's phenomenon (e.g. beta-blockers); a possible association with silicone breast implants seems to have been disproved.
3. Ask about treatment received (e.g. D-penicillamine) and side-effects thereof.
4. Inquire about degree of disability—function at home, ability to work, financial security.

Scleroderma may be classified as limited or diffuse. Limited disease means involvement of the skin up to the elbows (and may include the face) without chest, abdominal or internal organ involvement, except for the oesophagus. These patients are usually anticentromere positive. In CREST (typically a more benign form of scleroderma, usually with oesophageal involvement causing dysphagia), sclerodactyly is limited with changes extending only as far as the MCP joints. The signs are calcinosis (calcific deposits in subcutaneous tissue at the ends of the fingers), Raynaud's phenomenon (resulting in loss of tissue pulp at the ends of the fingers), sclerodactyly (tightening of the skin on the fingers) and telangiectasia. Progressive pulmonary fibrosis can occur.

Localised scleroderma is called *morphea*. It presents as single or multiple plaques of skin induration. Linear scleroderma involves the face or a limb.

The examination (Fig 6.17)

Figure 6.17   Systemic sclerosis.

1. **GENERAL APPEARANCE**
   'Bird-like' facies
   Weight loss (malabsorption)

2. **HANDS**
   CREST—calcinosis, atrophy of distal
     tissue pulp (Raynaud's),
     sclerodactyly, telangiectasia
   Dilated capillary loops
   Small joint arthropathy and tendon
     crepitus
   Fixed flexion deformity
   Hand function

3. **ARMS**
   Oedema (early) or skin thickening
     and tightening
   Pigmentation
   Vitiligo
   Hair loss
   Proximal myopathy

4. **HEAD**
   Alopecia
   Eyes—loss of eyebrows, anaemia,
     dryness (Sjögren's), difficulty with
     closing
   Mouth—dryness, puckered, difficulty
     with opening

   Pigmentation
   Telangiectasia

5. **DYSPHAGIA**
   Ask patient

6. **CHEST**
   Tight skin ('Roman breast plate')
   Heart—cor pulmonale, pericardial
     effusion, pericarditis, failure,
     arrhythmias, pulmonary
     hypertension
   Lungs—fibrosis, reflux pneumonitis,
     chest infections, lung carcinoma,
     vasculitis

7. **LEGS**
   Skin lesions
   Vasculitis
   Small joint arthropathy
   Patellar crepitus

8. **OTHER**
   Blood pressure (hypertension in
     renal involvement)
   Urine analysis (proteinuria)
   Temperature chart (infection)
   Stool examination (steatorrhoea)
   Cancer elsewhere (non-melanoma
     skin cancer, primary liver cancer)

Make a general inspection for weight loss (owing to malabsorption or dysphagia).

Look at the hands. Look for the signs of limited scleroderma. These include sclerodactyly (tightening of the skin of the fingers) with extension up to the elbow, telangiectasia, finger tapering, pitting scars, signs of calcinosis (calcific deposits in subcutaneous tissue at the ends of the fingers) and the effects of Raynaud's phenomenon (loss of tissue pulp at the ends of the fingers).

Nail-fold capillaroscopy is useful but few have the skill. The presence of dilated tortuous vessels always indicates an underlying connective tissue disorder of some sort. Assess hand function.

Look at the arms for skin changes and assess proximal weakness (myositis).

Examine the head. Note any alopecia. Look at the face for 'salt-and-pepper' pigmentation, loss of wrinkling, 'bird-like' or 'mouse-like' facies (because of puckering of the mouth) and telangiectasia. Check for any difficulty in closing the eyes, for dryness of the eyes (Sjögren's syndrome) and pale conjunctivae (anaemia). Check for any difficulty opening the mouth wide and for dryness and puckering of the mouth.

Look at the chest for the 'Roman breast plate' effect as a result of skin tightening. Examine the cardiovascular system for pericarditis, arrhythmias, cor pulmonale and cardiac failure (owing to myocardial fibrosis). Examine the respiratory system for pulmonary fibrosis, reflux pneumonitis, infection, lung carcinoma and vasculitis.

Look at the legs for vasculitis and ulceration.

The blood pressure must be taken. Also check the urine analysis and temperature charts.

Investigations

The ESR may be raised. Anaemia may be present owing to chronic disease, iron deficiency (secondary to bleeding from oesophagitis), folate or vitamin B_{12} deficiency (secondary to malabsorption), or a microangiopathic haemolytic anaemia, which is usually associated with renal disease. Hypergammaglobulinaemia (particularly IgG) is present in 50% of cases. Rheumatoid factor is present in 25% and ANA is found in 40% of cases. Anticentromere antibody is particularly associated with CREST (70%) (see Table 6.59). Investigations for malabsorption and dysphagia may be necessary. Assess visceral involvement with chest X-ray films, respiratory function tests, high-resolution computed tomography (CT) of the chest, gastroscopy or oesophageal manometry, depending on the clinical presentation.

Treatment

This debilitating chronic disease will expose the patient to the need for recurrent investigations and adjustments to treatment. These matters need careful explanation from the outset.

Symptomatic treatment includes avoiding vasospasm (by avoiding smoking, beta-blockers and cold weather). Aggressive treatment of reflux is important to prevent the formation of oesophageal strictures. Nifedipine, phenoxybenzamine, prazosin or methyldopa may help Raynaud's phenomenon. The prostacyclin analogue iloprost showed promise for Raynaud's phenomenon in scleroderma. Artificial tears are useful for dry eyes and NSAIDs may help with joint symptoms. Treat malabsorption (particularly bacterial overgrowth, with antibiotics) and reflux oesophagitis (with proton pump inhibitors).

D-penicillamine (an immunosuppressant drug that also interferes with collagen cross-linking) may be helpful for skin disease and may improve survival. It has been usual to start treatment with a low dose—250 mg/day—and increase this over several months to 1 g/day if tolerated. More recent studies have shown no advantage of higher doses over a regimen of 125 mg second daily. The drug has a number of severe side-effects (Table 6.61). Monthly full blood counts are usually recommended. Intravenous cyclophosphamide is used if there is lung involvement. Pericarditis, inflammatory myopathy and early interstitial lung disease may respond to steroids.

Many other drugs have been tried for patients with scleroderma, including angiotensin receptor blockers, selective serotonin reuptake inhibitors, serotonin antagonists, topical nitrates and platelet inhibitors. There are no controlled trials showing that treatment can reverse the course of the disease.

The endothelin receptor antagonist, bosentan, has been approved for the treatment of pulmonary artery hypertension associated with scleroderma for patients with WHO class III or IV symptoms.

Aggressive treatment of hypertension to prevent renal failure is vital—angiotensin-converting enzyme (ACE) inhibitors are the drug class of choice. Dialysis is not contraindicated. Captopril is often given to patients with normal renal function to prevent hypertensive renal crises.

Prognosis is worse in men and those with renal or late-onset disease. Skin and gut involvement without other organ disease has the best prognosis.

Table 6.61   Side-effects of D-penicillamine

Severe	More minor
Glomerulonephritis and nephrotic syndrome	Alteration of taste
Myasthenia gravis	Skin rashes
Thrombocytopenia	Fever
Leukopenia	Nausea
Aplastic anaemia	Anorexia

Endocrine system

Osteoporosis (and osteomalacia)

Osteoporosis, particularly in postmenopausal women and in patients taking cortico-steroids, is increasingly encountered in the examination. It will commonly form part of another medical problem. Osteoporotic fractures can affect 30% of postmenopausal women over their lifetime. Many older women have undergone screening bone densitometry and may be aware that they have asymptomatic osteoporosis. Patients who have had a history of a hip fracture, or who have evidence of an endocrine disorder, malabsorption, liver disease, Crohn's disease or bone marrow disease, or who are taking certain medications, should have the possibility of osteoporosis considered while they are being evaluated (Table 6.62).

The history

1. Ask about a history of fractures, particularly fractures of the hip, wrist, humerus or ribs, and vertebral compression fractures (especially T12), which may have occurred with minimal stress. Acute back pain that subsides over weeks to months and then recurs may be caused by compression fractures.
2. If a hip fracture has occurred, ask about any secondary complications, including pulmonary thromboembolism and nosocomial infections.
3. Ask about symptoms of bone pain, which may be diffuse, and proximal muscle weakness. These features may occur with osteomalacia (characterised by defective bone mineralisation in adults).
4. Ask the patient whether he or she has had skeletal X-ray examinations. Note that X-rays are insensitive for bone loss as a substantial reduction of bone mass must occur before changes on the X-rays will be visible.
5. Ask about risk factors for osteoporosis or osteomalacia, if suspected (Table 6.63). Determine the menstrual history and age of onset of menopause. Inquire about symptoms of thyroid excess or thyroid hormone replacement (thyroxine). Determine if there are symptoms or a history of anaemia (e.g. coeliac disease). Take a careful drug history. Medications that cause osteoporosis include alcohol, heparin, steroid use, thyroxine over-replacement, anticonvulsants (by affecting vitamin D metabolism), cyclosporin and chemotherapy.

Table 6.62   Major secondary causes of osteoporosis

1. Endocrine diseases
   (a) Hyperthyroidism
   (b) Hyperparathyroidism
   (c) Cushing's syndrome
   (d) Growth hormone deficiency
   (e) Hyperprolactinaemia
   (f) Hypogonadism
2. Gastrointestinal diseases
   (a) Malabsorption syndromes (e.g. coeliac disease, Crohn's disease)
   (b) Chronic cholestasis (e.g. primary biliary cirrhosis)
3. Malnutrition
   (a) Anorexia nervosa
   (b) Scurvy
   (c) Alcoholism
4. Bone marrow disorders
   (a) Multiple myeloma
   (b) Disseminated carcinoma
   (c) Lymphoma
   (d) Leukaemias
5. Connective tissue disease
   (a) Marfan's syndrome, Ehlers-Danlos syndrome
   (b) Osteogenesis imperfecta
   (c) Rheumatoid arthritis
6. Drugs
   (a) Chronic heparin therapy

Table 6.63   Causes of osteomalacia

1. Unavailability of vitamin D:
   (a) vitamin D malabsorption (e.g. coeliac disease, pancreatic insufficiency, cirrhosis)
   (b) abnormal vitamin D metabolism (e.g. chronic renal failure, pseudohypoparathyroidism)
   (c) decreased vitamin D bioavailability (e.g. inadequate sunlight, nephrotic syndrome, peritoneal dialysis)
2. Phosphate unavailability caused by phosphate binding antacids, hereditary hypophosphataemia, tumour-induced osteomalacia (e.g. fibrous dysplasia of bone), and Fanconi syndrome type 1 or 2
3. Metabolic acidosis (e.g. distal renal tubular acidosis)

6. Inquire about a poor diet (a low-fat diet often limits calcium intake) or inadequate sunlight exposure if a recent immigrant or nursing home resident, a history of renal disease or phenytoin use (all risk factors for osteomalacia). Ask about the patient's exercise history. Physical activity throughout life preserves bone mass. Cigarette smoking reduces skeletal mass.

7. Determine any risk factors for falls: a greater risk of falls increases the risk of fracture at any level of osteoporosis.
8. Determine the social impact of the disease (e.g. immobility).

The examination

There are usually no signs of osteoporosis unless a recent fracture has occurred. Examine for bone tenderness and proximal weakness. Look for signs of thyroid disease and Cushing's syndrome. Thoracic kyphosis may be a sign of vertebral fractures. Assess weight and general nutritional status.

Investigations

1. Bone densitometry using dual-energy X-ray absorptiometry (DEXA) of the lumbar spine and/or proximal femur remains the test of choice for evaluation of bone mineral density (Table 6.64). Osteopenia is used to refer to a bone mineral density between 1 and 2.5 standard deviations below peak bone mass; osteoporosis refers to a bone mineral density of more than 2.5 standard deviations below peak bone mass. The measurement is often given as a T score. This is the number of standard deviations by which the measured bone density falls below the average for a young normal person of the same sex. For example, a T score of <–2.5 means severe osteoporosis.
2. Review the serum calcium and alkaline phosphatase results. In osteoporosis, serum calcium and alkaline phosphatase levels should be normal. Alkaline phosphatase is usually elevated in all forms of osteomalacia. If there is vitamin D deficiency, then serum 25-OH vitamin D levels are usually low (e.g. vitamin D malabsorption, chronic liver disease). Assessment of calcium, parathyroid hormone and vitamin D levels will usually distinguish the most important causes of osteomalacia, and allow specific diagnostic tests to be appropriately directed (Table 6.65).

   A sustained elevation of alkaline phosphatase should lead to consideration of osteomalacia as well as Paget's disease and metastatic malignancy to bone. A full blood count and erythrocyte sedimentation rate (ESR) estimation should be ordered to look for evidence of myeloproliferative disease, and renal and liver function tests ordered to exclude renal or hepatic disease. Thyroid stimulating hormone should be measured to rule out thyrotoxicosis. If osteoporosis is unexpectedly severe, then an electrophoretogram (EPG) should be considered to rule out multiple myeloma. In men, a serum testosterone level is worthwhile.
3. Ask to review any skeletal X-rays. In osteoporosis of the spine, there is characteristic loss of trabecular bone in the vertebral body, including accentuation of the

---

Table 6.64   Indications for bone mineral density (BMD) assay

Fracture occurring after minimal trauma
Monitoring of known low BMD after at least 1 year
Monitoring of bone loss after prolonged steroid use, or as a result of hypogonadism
Monitoring of bone loss in primary hyperthyroidism, chronic liver disease, chronic renal disease, Crohn's disease, known malabsorption, and rheumatoid arthritis
Measurement of BMD 12 months after change in treatment for known low BMD

Table 6.65   Tests in bone disease

Disease	Calcium	Phosphate	25-OH vitamin D	Parathyroid hormone	Alkaline phosphatase (bone)
Osteoporosis	N	N	N	N	N
Osteomalacia or rickets owing to malabsorption or dietary lack	Low–N	Low–N	Decreased	Increased–N	Increased
Osteomalacia with renal bone disease	Variable	N–increased	Variable	Increased–N	Increased
Familial hypophos-phataemic rickets	N	Decreased	N	N	Increased
Primary hyperpara-thyroidism	Increased	Decreased–N	N	N	Increased
Paget's disease	N	N	N	N	Increased

N = normal.

vertebral endplates. The vertebral trabeculae become more prominent with the loss of horizontal trabeculae. Also look for collapse, anterior wedging and the codfish deformity (from expansion of the intervertebral disc).

In osteomalacia, X-rays may show some decrease in bone density with coarsening of trabeculae and blurring of the margins. A specific abnormality is Looser's zones (pseudo fractures) in the long bone shafts; these are ribbon-like zones of rarefaction. Other characteristic abnormalities may include a triangular (trefoil) pelvis and biconcave collapsed vertebrae. If there is secondary hyperparathyroidism present with osteomalacia, then bone cysts, erosion of the distal ends of the clavicles and subperiosteal resorption in the phalanges may be seen.

4. In difficult cases, an iliac crest bone biopsy with double tetracycline labelling can help distinguish osteoporosis from osteomalacia.
5. Consider undertaking tests for secondary causes of osteoporosis if the clinical picture suggests this may be helpful.

Treatment

Established osteoporosis is currently not reversible with medical therapy. Early intervention can prevent progression of osteoporosis and is of value. Secondary causes of osteoporosis should be identified and corrected if present.

1. *Calcium.* As calcium absorption decreases with age, calcium therapy has a modest benefit in both early and late postmenopausal women. Calcium intake of less than 400 g/day is unlikely to affect skeletal calcification. Consumption of 1500 mg of calcium daily in adults over the age of 65 is sensible.

2. *Bisphosphonates.* These drugs increase bone mineral density in postmenopausal women. They are currently indicated for use in Australia for patients with proven osteoporosis and fracture related to minimal trauma. These drugs can cause oesophageal ulceration that presents with odynophagia, usually within 1–2 months of commencing therapy. Patients unable to tolerate oral bisphosphonates can be given the drug as an infusion once every 3 months or, with some of the newer agents, once a year.

3. *Oestrogen.* Both oral and topical oestrogen will prevent loss of cortical and trabecular bone in postmenopausal women. Therapy is probably more effective if started earlier in menopause as bone loss is most rapid then. As oestrogen increases the risk of endometrial carcinoma, combination with progesterone is important unless a hysterectomy has been performed. A past history of endometrial cancer is a contraindication. There is an increased risk of breast cancer as well as deep venous thrombosis and pulmonary embolism. Cardiovascular risk is also increased, at least at first.

4. *Selective oestrogen receptor modulators.* Raloxifene, closely related to tamoxifen, reduces the risk of spine fractures. It increases the risk of deep venous thrombosis but has a lower risk of breast cancer. Tamoxifen is a mixed oestrogen receptor antagonist and agonist that prevents bone loss.

5. *Parathyroid hormone peptide.* This drug is very effective for osteoporosis but very expensive.

6. *Calcitonin.* There have been inconsistent results with calcitonin and any effect is smaller than with other therapies. The drug can be given subcutaneously or intranasally. Administration can cause nausea, flushing and inflammation.

7. *Vitamin D.* The role of vitamin D in postmenopausal osteoporosis is controversial but vitamin D is of definite value in patients with low levels of vitamin D. Serum calcium levels should be monitored when patients are given synthetic vitamin D.

8. *Men with osteoporosis.* In men who have osteoporosis and androgen deficiency, androgen replacement should be given unless there is a history of prostatic carcinoma. If there is secondary hypogonadism, human chorionic gonadotrophin or pulsatile gonadotrophin-releasing hormone may be worthwhile. The value of bisphosphonates and calcitonin as well as raloxifene is not clear in men.

9. *Steroid-induced osteoporosis.* This is very important because, if prednisone is considered likely to be needed for a number of months or longer, then measures to prevent bone loss are important from the time steroids are begun, particularly in postmenopausal women or when high doses are needed. Coadministration of bisphosphonates is of value here. Calcium and 25-OH vitamin D in combination has also been shown to be effective. These are the only drugs that have been shown to reduce fracture risk for patients on steroids. Other measures, such as cessation of smoking and an exercise regimen, are important and must be recommended strongly to the patient.

10. *Surgical treatment of fractures* is often required. Frail elderly patients with other medical problems will require careful assessment of anaesthetic risk. Vertebral fractures may cause severe pain that requires potent analgesics. Bed rest should be

as brief as possible. Injection of bone cement into the vertebral body (vertebro-plasty) is a new treatment that may relieve pain and possibly has other benefits.

Hypercalcaemia

Hypercalcaemia is a common medical problem and therefore can appear in a long case. It is most likely to be a diagnostic problem. Most patients (90%) have hyper-parathyroidism or malignancy (Table 6.66). The asymptomatic patient usually has hyperparathyroidism. A malignant condition that is advanced enough to cause hypercalcaemia is likely to have caused other symptoms.

Table 6.66   Causes of hypercalcaemia

1. Primary hyperparathyroidism (from a solitary adenoma, or multiple endocrine neoplasia rarely)
2. Malignancy (e.g. metastatic breast cancer, lung or renal cancer releasing humoral mediators, haematological malignancies)
3. Increased vitamin D (excess ingestion, granulomatous disease) (increased 25-OH vitamin D)
4. Increased bone turnover (e.g. hyperthyroidism, thiazide diuretics, vitamin A intoxication)
5. Renal failure (secondary hyperparathyroidism)
6. Familial hypocalciuric hypercalcaemia
7. Other (e.g. lithium)

The history

1. If the patient tells you that he or she has high calcium levels, inquire about the non-specific symptomatic manifestations. These include tiredness, weakness or episodes of confusion. Inquire about anorexia and constipation as well as nausea and vomiting: acute abdominal pain from acute pancreatitis may have occurred. Inquire about polyuria and polydipsia. Ask about a history of hypertension or a slow heart rate.
2. Inquire about a history of peptic ulcer or renal colic ('stones, moans, bones and abdominal groans' from primary hyperparathyroidism). Ask about joint pain from pseudogout (chondrocalcinosis in primary hyperparathyroidism). Inquire about a past history of hypertension (hyperparathyroidism).
3. Ask the patient if he or she was known to have a neck mass in the past or have had an operation to remove the parathyroid gland. In most cases a single adenomatous gland is found but they can be multiple. Surgical parathyroidectomy is the definitive treatment for primary hyperparathyroidism. Most neck masses will be coincidental thyroid nodules rather than a benign or malignant parathyroid tumour.
4. Ask the patient if he or she has had an examination of the eye and whether calcium was seen (band keratopathy). Also ask the patient if there have been X-rays of the bones. X-rays of the hand may show, in hyperparathyroidism, sub-periosteal reabsorption on the radial sides of the phalanges and in the distal phalangeal tufts (as well as in the distal clavicles).
5. Determine if there is any past history of malignant disease, including diseases that metastasise to bone (e.g. carcinoma or myeloma) or haematological disease such as lymphoma (ectopic vitamin D production).
6. Ask about drugs, including thiazide diuretics, lithium, and ingestion of calcium or vitamin D.

7. Inquire about known renal failure, a cause of secondary hyperparathyroidism because of resistance to parathyroid hormone and growth of the size of the glands. These enlarged glands then produce partly non-suppressible parathyroid hormone and hypercalcaemia.

8. Ask about symptoms of thyrotoxicosis or phaeochromocytoma. Ask about recent immobilisation.

9. Check if there is a family history of high serum calcium levels, such as familial hypocalciuric hypercalcaemia (autosomal dominant). Classically a patient with this condition has had hypercalcaemia since a relatively young age, with only a slight elevation in the serum parathyroid hormone level at most and with a personal or family history of unsuccessful neck exploration; it does not require any therapy. A family history of hypercalcaemia may also occur with the multiple endocrine neoplasia syndromes, MEN1 and MEN2A. These are both autosomal dominant conditions. These patients may have symptoms related to the other features of their MEN syndrome (e.g. peptic ulceration from the Zollinger-Ellison syndrome owing to excess gastrin secretion).

10. Many patients are asymptomatic and had hypercalcaemia detected on a routine set of biochemical tests. Hyperparathyroidism has been recognised much more commonly since automated biochemical analyses have become routine.

The examination

Look for any evidence of a neck scar from parathyroid surgery, as well as forearm scars from reimplantation of a parathyroid gland from the neck. Evaluate the patient for evidence of malignancy, including lymphadenopathy or organomegaly. Look for evidence of renal failure. Carefully evaluate the respiratory system for any evidence of sarcoidosis as well as tuberculosis or histoplasmosis.

Take the pulse for bradycardia, a result of a high serum calcium level. Measure the blood pressure for evidence of phaeochromocytoma. Examine for signs of thyrotoxicosis. Look for pigmentation from Addison's disease. Examine for proximal weakness and signs of pseudogout in the joints. Examine the cornea for band keratopathy (calcification at 3 and 9 o'clock).

Investigations

Look at the total serum calcium level. Remember that apparently high calcium levels can be the result of haemoconcentration while the blood is being collected. Correct for hypoalbuminaemia: add 0.02 mmol/L to the serum calcium concentration for every 1 g/L by which the serum albumin level is less than 40 g/L. The calcium level at which symptoms occur varies, but most patients have symptoms when the corrected calcium level reaches 3 mmol/L. Higher levels are associated with tissue calcification and the risk of renal failure, especially if the phosphate level is normal or increased by renal impairment. Once the calcium level approaches 4 mmol/L, unconsciousness and cardiac arrest can occur.

Measure the parathyroid hormone level. If elevated, primary hyperparathyroidism is the most likely diagnosis. If the patient is taking lithium or thiazide, the test should be repeated after discontinuing drug treatment because these drugs may influence both calcium and parathyroid hormone secretion. In a young otherwise asymptomatic person with a marginal elevation of parathyroid hormone, a 24-hour urine calcium examination should be asked for next to exclude familial hypocalciuric hypercalcaemia. The condition is caused by faulty calcium sensing by the parathyroid glands and renal tubules.

If there is a low or undetectable parathyroid hormone level, consider the possibility of granulomatous disease, including sarcoidosis and lymphoma. An increased level of 25-OH vitamin D supports this possibility. Ask first to review the chest X-ray.

Increased urinary cyclic AMP levels are suggestive of tumour secretion. Investigations to look for malignancy if suspected (e.g. protein electrophoresis, computed tomography [CT] scan, etc.) may then be required.

Treatment

If the diagnosis is hyperparathyroidism, surgical parathyroidectomy is usually indicated. If the patient is asymptomatic, then treatment is more controversial but younger patients with higher calcium levels will usually be offered surgery. Preoperative localisation is not required for the skilled surgeon, but if there is a need for a repeat procedure this can be evaluated using ultrasonography, CT or technetium-99m sestamibi scanning.

Note whether there has been hypocalcaemia after surgery. If there is no residual parathyroid tissue left, lifelong vitamin D therapy is necessary or, alternatively, autotransplantation of parathyroid tissue into the forearm may be offered.

In malignant hypercalcaemia, the underlying tumour should be treated. Steroids are often effective in lowering the serum calcium level. With granulomatous disease, steroids are also effective in lowering the calcium level; chloroquine may be useful in patients who cannot tolerate steroids.

Lithium treatment may need to be stopped. Hypercalcaemia does not necessarily mean lithium toxicity.

Familial hypocalciuric hypercalcaemia rarely causes symptoms and should not be treated with parathyroidectomy.

In an emergency, rehydration with intravenous saline and frusemide is indicated. Parenteral calcitonin lowers calcium levels only transiently. The use of intravenous bisphosphonates can be very effective but requires repeated doses.

There is evidence that asymptomatic patients with hyperparathyroidism who are not treated have increased bone loss compared with controls. Significant increases in fracture risk (especially of the wrist and spine) have been demonstrated.

Paget's disease of the bone (osteitis deformans)

This is usually a disease of the elderly but it may occur in younger patients. Less than 1% of the adult population is affected. The condition is characterised by excessive resorption of bone and increased formation of new bone in an irregular 'mosaic' pattern. Bone turnover may be increased 20 times early in the course of the disease. The aetiology is unknown but may be caused by a persistent paramyxovirus infection of osteoclasts. There are reports of familial occurrence with an autosomal dominant inheritance. It presents as a management problem.

The history

1. Ask about symptoms that led to the diagnosis:
   (a) isolated elevation of alkaline phosphatase on routine blood testing
   (b) an incidental finding on an X-ray
   (c) bone pain
   (d) secondary osteoarthritis
   (e) change in height or hat size
   (f) progressive bone deformity or pathological fracture; gait abnormalities associated with change in length of a long bone
   (g) neurological symptoms—hearing loss, neurological gait disturbance (suggestive of basilar invagination with long tract, or cerebellar involvement or spinal cord compression), cranial nerve symptoms, headache
   (h) symptoms of congestive cardiac failure
   (i) symptoms of renal colic (as there is an increased incidence of calcium nephrolithiasis in this disease, especially during the resorptive phase)

(j) gout, secondary to increased bone turnover
(k) sarcoma of bone (very rare—less than 1% of cases, occasionally multicentric)
(l) symptoms of hypercalcaemia—thirst, polyuria, nausea, coma (a rare occurrence even in immobilised patients or alternatively caused by coexisting primary hyperparathyroidism, which is common)
(m) pathological fractures, especially of the convex side of weight-bearing bones and can be multiple.

2. Inquire about articular pain, which may be caused by secondary osteoarthritis in joints adjacent to sites of pagetic involvement and true bone pain. Secondary osteoarthritis is characterised by pain and stiffness, which improves with joint movement; alternatively it may initially be exacerbated by weight-bearing and relieved by rest. True bone pain is more often constant or gnawing and is worse at night. A sudden exacerbation of bone pain may indicate a pathological fracture or the development of an osteosarcoma.
3. Ask about treatment, its effectiveness and side-effects.
4. Inquire about disability at home and work. Remember, though, that most patients are asymptomatic.

The examination (Fig 6.18)

Figure 6.18 Paget's disease.

1. GENERAL INSPECTION
    Short stature
    Limb deformity
    Obvious osteosarcoma (bony
       swelling)

2. FACE
    Skull diameter (measure)
    Auscultate skull (bruits)
    Fundi—angioid streaks, optic
       atrophy
    Hearing (ossicle or VIII nerve
       involvement)
    Other cranial nerves (foramina
       overgrowth or basilar invagination)

3. NECK
    Short neck (basilar invagination)
    Jugular venous pressure—cardiac
       failure (high output)

4. BACK
    Deformity

Tenderness
Warmth
Bruits

5. LEGS
    Bowing femur, tibia
    Tenderness, warmth, swelling
       bones
    Hip examination (movements)
    Knee examination

6. GAIT

7. NEUROLOGICAL ASSESSMENT
    OF LIMBS
    (spinal cord compression, basilar
       invagination)

8. OTHER
    Urine (blood)
    Height (measure)

Inspect generally for short stature and obvious deformity.

Look at the face. Measure the skull diameter (>55 cm is usually abnormal). Look for prominent skull veins, feel for bony warmth (actually caused by vasodilatation in the skin) and auscultate for systolic bruits. Examine the fundi for angioid streaks (Table 8.30) and for papilloedema or optic atrophy, which are rare. Also assess visual acuity and visual fields. Test to see if hearing is decreased as a result of ossicle involvement or eighth nerve compression. Remember, *all* the other cranial nerves (p 283) may rarely be affected owing to overgrowth of foramina or basilar invagination, so examine them carefully.

Look at the neck for basilar invagination. These patients have a short neck and low hairline, the head is held in extension and neck movements are decreased. Assess the jugular venous pressure and examine the heart for signs of cardiac failure owing to a hyperdynamic circulation (p 226).

Examine the back (p 282). Note any deformity, especially kyphosis. Tap for tenderness. Feel for warmth. Auscultate for systolic bruits over the vertebral bodies.

Look at the legs for anterior bowing of the tibia and lateral bowing of the femur. Feel for warmth. Note any changes of osteoarthritis in the hips and knees. There may be limitation of hip movements—especially of abduction, which suggests protrusio acetabulae—and fixed flexion deformity of the knees (p 281). Be careful, as the bones may be tender.

Sarcomas (a feared, but rare complication) should be looked for, particularly in the femur, humerus and skull; they usually present as tender, localised swellings. They can be multiple.

A full neurological examination is necessary for spinal cord compression and basilar invagination, which may even cause quadriparesis. If the patient is mobile, don't forget to assess walking for any disability (p 317). Cerebellar signs may also rarely occur with basilar invagination.

Check the urine analysis (for blood, as renal stone incidence is increased) and measure the patient's height (for serial follow-up).

Investigations

These are indicated in symptomatic patients requiring treatment and in asymptomatic subjects to determine the extent of skeletal involvement. Testing for hypercalcaemia may be worthwhile for any patient who is immobilised.

The serum alkaline phosphatase level is an indicator of disease activity, as is the urinary hydroxyproline level. Other biochemical markers of bone turnover will also be increased (e.g. osteocalcin, urine or serum cross-links of collagen).

Radiologically the bones most often involved are the pelvis, femur, skull and tibia. Look for bony enlargement, increased density, an irregular widened cortex and cortical infractions (incomplete pseudofractures) on the convex side of the bowed long bones. The early lytic phase of the disease, presenting with a flame-shaped osteolytic wedge advancing along the bones, is often overlooked. Secondary arthritic changes may occur (e.g. hips). Bone scanning is more sensitive than an X-ray in assessing the extent of disease. CT scanning or magnetic resonance imaging (MRI) may be useful in the investigation of an atypical lesion, especially if sarcoma is suspected.

Paget's disease is occasionally confused with osteoblastic bone secondaries (e.g. from prostate, Hodgkin's disease) or fibrous dysplasia.

Treatment

The indications for treatment are bone pain, progressive deformity, or complications such as neural compression or high-output cardiac failure, and as a prelude to orthopaedic surgery. Treatment of patients with pagetic involvement of weight-bearing bones may be indicated to attempt to prevent deformity and pathological fracture. Proof of benefit is not available, however.

Simple analgesics or non-steroidal anti-inflammatory drugs (NSAIDs), including cyclo-oxygenase 2 (COX-2) inhibitors, should be used first to control pain. Orthopaedic procedures such as total hip replacement may be indicated.

A number of drugs are available which reduce bone resorption. Calcitonin of salmon or human origin, given subcutaneously, often improves bone pain and may be useful in the treatment of neurological complications. Although side-effects (nausea, flushing and diarrhoea) are common and may limit treatment in up to 20% of patients, it is still regarded as first-line therapy. Resistance to salmon calcitonin after 1–2 years may indicate the development of neutralising antibodies. Serum alkaline phosphatase levels and urinary hydroxyproline levels are useful guides to the effect of treatment; a 50% reduction in either test value indicates a good response to treatment.

An oral bisphosphonate (e.g. alendronate) is usually effective at reducing hydroxy-proline excretion and often relieves symptoms but may exacerbate bone pain initially. It also impairs bone mineralisation and may cause osteomalacia. However, bone turnover is reduced and new bone is usually more normal in structure. The bisphosphonates should be given in combination with calcium supplements and vitamin D (400 IU/day). Ulcerating oesophagitis causing dysphagia is an important side-effect. Many now use this drug as first-line therapy; it is not generally indicated for asymptomatic patients. Intravenous infusions of the potent bisphosphonate pamidronate (APD, disodium-3-amino-1-hydroxypropylidenediphosphonate) may produce prolonged suppression of pagetic activity and may normalise bone turnover in patients with mild disease without adverse effects on bone mineralisation or bone formation.

Mithramycin, given intravenously, can be very effective. It is reserved for occasions when rapid remission is required (e.g. spinal cord compression). There may be significant increases in bone lysis and predisposition to fractures with this drug, as well as bone marrow depression.

Surgery, including osteotomy for misshapen femurs, may be useful. It is important for the patient to avoid immobilisation in the postoperative period because of the risk of hypercalcaemia.

The appearance of osteosarcoma is associated with a poor prognosis. Preoperative chemotherapy followed by amputation—the current treatment for spontaneously occurring tumours—is being evaluated.

Acromegaly

Although an uncommon condition, acromegaly is a chronic illness and common as a long or a short case (p 272).

The history

The patient will probably know the diagnosis, although if the condition has only recently been suspected investigations may still be underway. The patient may be in hospital for these tests because of a complication of the condition or, perhaps more likely, has been brought in for the clinical examinations.

1. Find out when the diagnosis was made and how long ago; in retrospect, the patient may have had symptoms for years. The average time taken to make the diagnosis is more than 10 years.
2. Ask why the diagnosis was suspected. The onset of abnormalities is usually very gradual. The common features of the condition are listed in Table 6.67. Ask what changes the patient has been aware of and whether these have improved with treatment. Bony and acral changes are irreversible and early diagnosis is worthwhile.
3. Ask about the associations and complications of the condition. The mortality rate for untreated acromegaly is about twice that of the age-matched population, mostly as a result of an increased risk of cardiovascular disease. There is also an increase in the incidence of colonic polyps and carcinoma of the colon.
4. There is now a recognised association with obstructive sleep apnoea, and questions should be asked about snoring, daytime sleepiness and the other relevant symptoms. The reason for the association is the enlargement of the tongue and swelling of the upper airway.

Table 6.67 **Symptoms and signs in acromegaly**

Acral enlargement*
Enlarged jaw and facial features*
Sweating*
Soft-tissue enlargement*
Headache*
Peripheral neuropathy
Paraesthesiae
Carpal tunnel syndrome
Symptoms of sleep apnoea
Impotence
Muscle weakness
Galactorrhoea

* In >50% of patients.

---

5. Ask if the patient knows what investigations have been performed (see investigations below).
6. Ask about current and past treatment and how helpful this has been. Pituitary surgery and radiotherapy have a number of complications.
7. As with any chronic illness, the effect of acromegaly on the patient's life may be severe. Ask about occupation and ability to work.

The examination

See page 265.

Investigations

The condition has been diagnosed in the past with a glucose tolerance test; here growth hormone (GH) suppression is measured in response to a glucose load. Failure of suppression is characteristic of acromegaly but the test is non-specific and may be abnormal in renal impairment, thyrotoxicosis and diabetes. The preferred test now is measurement of insulin-like growth factor I (IGF-I). Unlike GH, the level of IGF-I does not fluctuate and the absolute level reliably reflects the average GH level. There is physiological elevation of the level in pregnancy and during puberty, but otherwise elevation is very specific for acromegaly. In 25% of acromegalic patients, the prolactin level is elevated and this can be associated with galactorrhoea. Other pituitary hormone levels may be low because of interference with normal pituitary function by the large mass of the tumour. Baseline pituitary function should be assessed with measurements of prolactin, cortisol, thyroxine and either oestradiol or testosterone.

Imaging is performed once an elevated IGF-I is confirmed. MRI scanning is the modality of choice. It provides excellent anatomical definition of the tumour.

Treatment

The aim of treatment is to prevent excess GH production without interfering with normal pituitary function. Early diagnosis makes treatment easier and more effective, and IGF-I testing makes the diagnosis easier.

Acromegaly is cured when the IGF-I level is normal and is suppressed to less than 2 mIU/L after an oral glucose load. However, symptomatic relief can be obtained without complete cure.

Medical treatment

Long-acting somatostatin analogues, such as octreotide, are now available. These drugs mimic the inhibition of GH release by somatostatin. They have the advantage that they are long-acting enough to be effective when given by subcutaneous injection. The usual dose is 100 μg three times a day but this can be increased to up to 1500 μg/day. Unlike somatostatin they do not significantly inhibit insulin secretion. Unless surgery or radiotherapy has cured the disease, octreotide must be continued indefinitely. Symptoms such as headache, arthralgia and sweating improve after a few weeks. The drug will also cause a reduction in the size of the tumour, which can make surgery easier. Side-effects of treatment are usually relatively mild and include discomfort at the injection site, diarrhoea, anorexia, abdominal bloating and cholelithiasis. Long-acting depot injections are now available but expensive. For this reason they are usually reserved for patients in whom other treatment has not been completely successful or is contraindicated.

Bromocriptine is also available for treating acromegaly. It causes a paradoxical suppression of GH release in acromegalics but at tolerated doses remission is not usually obtained. Side-effects include nausea, anorexia and hypotension. The drug is most often used as adjunctive treatment after radiotherapy or surgery.

Newer dopamine agonists that are more effective than bromocriptine include cabergoline.

Surgery

Trans-sphenoidal pituitary surgery is effective at selectively resecting the benign adenoma and preserving pituitary function in 50–80% of surgically treated cases. If cure is defined as a return of IGF-I to the normal range, then surgical cure is less often obtained. Nevertheless, symptoms are almost always greatly relieved by surgery. The perioperative mortality rate should be less than 1%. Uncommon complications include cerebrospinal fluid rhinorrhoea, diabetes insipidus and stroke. Hypopituitarism follows eventually in about 10% of patients.

Radiotherapy

Conventional radiotherapy delivers about 5000 cGy to the pituitary over 5 weeks. It works only slowly. GH levels take a year to fall by 25%. Even after 10 years few patients achieve normal IGF-I levels. Hypopituitarism is common after radiotherapy but other side-effects are rare. Newer, more promising techniques use computerised MRI to deliver larger doses accurately to the gland ('stereotactic radiosurgery').

Overall, surgery remains the treatment of first choice. Medical treatment with somatostatin analogues is increasingly useful, both before surgery and afterwards if removal is incomplete.

Types 1 and 2 diabetes mellitus

This is a common subject for the long case as diabetic patients are always available. Diabetes presents usually a management rather than a diagnostic problem. The examiners like this disease because it tests very practical management skills. The classification of the types of diabetes has been revised. Juvenile diabetes (immune-mediated diabetes) is now called type 1 and maturity-onset diabetes (non-immune-mediated diabetes), type 2. Most type 1 diabetes (type 1A) is associated with autoimmune destruction of islet cells but a small proportion of these diabetics do not have these abnormalities (type 1B). The cause of diabetes in these patients is not known but it is more common in Asian populations. Type 2 diabetes is increasingly found in obese adolescents and children. Over 90% of diabetics have type 2 disease.

Don't forget the criteria for diagnosis of diabetes mellitus—a fasting (overnight) blood sugar level of 7.0 mmol/L or higher on at least two separate occasions or, in the absence of fasting hyperglycaemia, a 2-hour postprandial glucose level of 11.1 mmol/L or higher. Fasting blood glucose levels between 6.1 and 7.0 mmol/L are considered to represent impaired fasting glucose levels. There is evidence that complications of diabetes may occur in some populations when the fasting glucose level is over 6.1 mmol/L.

The history

1. Ask about the age at which diabetes was diagnosed and its manner of presentation—thirst, polyuria and polydipsia, weight loss, infection, ketoacidosis, asymptomatic glycosuria. Remember the rare causes of glucose intolerance (Table 6.68).

Table 6.68   Causes of glucose intolerance

1. Diabetes mellitus
2. Counter-regulatory hormone excess (rare)
   Acromegaly
   Cushing's syndrome
   Phaeochromocytoma
   Glucagonoma (associated with necrolytic erythema)
3. Pregnancy
4. Drugs
   Steroids or oral contraceptives
   Streptozotocin
   Thiazide diuretics (temporary and mild, secondary to hypokalaemia)
   Phenytoin, diazoxide (insulin secretion inhibited)
5. Pancreatic disease
   Chronic pancreatitis or carcinoma
   Haemochromatosis (decreased insulin production with or without increased insulin resistance)
6. Chronic liver disease (insulin resistance)
7. Syndromes:
   Lipoatrophic diabetes (generalised lipoatrophy, hepatomegaly, hirsutism, hyperpigmentation, hyperlipidaemia)
   Type A syndrome (usually young women with acanthosis nigricans and polycystic ovary disease)
   Type B syndrome (acanthosis nigricans and autoimmune disease)

---

2. Ask about the treatment initiated at diagnosis and major changes that have occurred over time (insulin is required for survival in type 1 diabetes, which usually has an onset below age 30 years; in type 2 diabetes, control typically becomes more difficult with time).
3. Ask about the diet prescribed (Table 6.69). The previous strict dietary rules using exchanges and portions have largely been abandoned but some patients may still use them (one exchange = 15 g of carbohydrate = 60 calories = 250 kilojoules [but the definition does vary]; e.g. for an average-sized male, 3 exchanges for each main meal and 2 exchanges for morning and afternoon tea and supper are

Table 6.69 Dietary recommendations for diabetics (type 1 and type 2)
Protein 10–20% kJ/day
Saturated fat <10% kJ/day
Polyunsaturated fat 10% kJ/day
Carbohydrate and monounsaturated fats for the rest
Artificial sweeteners as required
Fibre 30 g/day
Minimise cholesterol intake (<300 g/day)

required to provide an even carbohydrate distribution—50% of the diet). Ask if the patient knows about the glycaemic index (GI) factor.

4. Ask whether oral hypoglycaemic drugs have been used or are being taken.
5. Ask about insulin treatment—how much and when taken. Also ask where the insulin is injected and by whom, and find out the type of insulin syringe used (e.g. a pen injector).
6. Ask about the progress of the disease:
   (a) assessment of control adequacy—Does the patient test the urine or (more likely and desirable) use a home blood glucose monitoring meter? Which glucose reagent strip is used and which meter? (Remember that different meters require different reagent strips.); inquire how often the tests are done, the usual results, at what time of day the test is performed (pre- or postprandial, or both) and whether the dose is adjusted at other times (e.g. gastrointestinal upset); ask about recent glycosylated haemoglobin (HbA_{1c}) results; ask about symptoms of poor control:
      (i) hyperglycaemia—polyuria, thirst, weight loss, intermittent blurring of vision, hospital admissions with ketoacidosis (type 1 diabetics only)
      (ii) hypoglycaemia/hypoglycaemia awareness—ask the patient to describe the symptoms and how they are managed; ask specifically about morning headaches, morning lethargy and night sweats (symptoms suggestive of nocturnal hypoglycaemia), weight gain and seizures; ask about the time of day in relationship to food, alcohol, exercise and insulin injection
   (b) involvement of other systems:
      (i) vascular system—ischaemic heart disease, intermittent claudication, cerebrovascular disease
      (ii) nervous system—peripheral neuropathy, autonomic neuropathy (causing erectile dysfunction, fainting, nocturnal diarrhoea) (see Table 8.36), amyotrophy
      (iii) eyes—regular visits to an ophthalmologist or retinal photography at the diabetes clinic and treatment received (ask especially about laser treatment)
      (iv) renal system—dysuria, nocturia, oedema, hypertension
      (v) skin—boils, vaginitis and balanitis, Candida, necrobiosis lipoidica (p 276).
7. Ask about drug history—steroids, thiazides, oral contraceptives, beta-blockers.
8. Ask about associated other diseases—history of pancreatitis, Cushing's syndrome (p 269), acromegaly (p 272).
9. Inquire about social background—type of work, living conditions (living alone or with family), coping with giving insulin (associated blindness, etc.), eating habits, financial situation, work, driving (type of licence held).

10. Ask about variations in weight, regular exercise program.
11. Ask about cardiovascular risk factors, including family history, serum cholesterol level, smoking, hypertension and drug and non-drug attempts at control of these factors (except family history).
12. Inquire about family history of diabetes and obstetric history (e.g. big babies, stillbirths), other risk factors for type 2 diabetes (Table 6.70).

Table 6.70   Risk factors for type 2 diabetes
Family history (first-degree relatives)
Age over 45
Overweight (BMI >27 kg/m^2)
Race (Australian Aboriginals—at risk with BMI >22 kg/m^2), Pacific Islander
Previous abnormal fasting glucose (6.1–7.0 mmol/L)
Gestational diabetes
Hypertension
Polycystic ovaries
BMI = body mass index.

The examination

Detailed examination is essential, looking specifically for complications of the disease. If obese, assess body mass index.

Management

The general aim is to regulate diet, exercise and insulin so as to allow the patient to lead a normal life while avoiding short- and long-term complications. In adults with type 1 diabetes, multiple injection regimens are preferred because the improved control prevents or retards the progression of complications.

The newly diagnosed diabetic

The major management decision here is whether insulin is required. This will, in some cases, be obvious (e.g. for the type 1 patient with ketoacidosis) but for many elderly, obese diabetics the position is not so clear. If insulin is not indicated at presentation, attempt to gain control first by weight loss and diet, followed by oral hypoglycaemic agents.

1. Weight loss to achieve ideal body weight increases insulin sensitivity. Abdominal obesity (waist–hip ratio >0.9 for women and >0.8 for men) increases the risk of metabolic complications.
2. Realise that there is some disagreement about the ideal diet but achieving ideal weight is essential. The recommended diet (Table 6.69) should be tailored to the patient's requirements and activities. For example, kilojoule recommendations for 20-year-old men undertaking normal activities are 175 kJ/kg of body weight and for a 75-year-old man are 140 kJ/kg. Distribution of carbohydrate should be worked out on an individual basis. Fat intake should be kept to 30% or lower of the kilojoules for patients who are not overweight and considerably less for obese patients. The distribution of kilojoules is more important for insulin-requiring patients, who should usually have about 20% for breakfast, 35% for lunch, 30% for

dinner and 15% for supper. Patients who use short-acting insulin before each meal may be able to vary the insulin dose to suit the meal. The diet should include high-fibre foods and monounsaturated fats. Polyunsaturated fats can raise triglyceride levels but monounsaturates tend to reduce them. Patients with nephropathy may be advised to restrict protein intake, usually to about 10% of caloric intake.

3. The use of oral hypoglycaemic agents is generally accepted.

   (a) Metformin is the only available biguanide and is regarded as the agent of choice in the obese patient with type 2 diabetes. Side-effects of biguanides include:

   (i)   diarrhoea, anorexia, nausea and occasionally vomiting

   (ii) vitamin B_{12} malabsorption

   (iii) lactic acidosis (the risk is increased in the elderly and in patients with cardiovascular, liver and renal disease).

   Metformin rarely causes hypoglycaemia and there is a synergistic effect when it is used in combination with sulfonylureas.

   (b) Sulfonylureas include first-generation drugs (e.g. chlorpropamide and tolbu-tamide) and second-generation drugs (e.g. gliclazide, used for obese patients; glipizide, used for thin patients; and glibenclamide). Second-generation drugs are as effective as the first-generation ones and are associated with fewer drug interactions. Side-effects of sulfonylureas include:

   (i)   possibly an increase in cardiovascular death rate—this fear seems not to have been well founded, as the UKPDS trial (see below) did not find any increase in cardiovascular mortality for patients on these drugs

   (ii)   prolonged hypoglycaemia—this is greatest with glibenclamide, which is therefore not recommended for those over the age of 60; gliclazide and glipizide are as effective and safer

   (iii) weight gain (owing to increase in appetite and mild hypoglycaemia)

   (iv)   bone marrow depression

   (v)   cholestatic jaundice

   (vi)   skin rash

   (vii) alcohol intolerance, causing flushing

   (viii) water retention and hyponatraemia (syndrome of inappropriate anti-diuretic hormone [SIADH]).

   The effectiveness of the sulfonylureas is variable and rates of secondary failure vary between agents. Primary failure occurs in 40% of cases, secondary failure in 3–30%; only 20–30% of patients continue with satisfactory control. Substitution of one drug for another may be worth trying before abandoning oral hypoglycaemic therapy.

   The mechanism of action of sulfonylureas is to increase insulin action peripherally, and to increase insulin secretion.

   (c) The thiazolidinediones are a newer class of oral hypoglycaemic drugs. They reduce insulin resistance, blood sugar levels and triglycerides. Pioglitazone and rosiglitazone are available in Australia. Their use is restricted to patients whose HbA_{1c} is over 7% during the previous 3 months and who are on maximum tolerated doses of metformin and a sulfonylurea. Patients on insulin must also be on metformin and have a raised HbA_{1c}. Liver function tests must be performed 2 monthly for the first year and the drug stopped if the alanine aminotransferase (ALT) level rises above 2.5 times normal. The drugs are associated with small rises in high-density lipoprotein (HDL) and low-density lipoprotein (LDL) cholesterol and with peripheral oedema. They are contraindicated for patients with class III or IV heart failure.

   (d) Acarbose inhibits intestinal alpha-glucosidase, slowing polysaccharide degradation and absorption. It is a useful agent taken before meals with other treatment. Side-effects include flatulence, diarrhoea and abdominal pain, but there is no major toxicity.

Insulin therapy

1. Insulin requirements initially are generally between 0.4 and 1.0 U/kg/day. An anorectic agent should be considered when requirements exceed 1.5 U/kg/day. Insulin therapy is now often begun on an outpatient basis and under these circumstances small doses (e.g. 0.25 U/kg/day), sufficient to prevent ketosis, are used with a view to avoiding hypoglycaemia. Possible insulin regimens include: the basic bolus regimens, using a short-acting insulin at mealtimes (actrapid or humulin R) with an intermediate or long-acting insulin at suppertime (isophane, lente or ultralente insulin); twice-daily double mix, using a combination of short- and intermediate-acting insulin (premixed ratios—short:intermediate 15:85, 20:80, 30:70 and 50:50—are commercially available, or the patient may mix insulins in a syringe). In patients with type 2 diabetes a combination of oral hypoglycaemic agents at mealtimes with an intermediate- or long-acting insulin at supper. Continuous subcutaneous insulin infusion is a treatment option but infusion devices remain beyond the means of most patients with diabetes and may be associated with an increased risk of morbidity and mortality related to hypoglycaemia. Intraperitoneal insulin administration in the dialysate is useful in the management of patients on continuous ambulatory peritoneal dialysis (CAPD), and continuous intraperitoneal infusion has been attempted in some centres.

   Human insulin has replaced the highly purified (monocomponent) insulins but bovine insulin is still available. When a patient is changed from bovine to human insulin, the insulin dosage should be reduced by about 20% because of differences in insulin kinetics. Many patients report altered symptoms of hypoglycaemia and a more rapid onset of symptoms after changing to human insulin. Aim for euglycaemia: ideally the glucose level should be between 3.5 and 7.0 mmol/L throughout the day and night.

2. Insulin resistance is defined as a requirement of more than 200 units per day. Causes of insulin resistance are:
   (a) obesity (decreased receptor number)
   (b) insulin antibodies (uncommon, and an indication for a more purified insulin)
   (c) circulating antagonist hormones—growth hormone (e.g. in puberty), cortisol, thyroxine, glucagon
   (d) association with acanthosis nigricans (e.g. receptor abnormalities, lipodystrophies). Remember, injecting into a lipoatrophied site may cause poor control because of unpredictable absorption.

3. Insulin allergy is now uncommon since the widespread introduction of human insulins but they can cause immediate local reactions (e.g. pruritus, local pain) or delayed reactions (e.g. swelling). Urticaria and anaphylaxis can also occur. Treatment in mild cases is with antihistamines and local steroids, but in severe cases desensitisation is important. Insulin allergy is more common in patients who stop and start insulin therapy.

4. Fasting hyperglycaemia is a major management problem. The 'Somogyi effect' refers to rebound morning hyperglycaemia following nocturnal hypoglycaemia, which is thought to be caused by release of counter-regulatory hormones. This is now, however, a matter of considerable debate. The treatment is to reduce the evening insulin dose. The 'dawn' phenomenon is early morning hyperglycaemia in the *absence* of nocturnal hypoglycaemia; here the treatment is to increase the insulin coverage without inducing hypoglycaemia.

5. Causes of hypoglycaemia in a previously stable diabetic on insulin therapy are:
   (a) decreased food intake, increased exercise or weight loss
   (b) injection errors
   (c) diabetic renal disease

    (d)   rare causes—high level of insulin antibodies, malabsorption, intestinal hurry, hypothyroidism, autoimmune adrenal insufficiency, panhypopituitarism or an insulinoma.

6. Haemoglobin A_{1c} gives an indication of control over the preceding 3 months and one should aim for a level of 7% or less, although the numbers may be distorted by one or two high blood sugar levels. Spurious readings may occur in renal failure, iron deficiency, haemoglobinopathies and pregnancy.

Diabetes education

As diabetes is a lifelong disease, detailed education by the team looking after the patient is important. Regular follow-up is essential. Blood glucose monitoring with a glucose meter is essential for all patients who can manage it—initially, testing several times a day before and 2 hours after meals, and before bed, may be necessary; later in stable diabetes twice-daily may be enough. Exercise promotes glucose utilisation; in the well-controlled diabetic it is important to reduce the dose of regular insulin before exercise or supplement with glucose. (*Note*: Exercise in the poorly controlled diabetic may precipitate ketoacidosis because of increased release of counter-regulatory hormones.)

Management of chronic complications

Complications are probably a result of damage caused by glycosylated proteins. Convincing evidence that tight control prevents or reverses complications is now available. Following the Diabetes Control and Complications Trial published in 1994 and the more recent United Kingdom Prognosis in Diabetes Study (UKPDS), clinicians now agree that rigorous control of blood sugar levels and aggressive control of blood pressure and other cardiovascular risk factors is essential. The blood pressure can be managed with any antihypertensive but the use of an angiotensin-converting (ACE) inhibitor or angiotensin II receptor blocker is strongly indicated when proteinuria has been detected, and is used routinely by some endocrinologists. Lipid control with the statins is being assessed in a number of trials. The high cardiovascular risk of these patients suggests that aggressive lipid-lowering with one of these drugs will be of value. Remember to control other risk factors, such as smoking (for retinopathy and vascular disease) and alcohol intake (for neuropathy and hypertriglyceridaemia).

Ideally, all patients are assessed every 2 years by an ophthalmologist. Less sophisticated fundoscopy may miss early diabetic retinopathy (see Table 8.37). Retinal cameras can now be used at the clinic to take clear retinal photographs, which can be repeated often and 'read' by an ophthalmologist.

Diabetic nephropathy is a common cause of chronic renal failure and results from arteriolar disease or glomerulosclerosis (classic Kimmelstiel-Wilson lesion or, more commonly, diffuse intercapillary glomerulosclerosis). The evolution of diabetic nephropathy has been well studied and can be divided into the following stages: (i) glomerular hyperfiltration; (ii) microalbuminuria; (iii) dipstick proteinuria; (iv) proteinuria in the nephrotic range; and (v) end-stage renal failure. Microalbuminuria is defined as a urinary albumin excretion in excess of 200 µg/min (measured using sensitive immunoassays) on more than two occasions in the absence of urinary tract infection and intercurrent illness. The albumin-to-creatinine ratio may be a more sensitive way of assessing the presence of significant proteinuria. Regular screening for microalbuminuria is now considered an important component of good diabetes management. The microalbuminuria stage is probably reversible with a combination of ACE inhibitor therapy, strict metabolic control and possibly dietary protein restriction. Once proteinuria develops, progression to end-stage renal failure appears inevitable over a period of about 5–10 years. The rate of progression may be modified by: control of hypertension—ACE inhibitors are the agents of choice but it is important to be aware of the risk of hyperkalaemia as a result of hyporeninaemic hypoaldosteronism and deteriorating renal function in patients with renovascular disease; treatment of urinary tract infections; dietary protein restriction; and possibly improving glucose control. ACE inhibition is indicated as soon as proteinuria is detected. There is an increased incidence of papillary necrosis with urinary tract infection. The best form of management for end-stage chronic renal failure in a diabetic is peritoneal dialysis and early renal transplantation. Remember that diabetics with chronic renal failure almost invariably also have retinopathy, which may be worsened by haemodialysis.

For those with severe systemic complications or end-stage renal disease, whole-organ pancreas (with or without kidney) transplantation is a promising therapeutic option. A number of successful kidney/pancreas transplants have been performed. Patients are generally euglycaemic without hypoglycaemic treatment. This is the treatment of choice for diabetics with renal failure.

The pregnant diabetic

Remember that blood sugar levels are normally lower in pregnancy. A woman with no diabetic history should be screened for gestational diabetes in the 24th–28th week. A 50-g glucose load is given and the blood sugar is measured 1 hour later. The normal result is <7.0 mmol/L. Between 7.0 and 7.8 mmol/L is borderline (repeat) and ≥7.8 mmol/L means that a formal 75-g glucose tolerance test is required. A fasting level of ≥5.5 mmol/L or a 2-hour level of ≥8.0 mmol/L indicates gestational diabetes mellitus.

Insulin requirements vary during pregnancy owing to the effects of human placental lactogen (HPL). In the first trimester, insulin requirements usually remain unchanged or may decrease, but in the second trimester some increase in insulin requirements occurs owing to rising HPL levels. By the third trimester insulin requirements are usually at least 50% higher than before pregnancy, but after delivery there is a dramatic decrease in insulin requirement.

Blood glucose control should be improved as much as possible before conception in a diabetic woman wanting to undertake pregnancy. Haemoglobin A_{1c} should be normalised, as strict metabolic control at the time of conception has been shown to prevent the otherwise increased incidence of congenital malformations in the offspring of diabetic mothers. The complications of poor control seen in the infant are: congenital malformations (incidence about 6%, double the normal rate), such as spina bifida; macrosomia; intrauterine fetal death in the later stages of pregnancy; hypoglycaemia after delivery; and complications related to immaturity (e.g. respiratory distress syndrome, hypocalcaemia, jaundice).

Use of home blood glucose monitoring, with testing of both preprandial and postprandial glucose levels, is essential. Strict glucose control must be maintained during labour and delivery. Paediatric services and a neonatal intensive care unit should be available.

Renal system

Chronic renal failure

Chronic renal failure is not a particularly common subject for the long case. However, it is a difficult and important one. The patient will usually know he or she has renal disease. Methodical questioning to establish the diagnosis, cause, management and complications is necessary.

The history

Questions regarding symptoms, diagnosis and aetiology

1. The earliest symptoms of renal failure include nocturia, lethargy and loss of appetite. The first episode of overt renal failure may have been precipitated by a further insult,

such as use of non-steroidal anti-inflammatory drugs (NSAIDs), radiocontrast injections, infection, angiotensin-converting enzyme (ACE) inhibitors or angiotensin II receptor (AR) blockers, dehydration or anaemia.

2. Glomerulonephritis (Tables 6.71 and 6.72). Determine whether there is a history of proteinuria, haematuria, oliguria, oedema, sore throat, sepsis, rash, haemoptysis or renal biopsy. Ascertain treatment details (e.g. antihypertensives, immunosuppressives, antiplatelet therapy, dialysis).

3. Analgesic nephropathy. Ask about the number, type and duration of analgesics consumed, urinary tract infections, hypertension, haematuria, gastrointestinal blood loss, nocturia, renal colic (sloughed papillae, stones), transitional cell cancer and anaemia. This cause of renal failure is now very uncommon following the withdrawal of compound analgesics containing aspirin and phenacetin.

4. Polycystic kidneys (see Table 8.17). Ask about family history, how the disease was diagnosed, haematuria, polyuria, loin pain, hypertension, renal calculi, headache, subarachnoid haemorrhages and visual disturbance (intracranial aneurysm).

5. Reflux nephropathy. Ask about childhood renal infections, cystoscopy, operations, treatment (e.g. regular antibiotics) and enuresis.

6. Diabetic nephropathy (or other complaints), use of ACE inhibitors or AR blockers.

7. Hypertensive nephropathy. Ask how the disease was diagnosed, duration and control of hypertension, treatment and compliance with medication, angiography, family history.

8. Connective tissue disease, especially systemic lupus erythematosus and scleroderma.

9. Is the patient aware of the long-term prognosis? If he or she is not on dialysis yet, has this been discussed? Is the patient likely to be eligible for dialysis or the transplant list?

Table 6.71 **The nephrotic syndrome**

Clinical features
1. Proteinuria (>3.5 g/24 h)
2. Hypoalbuminaemia (serum albumin <30 g/L)
3. Oedema
4. Hyperlipidaemia (increased LDL and cholesterol levels)

Causes
1. Primary (80%)
   Idiopathic membranous glomerulonephropathy is the commonest cause in adults over 40 years of age. Other primary causes include focal glomerular sclerosis, membranoproliferative glomerulonephritis and minimal change nephropathy
2. Secondary
   Systemic disease—SLE, diabetes mellitus, Hodgkin's disease (minimal change), solid tumours (membranous)
   Infection—hepatitis B, HIV (focal sclerosis), infective endocarditis, quartan malaria
   Drugs—gold, D-penicillamine, probenecid, high-dose captopril, non-steroidal anti-inflammatory drugs, heroin

Note: Renal vein thrombosis is a complication and rarely a cause of the nephrotic syndrome.

HIV = human immunodeficiency virus; LDL = low-density lipoprotein;
SLE = systemic lupus erythematosus.

Table 6.72   Classification of glomerulonephritis

Primary
Diffuse
1. Minimal change
2. Membranous
3. Proliferative
   Post-streptococcal (and after other infections)
   Mesangiocapillary
   Crescentic
   Mesangioproliferative

Focal
1. IgA nephropathy
2. Focal glomerulosclerosis

Glomerulonephritis as part of a systemic disease
   1. Systemic lupus erythematosus (SLE)
   2. Wegener's granulomatosis
   3. Polyarteritis nodosa (PAN)
   4. Goodpasture's syndrome
   5. Henoch-Schönlein purpura
   6. Infective endocarditis
   7. Cryoglobulinaemia ± hepatitis C
   8. Myeloma
   9. Diabetes mellitus
  10. Haemolytic uraemic syndrome

Ask when the underlying condition was diagnosed and how it is being treated. The progression to end-stage renal disease may be rapid or very prolonged, and this needs to be documented.

Questions regarding management

1. Conservative management. Ask about follow-up, medications, diet, salt and water allowance, investigations performed (particularly renal biopsy), effect on the quality of life and whether erythropoietin has been given subcutaneously in an attempt to elevate the haemoglobin. Has the patient been advised to restrict protein intake? There is controversy about the value of protein restriction in delaying end-stage renal failure. There is some evidence that restriction to 40–59 g a day may be helpful. Patients with nephrotic syndrome should be much less restricted. The concern about protein restriction is that it leads to more rapid loss of muscle mass without much delay in end-stage renal failure.
2. Dialysis (Table 6.73). Ask about haemodialysis or peritoneal dialysis, including where performed, how often, how many hours per week, relief of symptoms with treatment and subsequent complications. Also ask about shunts, other operations (e.g. renal tract operations, parathyroidectomy) and medications taken.
3. Transplant work-up and management. Ask when and how many, whether living relative or cadaver, postoperative course, improvement, symptoms since transplantation, medications, follow-up and long-term complications (e.g. neoplasia, steroid complications).
4. Bladder management for reflux or neurogenic bladder.

Table 6.73	Dialysis

Peritoneal dialysis (CAPD or APD)	
Advantages	Simple, reliable and safe (from a cardiovascular point of view). Removes large fluid volumes. Allows greater freedom of diet and fluid intake. Preferable for diabetics.
Disadvantages	Peritonitis, exit-site infections (around catheter). Protein loss (7–10 g/day usually; 30–40 g/day with peritonitis). Basal atelectasis. Abdominal hernias. Does not control uraemia in hypercatabolic patients. Hyperglycaemia. Catheter displacement. 'Peritoneal membrane failure'. Perforation of bladder and bowel (rare). Hydrothorax (rare).
Haemodialysis	
Advantages	Takes approximately 18 hours per week (5 hours three times/week plus set-up time). No protein loss. Large volumes can be ultrafiltrated.
Disadvantages	Circulatory access problems (thrombosis, infection of vascular access). Heparin may increase bleeding. Increased cardiovascular instability. Anaemia. Osteodystrophy. Dialysis dementia (aluminium).

Note: Mortality from dialysis is caused by myocardial infarction (60%) or sepsis (20%) in most cases. Acquired cystic disease in native kidneys may occur; <5% are malignant. Arthropathy and carpal tunnel syndrome may occur in long-term dialysis patients owing to amyloid (beta$_2$-microglobulin) deposition.

APD = automated peritoneal dialysis (exchanges done at night); CAPD = chronic ambulatory peritoneal dialysis.

5. Social arrangements and activities of daily living. Ask about employment, the family's ability to cope, travel, sexual function and financial situation.

Questions regarding complications

1. Conservatively treated patients. Ask about symptoms of anaemia, bone disease, secondary gout or pseudogout, pericarditis, hypertension, cardiac failure, peripheral neuropathy, pruritus, peptic ulcers, impaired cognitive function and poor nutrition. Have the doses of renally excreted drugs given for other conditions been reduced? Remember that although most drugs that require a loading dose are begun at their usual dose (and then continued at a reduced maintenance dose), digoxin, which has an altered volume distribution, must have its loading dose reduced.
2. Dialysis patients. Ask about shunt blockage and access problems, infection, pericarditis, peritonitis, etc.
3. Transplant patients. For patients with recent transplants ask about graft pain or swelling (failure of graft function, rejection), infection, urine leaks, steroid side-effects. For those with long-term renal grafts, ask about serum creatinine levels, proteinuria, recurrent glomerulonephritis (dense deposit disease), avascular necrosis, skin cancer and reflux nephropathy. Find out about compliance with drugs and whether the patient knows about rejection episodes and treatment, for example, with muromonab–CD3.

The examination (Fig 6.19)

Figure 6.19 Chronic renal failure.

1. **GENERAL INSPECTION**
   Mental state
   Hyperventilation (acidosis), hiccups
   Sallow complexion
   Hydration
   Fever

   Bladder
   Liver
   Lymph nodes
   Ascites
   Bruits
   Rectal (prostatomegaly, bleeding)

2. **HANDS**
   Nails—Terry's nails, brown lines
   Vascular shunts
   Asterixis
   Neuropathy

3. **ARMS**
   Bruising
   Pigmentation
   Scratch marks
   Urea frost (whole crystal
     deposits—terminal uraemia)
   Myopathy

4. **FACE**
   Eyes—anaemia, jaundice, band
     keratopathy
   Mouth—dryness, fetor
   Rash (vasculitis etc.)
   Facial hair—cyclosporin
   Saddle nose (Wegener's
     granulomatosis)

5. **CHEST**
   Heart—pericarditis, failure
   Lungs—infection

6. **ABDOMEN**
   Scars—dialysis, operations
   Kidneys—transplant kidney, renal
     mass
   Tenckhoff catheter, exit-site
     infection

7. **LEGS**
   Oedema—nephrotic syndrome,
     cardiac failure etc.
   Bruising
   Pigmentation
   Scratch marks
   Gout
   Neuropathy
   Vascular access

8. **BACK**
   Tenderness
   Oedema
   Spina bifida scar

9. **URINE ANALYSIS**
   Specific gravity, pH
   Glucose—diabetes
   Blood—'nephritis', infection,
     stone etc.
   Protein—'nephritis' etc.

10. **URINE SEDIMENT**
    Red cells
    Casts

11. **OTHER**
    Blood pressure—lying and
      standing
    Fundoscopy—hypertensive and
      diabetic changes etc.
    Vasculitis

A complete physical examination is always essential. Look particularly for the following.

1. General appearance. Mental state, hyperventilation, Kussmaul's breathing, hiccupping and the state of hydration.
2. Hands. Nails—white transverse opaque bands or lines in hypoalbuminaemia; a brown arc near the ends of the nails (Terry's nails) in renal failure. Also, palmar crease pallor, vasculitis, vascular shunts at the wrist, asterixis and peripheral neuropathy.

3. Arms—bruising, pigmentation, scratch marks, subcutaneous calcification, myopathy, fistulae and skin cancers, especially squamous cell carcinomas.
4. Face—eyes for jaundice, anaemia and band keratopathy (caused by hypercalcaemia); mouth (dry, fetor); rash (e.g. SLE) and a Cushingoid appearance.
5. Chest—pericardial rub, cardiac failure, lung infection, pleural effusion, venous hum (shunt).
6. Abdomen—costovertebral angle tenderness (push with the thumb), palpable kidney, scars (owing to dialysis or transplants), renal artery bruit (a systolic bruit or occasionally a systolic–diastolic bruit in the upper abdomen suggests possible renal artery stenosis), bladder enlargement, rectal examination (for prostatomegaly, urethral mass and signs of blood loss), nodes (lymphoma, cytomegalovirus or other infections if the patient is immunosuppressed), ascites (dialysis or other causes) and femoral bruits and pulses.
7. Urine for blood, protein, specific gravity, pH, glucose, urine microscopy, and examination of the urinary sediment for casts.
8. Legs—oedema, bruising, pigmentation, scratch marks, peripheral neuropathy, vascular access (for shunts) and myopathy.
9. Back—bone tenderness and sacral oedema.
10. Blood pressure lying and standing. Fundoscopy.

Investigations

1. Determine renal function:
   (a) glomerular filtration rate (GFR)—24-hour creatinine clearance (creatine clearance levels of <10 mL/min are considered indications for dialysis) and plasma creatinine/urea level
   (b) tubular function—plasma electrolyte levels, urine specific gravity and pH, glycosuria, serum phosphate and uric acid, aminoaciduria, serum calcium and plasma albumin levels
   (c) urine analysis and 24-hour urinary protein excretion
   (d) others if necessary—DTPA (diethylenetriamine penta-acetate) scan for renal artery stenosis or urinary tract obstruction.
2. Determine renal structure:
   (a) ultrasound—renal size and symmetry, signs of obstruction; small kidneys suggest chronic disease
   (b) plain X-ray film of the abdomen (KUB—kidneys, ureters, bladder)
   (c) intravenous pyelogram (IVP) under good hydration (but avoid in patients with diabetes mellitus or myeloma or when the creatinine level is >150 mmol/L—it has largely been replaced by less invasive tests)
   (d) computed tomography (CT) scan (same restrictions as for IVP if contrast is to be used; the use of oral N-acetylcysteine before and after the use of contrast material has become popular and may offer some renal protection)
   (e) cystoscopy and retrograde pyelography
   (f) other—renal artery Doppler study, renal angiography.
3. Investigations aimed towards the likely underlying disease process—renal biopsy, measurement of antinuclear antibody, hepatitis B surface antigen, hepatitis C, HIV, complement, immune complexes, immunoelectrophoresis, micturating cystogram, urine cytology.
4. Investigations aimed at assessing the widespread effects of renal failure—blood count, serum ferritin and iron saturation level, midstream urine examination, calcium, phosphate and alkaline phosphatase levels, parathyroid hormone level, nerve conduction studies, arterial Doppler studies.
5. The following features favour chronic over acute renal failure: nocturia, polyuria, longstanding hypertension, renal osteodystrophy, peripheral neuropathy, anaemia,

hyperphosphataemia and hyperuricaemia. The differentiation of acute and chronic renal failure is also aided by determining kidney size. They are usually small in chronic renal failure, but the exceptions to this rule include:

(a) diabetic nephropathy (early)
(b) polycystic kidneys
(c) obstructive uropathy
(d) acute renal vein thrombosis
(e) amyloidosis
(f) rarely other infiltrative diseases (e.g. lymphoma), which can all produce chronic renal failure but maintain normal kidney size.

In general, however, kidneys enlarge or maintain normal size in acute renal failure and are small in chronic renal failure.

Anaemia and burr cells in the peripheral blood film are usually evidence of chronic renal failure but may occur in acute renal failure (e.g. in SLE), thrombotic thrombocytopenic purpura, and the haemolytic uraemic syndrome.

Always ask about previous urine analyses, such as insurance examinations in which proteinuria may have been detected and followed up, thus giving a clue about chronic glomerulonephritis.

Treatment

This most chronic disease (Table 6.74) has profound affects on the patient and his or her relatives. The association between the patient and the renal physician and nursing staff becomes a very intense one, often over many years. It is important to ask detailed questions about: the way the patient copes with the condition; whether work or travel are possible; and what the patient feels about the long-term prospects. Has a dialysis patient considered accepting a kidney from a live donor?

1. Treat reversible causes of deterioration. These include:
   (a) hypertension
   (b) urinary tract infection
   (c) urinary tract obstruction
   (d) dehydration
   (e) cardiac failure
   (f) drug use (e.g. radiocontrast, NSAIDs, aminoglycosides, cyclosporin)
   (g) hypercalcaemia
   (h) hyperuricaemia with urate obstruction
   (i) hypothyroidism or rarely hypoadrenalism.
2. Monitor and control the blood pressure very carefully.
3. Carefully attend to salt and water balance, and acidosis.
4. Normalise the calcium and phosphate levels with diet, phosphate binders or calcitriol.
5. Restrict dietary protein. Although this may delay slightly the need for dialysis, it leads to wasting and protein malnutrition. It is no longer universally recommended.
6. Dialyse when indicated (see below).
7. Consider transplantation.

The absolute indications for dialysis are (see Table 6.73):

1. uraemic symptoms despite conservative management (GFR <20 mL/min; creatinine level >0.7 mmol/L)
2. volume overload despite salt and water restriction and diuretic use
3. hyperkalaemia unresponsive to conservative measures
4. progressive deterioration of renal function (dialyse before symptoms develop)
5. acute renal failure (dialyse early).

Note: Dialysis may be started earlier to avoid the above complications.

Table 6.74 Complications and treatment of chronic renal failure

Anaemia
Causes include: erythropoietin deficiency, poor nutrition (especially folate
deficiency), blood loss, haemolysis, bone marrow depression, chronic disease
and aluminium toxicity.
   Treatment should include prophylactic folate supplements for dialysis patients.
Erythropoietin is very effective for the chronic anaemia of renal failure and can
normalise the haematocrit. Erythropoietin is commonly used in conjunction with intravenous iron supplements (as oral iron is poorly absorbed in end-stage renal disease).

Bone disease
Maintenance of normal calcium and phosphate levels is the key to preventing the
problem. Treatment with calcium carbonate (to bind phosphate in the gut), vitamin D
analogues and low calcium concentration in dialysis fluids is necessary.
1. Osteomalacia—diagnosis by:
    (a) X-ray films (decreased density, Looser's zones)
    (b) low calcium, phosphate and vitamin D levels
    (c) high serum alkaline phosphatase level
    (d) bone biopsy (tetracycline-labelled)
2. Tertiary hyperparathyroidism—diagnosis by:
    (a) X-ray film (microcysts on radial side of the middle phalanx, erosion of the
        clavicular ends, 'Rugger jersey' spine, telescoped terminal phalanges,
        metastatic calcification of vessels)
    (b) high phosphate and parathyroid hormone levels, and a high calcium level
    (c) bone biopsy (tetracycline-labelled)
3. Osteoporosis
4. Osteosclerosis
5. Aluminium-induced bone disease and adynamic bone
6. Hypercalcaemia and hyperphosphataemia is a common problem

Peripheral neuropathy
This is now uncommon in patients receiving adequate dialysis. It is more often a
result of diabetes than of renal failure itself. Combined pancreatic islet and renal
transplant may help.

Hypertension
This needs careful monitoring and control of salt and fluid balance as well as
judicious use of antihypertensive drugs.

Infection
Predisposed to the disease and the immunosuppressive drugs given to treat
glomerulonephritis, and the need for frequent intravenous vascular access.

Acidosis
This is often treated with dialysis and carefully monitored. Calcium carbonate often
helps.

Hyperkalaemia
This should be treated with a low-potassium diet and ion-exchanging resins if
necessary. Dialysis is very effective.

Renal transplantation

Renal transplantation is now a widely accepted, commonly performed treatment for end-stage renal failure. Patients unfortunately continue to have a number of chronic problems, which may bring them into hospital and make them available for examinations. Cadaveric transplantation is generally more common than the use of matched family donors. Specific contraindications to renal transplantation include recent malignancy, an untreatable focus of infection and severe external disease. The prognosis continues to improve and the introduction of cyclosporin and other immunosuppressives has made a substantial difference to survival rates in both groups of patients. The 1-year graft survival rate is now over 90% in experienced centres. The selection of patients for transplant is difficult. Shortages of donor organs mean that transplant is not offered to elderly patients, those with other serious illnesses or those with unrevascularised coronary artery disease.

The history

1. Ask the patient about the cause of the original renal failure (p 196). Find out how long the transplant has been in situ and whether this is the first transplant. Ask whether the kidney came from a relative or was a cadaveric graft.
2. The patient should be well informed about previous rejection episodes and how these have been managed. Find out whether this is the reason for the current admission. Clinically, rejection may be marked by fever, swelling and tenderness over the graft. The patient should be aware of all these signs. There is also often a reduction in urine volume. A rise in creatinine level is usual. Ask about recent graft biopsies, which may have been necessary to assess rejection, or recurrence of disease or drug toxicity.
3. Find out what immunosuppressive drugs the patient is taking and in what doses. He or she should know whether changes in doses have been required recently because of problems with any of the drugs.
4. Ask about specific complications of immunosuppression. Cyclosporin can result in significant side-effects. The drug can be associated with an increase in hirsutism, tremor, gout, renal impairment, increased liver function tests (especially bilirubin), hypertension, hyperkalaemia, gingival hypertrophy and rarely haematological malignancy. Ask about ischaemic heart disease and peripheral vascular disease, infections and malignancy, as the incidence of these conditions remains higher than in the general population.

The examination

Look particularly at the skin for squamous and basal cell carcinomas. Note any signs of Cushing's syndrome and hirsutism (e.g. cyclosporin). Examine the abdomen carefully, noting the position and site of the allograft and whether it has any tenderness or bruits. Look for old vascular access sites for haemodialysis and decide whether there will be problems finding sites for access for further dialysis if this is required.

Examine the lungs for signs of infection and the mouth for *Candida*. Inspect the gums. Note gouty tophi. Look at the temperature chart.

Investigations

1. It is important to obtain the serum creatinine level and, if possible, establish whether the serum creatinine level has been rising or falling since the time of the transplantation. A slightly elevated creatinine level is considered acceptable in patients on cyclosporin treatment as this drug interferes with renal function.

2. The electrolyte levels and liver function test results are important. Cyclosporin can cause hepatotoxicity and renal impairment, as can cytomegalovirus (CMV) infection of the liver.
3. A white cell count should be obtained to look for leukocytosis (infection or steroids) and leukopenia (e.g. excessive doses of azathioprine). The azathioprine dose is usually adjusted according to the neutrophil count. The haemoglobin is usually normal in patients with a successful transplant and good function.
4. The results of blood cultures should be sought if there has been any suggestion of recent infection. Urinary tract infection must also be considered, and early urine microscopy is helpful.
5. Exclude prerenal and postrenal disease. A renal scan and ultrasound with measurement by Doppler is useful for estimating renal artery blood flow.

Management

The majority of patients receiving chronic dialysis are candidates for renal transplantation. The donor's kidneys must be ABO-compatible. Typing by human leucocyte antigens (HLA) -A, -B and -DR improves graft survival. Three HLA antigens are inherited from each parent. A complete match is for six antigens. The graft survival rate for these patients is 50% at 20 years. The long-term graft survival rate declines with a decrease in the number of matches. The recipient is usually screened for antibodies to class 1 antigens (HLA-A and -B) before receiving the transplant. Their presence is associated with hyperacute rejection.

Management problems include acute tubular necrosis, infection, cyclosporin nephrotoxicity (acute vasoconstriction, haemolytic uraemic syndrome or dose-related nephrotoxicity) and rejection episodes.

Rejection is prevented by the use of steroids, azathioprine (or mycophenolate) and cyclosporin. Acute rejection episodes are treated with three pulse doses of 0.5–1 g intravenous methylprednisolone, or monoclonal antibody (e.g. muromonab–CD3) if the episode is resistant to steroids. Azathioprine is given in doses of 1.5–3 mg/kg/day; it is metabolised by the liver so its dose does not need to be varied according to renal function, but the dose is usually adjusted according to the neutrophil count. The use of allopurinol should be avoided because it interferes with azathioprine excretion and increases bone marrow toxicity. Prednisone is given in maintenance doses of approximately 7.5–10 mg daily after about 6 months. A gradually rising creatinine level may be a sign of cyclosporin toxicity (which, if caused by interstitial fibrosis, is not reversible) or of chronic rejection. This is a difficult clinical problem but graft biopsy can be used to decide whether the cyclosporin should be stopped or immunosuppression increased.

Opportunistic infections typically occur a month or more post-transplant. *Toxoplasma*, *Nocardia* and *Aspergillus* are now less common with current immunosuppressive protocols; viral infections (especially CMV) dominate. Infection must be aggressively diagnosed (e.g. by blood cultures and lung biopsy) and treated. When infections are life-threatening, immunosuppressive treatment, apart from prednisone, should be suspended.

The major cause of graft loss is chronic rejection. Recurrence of glomerulonephritis in the transplanted kidney occasionally occurs and is most common with focal glomerulosclerosis. IgA nephropathy, Goodpasture's syndrome and membranoproliferative glomerulonephritis (especially type II) can also recur.

Central nervous system

Multiple sclerosis

This is a common chronic disease. Patients suffering from multiple sclerosis (MS) are easily available for the clinical examinations. They are mostly very well informed about, and interested in, their disease. MS usually begins in early adult life and is more common in women (2:1).

The history

Diagnosis requires at least two neurological events separated in time and place within the central nervous system (CNS). MS is primarily a clinical diagnosis.

1. Presenting symptoms (listed in approximate order of importance):
    (a) episodes of spastic paraparesis, hemiparesis or tetraparesis (may present as gradually progressive disease in late-onset MS)
    (b) episodes of limb paraesthesiae (owing to posterior column, medial lemniscus or internal capsule involvement)
    (c) episodes of visual disturbance—loss of acuity, pain on eye movement, loss of central visual field (optic neuritis)
    (d) episodes of ataxia (owing to cerebellar or posterior column involvement)
    (e) band sensations around trunk or limbs
    (f) less common symptoms, such as vertigo, symptoms of cranial nerve disorders (e.g. tic douloureux), urinary urgency, incontinence of faeces, impotence, depression, euphoria, dementia, seizures, bulbar dysfunction (pseudobulbar palsy).
2. Ask about precipitating factors, such as heat (hot baths, etc.), infection, fever, pregnancy and exercise.
3. Ask about family history (MS is eight times more common in immediate relatives and occurs more often in subjects with human leucocyte antigen (HLA) -B7 and -DW2 and less often in subjects with HLA-B12).
4. Ask about social disability—sexual function, work, financial problems.
5. Ask about place of birth (MS is 10 times more common in subjects who spent their childhood in temperate latitudes than in tropical regions).
6. Find out what treatments have been tried and with what success and side-effects. Various unproven treatments are often tried by patients with this incurable disease. Ask if any of these have been used.

The examination

The signs can be very variable. Look particularly for signs of spastic paraparesis and posterior column sensory loss as well as cerebellar signs.

Examine the cranial nerves. Look carefully for loss of visual acuity, optic atrophy, papillitis and scotomata (usually central). Internuclear ophthalmoplegia is an important sign and is almost diagnostic in a young adult. It can also occur in patients with systemic lupus erythematosus (SLE) or Sjögren's syndrome who may have disease confined to the CNS, or with brain stem tumours or infarcts. Internuclear ophthalmoplegia is weakness of adduction in one eye as a result of damage to the ipsilateral medial longitudinal fasciculus; there may be nystagmus in the abducting eye. In MS, internuclear ophthalmoplegia is often bilateral. Other cranial nerves may rarely be affected (III, IV, V, VI, VII, pseudobulbar palsy) by lesions within the brain stem. Charcot's triad consists of nystagmus, intention tremor and scanning speech, but occurs in only 10% of patients.

Look for Lhermitte's sign (an electric shock-like sensation in the limbs or trunk following neck flexion). This can also be caused by other disorders of the cervical spine, such as subacute combined degeneration of the cord, cervical spondylosis, cervical cord tumour, foramen magnum tumours, nitrous oxide abuse and mantle irradiation.

Rarely, Devic's disease, usually seen in children or young adults, is present (bilateral optic neuritis and transverse myelitis occurring within a few weeks of one another) and may be a variant of MS.

Investigations

The differential diagnosis of multiple CNS lesions includes SLE, Sjögren's syndrome, Behçet's disease, acute disseminated encephalomyelitis, meningovascular syphilis, paraneoplastic effects of carcinoma, sarcoidosis, Lyme disease, and multiple emboli from any source.

It is important to distinguish MS affecting predominantly the spinal cord from other diseases—especially subacute combined degeneration of the cord (more common in the older population) and spinal cord compression presenting with root pain and persistent levels of sensory loss.

MS is essentially a clinical diagnosis but the following tests may be helpful.

1. Magnetic resonance imaging (MRI) is the imaging modality of choice. Typical changes are present in the great majority of patients with MS. Gadolinium contrast studies show leakage into the brain from blood vessels for up to months after the formation of a new lesion. T2-weighted images will show persisting changes probably owing to a combination of oedema, gliosis and inflammation. The extent of these abnormalities does not correlate well with the clinical picture but T1-weighted images may show hypodense areas whose extent does correspond to the patient's symptoms. These probably represent irreversible damage and axonal loss. Computed tomography (CT) scan may reveal low-density, sometimes contrast-enhancing, plaques in white matter (subcortical or periventricular, but only in 10–50% of cases). CT scanning is no longer in routine use for diagnosis of MS.
2. Cerebrospinal fluid in chronic MS contains oligoclonal IgG bands (70%) and an altered IgG:albumin ratio. Myelin basic protein may be elevated in acute demyelination. There are usually fewer than 50 white cells per millilitre in the cerebrospinal fluid but acute severe demyelination may result in a cell count exceeding 100/mL.
3. Visual-evoked responses are delayed in 80% of established cases and indicate past optic neuritis (important if there is only one other clinically detectable lesion present). Other helpful tests are auditory-evoked responses and somatosensory-evoked responses, which may indicate lesions elsewhere in the white matter. However, evoked potentials are less reliable than studies on cerebrospinal fluid and MRI.
4. Antimyelin antibodies are of uncertain value.

A definite diagnosis is not possible without the presence of two or more CNS episodes, usually separated in time. The first may be a clinical abnormality and the second detected by MRI or visually evoked responses. These include objective CNS changes usually involving long tract signs and symptoms: pyramidal, cerebellar, optic nerve, posterior columns and medial longitudinal fasciculus. Gradual progression of symptoms may be used to make the diagnosis if typical cerebrospinal fluid abnormalities are present. The MRI should show four distinct areas of abnormality at least 3 mm in diameter. There should be no other explanation for the symptoms (see above).

Treatment

There are two aspects to treatment of these patients—supportive and symptomatic treatment—and attempts to alter the disease progression.

1. General support is essential. During exacerbations, bed rest with meticulous nursing is vital. Treatment of bladder dysfunction, severe spasticity (e.g. with baclofen), tic douloureux and facial spasm (e.g. carbamazepine and physiotherapy) is important.
2. Interferon beta 1a and interferon beta 1b have been shown to reduce the frequency of exacerbations by about a third when used at an early stage of disease and to reduce the accumulation of CNS white matter lesions. They are possibly more effective for the relapsing forms of the disease (see below).

Copolymer I (glatiramer) (a polymer of myelin basic protein) may be used for patients with relapsing disease.

High-dose intravenous corticosteroids or adrenocorticotrophic hormone (ACTH) given during acute exacerbations may lessen the severity of symptoms and speed recovery. The final extent of disability is not affected, however. Methotrexate given in weekly doses of 7.5 mg reduces the progression of disability and the MRI signs of disease activity for up to 2 years. Azathioprine (2–3 mg/kg/day) is sometimes used for chronic progressive disease, and appears to have a modest beneficial effect. Cyclophosphamide may slow progression in patients under the age of 40. Its side-effects make it difficult to use. Plasmapheresis and intravenous gammaglobulin may also help exacerbations.

There are many support groups and organisations for patients with MS. These often give sensible advice to these distressed people and should be recommended to patients. It is most important, however, that the diagnosis is secure before patients are labelled with this condition with its numerous long-term implications.

Most patients have a sudden onset of their symptoms. Thereafter, four patterns of disease are recognised.

1. *Relapsing–remitting MS*: relapses with or without complete recovery but stable between episodes.
2. *Secondary progressive MS*: about half of the patients with relapsing–remitting MS develop secondary progressive MS within 10 years. They experience gradual progression of their symptoms without distinct episodes.
3. *Primary progressive MS*: these patients (10%) have increasing symptoms without distinct episodes from the start.
4. *Progressive relapsing MS*: in these patients there is gradual worsening with episodes of deterioration occurring later in the course of the illness.

At 15 years after the first episode, 80% of patients have significant symptoms that prevent work and require help with normal activities. If the initial episode is limited to a single abnormality and the MRI is normal, only 10% will go on to develop a second episode over the following 10 years. If the MRI is abnormal, up to 80% will experience further episodes.

Myasthenia gravis

This disease presents both diagnostic and management problems. Peak incidence in women is in the third decade but in men it is in the seventh decade. Overall it is more common in women (2:1). Exacerbations and remissions (incomplete) are common.

The history

1. Ask about symptoms at presentation:
   (a) ocular—diplopia (90%), drooping eyelids
   (b) bulbar—choking (weakness of pharyngeal muscles), dysarthria, difficulty (especially fatigue) when chewing or swallowing
   (c) limb girdle—proximal muscle weakness; there is fatigue on exertion and prompt partial recovery on resting.
2. Ask about a history of difficult anaesthesia (owing to prolonged weakness after muscle relaxation) and past episodes of pneumonia (as a result of bulbar and respiratory weakness).
3. Ask about how the diagnosis was made, including whether an edrophonium test was performed, whether electrodiagnostic studies were done, and whether the patient had blood tests for acetylcholine receptor antibodies.
4. Ask about a history of thymectomy.
5. Ask about other treatment—including drug dose and when the last dose was taken, plasma exchange or immunosuppressive therapy.

6. Ask about drug use, which may interfere with neuromuscular transmission (see below).
7. Ask about other organ-specific autoimmune disease associations (SLE, rheumatoid arthritis).
8. Inquire about the social history.

The examination

Examine for muscle fatigue, particularly the elevators of the eyelids and the oculo-motor muscles (tested by sustained upward gaze), bulbar muscles (tested by counting or reading aloud) and the proximal limb girdles (tested by holding the arms above the head). Look for the Peek sign (orbicularis oculi weakness—close the eyelids: within 30 seconds in myasthenia they will begin to separate and you will see the lower sclera). Asking the patient to smile may produce a snarling expression. Speech on prolonged speaking may sound dysarthric or nasal because of weakness of the palate. Weakness of neck flexion may be prominent. Reflexes are preserved. There is no sensory loss. Muscle atrophy is usually minimal. Look for a thymectomy scar.

Investigations

Tests for myasthenia gravis include the following.
1. *Edrophonium test.* Edrophonium (a short-acting anticholinesterase inhibitor) is given intravenously; if muscle strength improves dramatically, myasthenia gravis is likely.
2. *Acetylcholine receptor antibodies* (anti-AChR). These occur in 80–90% of cases, with false-positive results being rare (but the frequency of positive tests is lower in pure ocular and inactive myasthenia gravis). The titre is not directly related to disease severity. Antistriated muscle antibody is detectable in 90% of patients with a thymoma but is also common in elderly patients without a thymoma; muscle specific kinase antibodies (MuSK) are present in 20% of 'seronegative' (ACh antibody negative) patients.
3. *Electromyogram* (EMG). In myasthenia gravis, repetitive stimulation at low frequencies causes an asymptotic reduction (there is progressively less reduction with each shock) in muscle action potential amplitudes if that particular muscle is affected. Needle examination of affected muscles shows motor unit potential variation and, sometimes, fibrillation potentials and myopathic change. Single-fibre EMG shows increased jitter and blocking.
4. *Thymoma investigations*—chest X-ray film, thoracic CT scan or MRI.
5. *Associated conditions*—hyperthyroidism and autoimmune diseases (check thyroid function tests, rheumatoid factor and antinuclear antibodies).
6. *Respiratory function tests.* These patients may have severe respiratory impairment.

Treatment

Symptomatic

Anticholinesterases are the mainstay of treatment in mild cases. Pyridostigmine is the usual one prescribed. Potassium supplements and potassium-sparing diuretics (e.g. spironolactone) may give additional improvement but are rarely used these days. It is important to avoid drugs that interfere with neuromuscular transmission, including streptomycin, gentamicin, quinidine and procainamide. Sudden worsening of the patient's symptoms so as to be life-threatening (because of respiratory failure) is called a myasthenic crisis. They are often precipitated by infection, which must be treated aggressively with antibiotics (not aminoglycosides) and intensive respiratory support. Mechanical ventilation and a course of plasmapheresis may be required. Sometimes the problem may be excessive anticholinesterase inhibitor treatment (cholinergic crisis). Temporary suspension of drug treatment and monitoring of muscle strength may be all that is required for these episodes.

Disease-suppressing

Steroids are indicated for generalised severe disease when anticholinesterases are inadequate. They are then needed in the long term. They may aggravate disease initially (in the first week to 10 days), so all patients should be observed closely when treatment is commenced. Failed steroid treatment in patients with severe disease is an indication for immunosuppressive drug therapy (e.g. azathioprine, cyclosporin, mycophenolate). Rituximab has been tried in desperate cases. This chimeric antibody attaches to the CD20 membrane site of B lymphocytes and attracts killer T cells and antibodies that destroy the lymphocytes which make the pathological antibodies. A course of treatment is very expensive.

Thymectomy is advisable early for many patients with generalised myasthenia gravis if they are ACh-antibody positive. The exceptions are elderly patients or those with an easily inducible remission. Thymomas occur in 10% of cases (and of these 25% are malignant) and thymic hyperplasia occurs in 65%. Of such patients, after resection, 70% show improvement and 25% of those who improve undergo remission. Causes of failed response to thymectomy include incomplete removal, ectopic tissue and fulminant disease.

Plasmapheresis is useful in acute situations such as in myasthenic crisis, preparation for surgery or in the peripartum period. Very ill patients may need repeated treatments.

The prognosis of myasthenia gravis is good: 50% of patients have a remission, although 5–10% die from respiratory failure.

Differential diagnosis

The differential diagnosis of proximal muscle weakness is important. The ocular muscle dystrophies also need to be considered.

The Lambert-Eaton syndrome is occasionally confused with myasthenia gravis. This syndrome results from presynaptic failure of release of acetylcholine, caused by small cell carcinoma of the lung (in 50% of cases) or autoimmune disease. There is proximal muscle weakness and pain, and power may increase on repeated effort. Reflexes are reduced or absent. The ocular and bulbar muscles are usually spared. The EMG is helpful (high-frequency stimulation causes an increment, while low-frequency stimulation causes a decrement, and muscle action potential amplitudes are low). Symptoms may be reduced by guanidine or 3,4-diaminopyridine; steroids and plasma-exchange therapy can also be effective. Some patients with small cell carcinoma of the lung have a neurological remission if the tumour is completely removed.

Treatment with D-penicillamine may cause a mild reversible form of myasthenia.

Guillain-Barré syndrome

This disease is not uncommon in the examination, as patients may be in hospital for an extended period and present management difficulties. It is the most common acute polyneuropathy and can affect both sexes and all ages.

The history

1. Ask about the presenting symptoms of ascending motor weakness, their time course, and whether decreasing or increasing. The patient may report difficulty breathing. Other symptoms include paraesthesiae or sensory loss (sensory neuropathy is usually minimal) and symptoms of cranial nerve palsies, particularly bulbar lesions (all cranial nerves except I, II and VIII can be affected).

2. Ask about a preceding respiratory or gastrointestinal infection (which occurs in up to 50% of cases 1–3 weeks before). Other precipitating events, such as surgical operation, vaccination, intercurrent malignant disease (e.g. Hodgkin's disease), SLE and HIV infection should be inquired about.
3. Ask about previous episodes of disease (in chronic relapsing polyneuropathy).
4. Ask about evidence of autonomic neuropathy, such as postural hypotension, labile blood pressure, difficult to control arrhythmias and, rarely, sphincter dysfunction (see Table 8.36).
5. Inquire about the social history.

The examination

Predominantly, distal muscle weakness without atrophy is present, although 25% have more proximal than distal weakness. The upper limbs may be more affected than the lower limbs. Tendon reflexes are reduced or absent concomitant with the degree of weakness. Muscle tenderness is common (one-third of cases). Signs of autonomic neuropathy (severe postural changes in blood pressure and cardiac arrhythmias) must be looked for. Sensory loss is usually minimal but if present affects the posterior columns (vibration and proprioception) more than the spinothalamic tracts. Always measure forced expiratory time.

Differential diagnosis

Infections such as glandular fever, acute viral hepatitis, *Mycoplasma* pneumonia, *Campylobacter jejuni* or HIV can cause the Guillain-Barré syndrome. Post influenza vaccine disease is rare. The differential diagnosis of acute ascending motor paralysis includes diphtheria, polio, polyarteritis nodosa, acute intermittent porphyria, tick or snake bites and rhabdomyolysis, arsenic poisoning, botulism and other diseases affecting the neuromuscular junction. Remember that diphtheria, botulism and myasthenia gravis usually begin with bulbar symptoms.

The differential diagnosis of autonomic neuropathy includes diabetes mellitus, alcoholism, acute intermittent porphyria and amyloidosis.

Investigations

Guillain-Barré syndrome is a clinical diagnosis. Helpful tests include:
1. identifying the immune stimulus—by Monospot test, cold agglutinins, tests for cytomegalovirus, HIV or *Campylobacter*
2. cerebrospinal fluid examination—look for a raised protein level and the relative lack of white blood cells in 90% of cases; 10% have 10–50 mononuclear cells/mL
3. respiratory function tests (FEV_1, FVC) to assess progressive involvement of respiratory muscles; the patient can progress rapidly (even over hours) to respiratory failure requiring intubation and should be admitted to hospital, even if only mildly affected
4. nerve conduction and EMG studies—many nerves may have to be studied to find abnormalities because this disease is patchy but abnormalities include slowed motor conduction, conduction blocks, increased distal motor latencies, reduced sensory action potentials and increased F wave latencies; EMG evidence of denervation takes 10 days to 3 weeks to appear and may indicate axonal involvement with a worse prognosis.

Treatment

Physiotherapy is used to prevent contractures. Respiratory support in an intensive care unit is essential if the vital capacity is less than 1 L.

Plasmapheresis or intravenous gammaglobulin shorten the time to recovery from respiratory paralysis and hasten the return of mobility. They are equally effective and combined treatment offers no additional benefit. Treatment should be begun as soon as possible. Rapid improvement is much more likely if treatment is begun within 2 weeks of the first symptoms. Relapses may occur and are more common after intravenous gammaglobulin than after plasmapheresis. Steroids (and ACTH) are not beneficial.

Prognosis is good—most patients make a complete recovery over time (up to a year), but 2% die (usually of respiratory complications, pulmonary emboli, cardiac arrhythmias) and 10% have a major residual deficit. If the deficit does not diminish in 3 weeks or the patient has autonomic neuropathy, a poorer prognosis is more likely.

Transient ischaemic attacks and 'funny turns'

Patients presenting with a 'funny turn' can pose a difficult diagnostic problem as there are many possible explanations. The problem may be neurological, cardiac, endocrinological or psychiatric. A careful history and physical examination should enable the candidate to produce a sensible differential diagnosis and management plan. Treatment is usually fairly straightforward once the diagnosis is made.

The history

1. It may be possible from the history to establish whether cerebrovascular disease and, in particular, transient ischaemic attacks (TIAs), explain the funny turns. TIAs occur suddenly; there is focal neurological loss that is maximal at onset and does not spread or intensify. By definition the symptoms must resolve within 24 hours. Specific inquiry should be made about unilateral weakness or clumsiness, difficulty understanding or expressing spoken language, altered sensation unilaterally, and partial or complete loss of vision in one eye or bilateral blindness. Faintness, confusion, simultaneous bilateral weakness, slurred speech and spinning sensations are not localising symptoms and are less suggestive of a TIA.

2. Neurological deficits that have lasted for longer than 24 hours are consistent with the syndrome of a completed stroke. The absence of focal symptoms in a patient with severe headache and vomiting suggests subarachnoid haemorrhage. Vomiting and focal symptoms may occur with intracerebral haemorrhage but headache is present in less than 50% of these patients. In ischaemic stroke, the symptoms typically begin abruptly, often during sleep, and are not usually associated with headache or vomiting.

3. Presyncope refers to a sense of impending loss of consciousness, manifest as faintness or light-headedness and often associated with sweating, nausea, anxiety and visual dimming. Causes of this condition can include cardiac arrhythmias, postural hypotension, cough syncope and micturition syncope.

4. Epilepsy needs to be considered in the differential diagnosis. Partial epilepsy is usually accompanied by an aura or warning (e.g. flashing lights, twitching of the face or a limb, unilateral tingling or numbness, buzzing noises or humming). Primary generalised epilepsy begins with loss of consciousness; eyewitness accounts are crucial in making a diagnosis. Tongue-biting and incontinence with tonic–clonic movements suggest primary generalised epilepsy. Remember that seizure activity may accompany cerebral hypoxia of any cause (e.g. Stokes–Adams attacks). A long period of drowsiness often follows a major seizure.

5. Vertigo is the illusion of movement of self or of the environment. The sensation may be rotational. Often nausea, vomiting, imbalance and anxiety are associated. Causes of this condition include vestibular neuronitis, acute labyrinthitis, benign positional vertigo, Ménière's disease, vertebrobasilar insufficiency, posterior fossa

neoplasms, cerebellar haemorrhage and MS. Ask whether the vertigo is related to the position of the head (e.g. made worse by turning over in bed or by looking up). This symptom suggests labyrinthine disease, most commonly benign positioning vertigo.

6. Unsteadiness of gait may be secondary to a number of disorders of the peripheral or central nervous system. Drug side-effects, neoplasms, cerebellar and extrapyramidal diseases can present in this way.

7. Hypoglycaemia is an important, albeit rare, cause of funny turns and must always be considered in the differential diagnosis of suspected cerebrovascular disease. It is associated with hunger, sweating, tremor and tachycardia (owing to catecholamine release) as well as neurological dysfunction. Causes of hypoglycaemia include: too much insulin or oral hypoglycaemic agent and not enough food; reactive or postprandial, usually among patients with gastric surgery; or fasting (especially among patients with hypopituitarism, adrenal insufficiency, cirrhosis, alcoholism or rarely an insulinoma).

8. There are a number of cardiac causes of funny turns or syncope. A dizzy feeling related to standing up and without any component of true vertigo suggests postural hypotension. This can be a complication of antihypertensive treatment, especially with vasodilating drugs, and occasionally occurs in patients with single-chamber ventricular pacemakers (pacemaker syndrome). Orthostatic hypotension is common in the elderly and in patients with autonomic neuropathy (e.g. secondary to diabetes). Episodes of complete heart block may complicate ischaemic heart disease or be caused by degenerative disease of the conducting system. Ventricular and supraventricular tachyarrhythmias may cause dizziness or syncope, possibly associated with palpitations. Remember that antiarrhythmic drugs can cause bradycardia and are associated in some cases with dangerous proarrhythmic effects. Patients with severe aortic stenosis may present with exertional syncope, which is usually associated with ischaemic sounding chest pain.

9. Other conditions that need to be considered include episodes of hyperventilation or panic attacks. Patients who sigh often because of anxiety are rarely aware of any abnormality of their breathing. Their dizziness is often accompanied by a sensation of swaying. Transient global amnesia sometimes presents as a funny turn involving temporary disorientation and loss of memory.

10. Find out about risk factors and associated symptoms. If a TIA or stroke is suspected, inquire about risk factors for vascular disease (in particular, smoking, hypertension, diabetes and hyperlipidaemia). Neck pain may indicate arterial dissection. Symptoms of connective tissue disease or thrombotic episodes may be relevant. Ask for a list of all the drugs that the patient has been taking. Medications increasing the risk of vascular episodes, including oral contraceptives and some peripheral vasodilator drugs that can lower blood pressure, must be asked about. Also ask specifically about sedatives, hypoglycaemic agents, anticonvulsants and drugs affecting cardiac conduction.

The examination

A complete examination of the neurological and cardiovascular systems is essential.

1. The fundi should be carefully examined for evidence of emboli, hypertensive changes, diabetic changes and ischaemic retinopathy. Test the visual fields (e.g. left or right half visual field loss in a carotid territory stroke). Look for nystagmus.

2. Bruits should be listened for but their absence does not exclude tight carotid stenosis. Unfortunately, even if a bruit is present this does not necessarily indicate tight common or internal carotid artery stenosis, as external carotid artery stenosis can also cause a bruit.

3. If indicated, perform the Hallpike test for benign paroxysmal positional (positioning) vertigo (BPPV).
4. Check all the pulses. Decide whether atrial fibrillation is present. Test the blood pressure lying and standing for postural hypotension. Listen for murmurs (e.g. as a result of aortic stenosis, infective endocarditis, rheumatic heart disease or a prosthetic valve). Examine for peripheral vascular disease. Note the presence of an electronic pacemaker.
5. Palpate over the temporal areas for the tenderness of giant cell arteritis.

Investigations

1. In patients with a suspected, but not typical, TIA it is worthwhile checking a full blood count, erythrocyte sedimentation rate (ESR, elevated in temporal arteritis and in connective tissue disease), fasting plasma glucose (for evidence of diabetes or hypoglycaemia), cholesterol (for hypercholesterolaemia), serological testing for tertiary syphilis (*Treponema pallidum* haemoglutination test [TPHA]), urinalysis (for evidence of renovascular disease), and an ECG (for evidence of ischaemic heart disease, arrhythmia or heart block). Look for a long QT interval. Patients in sinus rhythm but with bifascicular or trifascicular block may be having episodes of complete heart block.
2. A CT or MRI scan of the head should be performed for all patients with TIA or stroke, as 5% of TIAs are caused by structural lesions. A CT scan is also worth performing in patients with established stroke to exclude haemorrhage, as this may alter management.
3. A carotid ultrasound should be performed in patients who have carotid territory TIAs. Suggestive features of a carotid artery TIA include monocular visual loss, unilateral sensory disturbances or weakness. Dysphagia and dysarthria can be caused by anterior or posterior circulation deficits. Vertebrobasilar TIAs, on the other hand, may cause bilateral visual loss, weakness or sensory disturbance, and crossed sensory and motor loss. If a greater than 60% stenosis of the origin of the internal carotid artery on the symptomatic side is found, carotid angiography should be considered with a view to endarterectomy or angioplasty, which is of value in otherwise fit patients.
4. Transoesophageal echocardiography (TOE) should be considered in any stroke patient with abnormalities on examination of the heart, or with abnormalities on the ECG (or chest X-ray). It is also recommended when no other cause has been found for the episode. A TOE with contrast injection may reveal a patent foramen ovale. This known cause of paradoxical embolism is present in up to 30% of people. Trials are underway to establish the benefits (if any) of catheter-based closure of these when they are detected in patients with otherwise unexplained stroke.
5. Patients with atrial fibrillation should have their thyroid function checked and an echocardiogram performed to look at left atrial size—a predictor of risk of embolic events.
6. In relatively young patients with a TIA (<50 years of age), careful attention to the possibility of a connective tissue disease is worthwhile. Check an antinuclear antibody, anticardiolipin antibody (because of antiphospholipid antibody syndrome) and procoagulation profile.

Management

This will of course depend on the diagnosis in the particular case. If a TIA is likely, you should plan to discuss vascular risk factor treatments, antiplatelet therapy and the role of carotid endarterectomy.

1. There is a direct relationship between high blood pressure, smoking and cholesterol level and an increased risk of ischaemic stroke as well as coronary artery disease. Therefore, management of risk factors by conservative means or with drugs is essential.

2. Antiplatelet therapy reduces the risk of stroke in patients prone to TIAs. Low-dose aspirin (between 75 and 150 mg per day) is a reasonable regimen to use. Clopidogrel is an adenosine diphosphate (ADP) inhibitor and an expensive alternative to aspirin. Recent studies have suggested a reduction in cerebral events when the combination of aspirin and dipyridamole is used. At least 2 years of treatment after a TIA is necessary but many would recommend the lifelong use of antiplatelet agents.

   In those with atrial fibrillation not caused by rheumatic heart disease, aspirin reduces the risk of a recurrent event by one-fifth and warfarin by one-half. The risk of major haemorrhage with warfarin use is less than 2% per year, especially if the international normalised ratio (INR) is kept below 2.5. Most cardiologists would recommend warfarin to any patient in atrial fibrillation who has had a definite or even a possible embolic event and in patients over 65, or those with hypertension or left atrial enlargement. In those who have rheumatic heart disease, mechanical prosthetic heart valves or other cardiac sources of emboli, long-term anticoagulation is strongly recommended.

3. Surgery. Carotid endarterectomy or angioplasty is worth considering in patients with a TIA in the carotid territory within the previous 6 months who have documented severe (>60%) stenosis of the origin of the internal carotid artery on the symptomatic side. Surgery in such cases is definitely superior to medical therapy. A decision to operate should be based on the availability of surgical expertise and the complication (stroke) rate of a particular surgical unit.

4. Other treatment will depend on the final diagnosis and can range from anticonvulsants to pacemaker insertion. It is usually unwise to treat these patients without an established diagnosis.

Infectious disease

Pyrexia of unknown origin (PUO)

While not a common long case, this problem presents both diagnostic and management problems. The term 'pyrexia of unknown origin' is used only for patients with a fever >38.3°C for more than 3 weeks when no diagnosis has been made during a week of intensive study. The common causes are listed in Table 6.75.

The history

1. Ask about chronological development of symptoms. Gastrointestinal tract symptoms should be sought (e.g. subphrenic abscess, diverticular abscess, cholangitis, appendiceal abscess, liver abscess, Crohn's disease, metastatic cancer in the abdomen, Whipple's disease). Note any preceding acute infections (e.g. diarrhoeal illness, boils). Chest pain may suggest pericarditis, multiple pulmonary emboli or rarely intraluminal dissection of the aorta. Joint pain may suggest rheumatoid arthritis, systemic lupus erythematosus (SLE), vasculitis, atrial myxoma or endocarditis. Dysuria or rectal pain may indicate prostatic abscess or urinary tract infection. Headache and joint or muscle pain may indicate giant cell arteritis. Night sweats may indicate lymphoma, tuberculosis, brucellosis, endocarditis or an abscess.

2. Ask about places of residence and overseas travel (e.g. malaria, amoebiasis, fungal infections).

Table 6.75   Important causes of pyrexia of unknown origin

1. Neoplasms:
   (a) lymphoma, leukaemia, malignant histiocytosis
   (b) solid tumours
       primary—renal, lung, atrial myxoma, large bowel, pancreas, liver
       secondary—metastatic disease (including melanoma, sarcoma)
2. Infections:
   (a) bacterial—tuberculosis, atypical mycobacteria, abscess (e.g. pelvic, abdominal), brucellosis, endocarditis, pericarditis, osteomyelitis, cholangitis, pyelonephritis, leptospirosis
   (b) viral, rickettsial and chlamydial—hepatitis, HIV, cytomegalovirus, Q fever, psittacosis
   (c) parasitic—malaria, amoebiasis, trichinosis, toxoplasmosis
3. Connective tissue diseases:
   (a) rheumatoid arthritis, systemic lupus, rheumatic fever, adult Still's disease
   (b) vasculitis—polyarteritis nodosa, temporal arteritis, Wegener's granulomatosis
4. Miscellaneous:
   (a) drug fever
   (b) inflammatory bowel disease, Whipple's disease
   (c) granulomatous disease—granulomatous hepatitis, sarcoidosis (uncommon)
   (d) multiple pulmonary emboli, intraluminal aortic dissection
   (e) thyroiditis
   (f) haematomas—retroperitoneal space (consider especially if on anticoagulants)
   (g) haemolysis
   (h) habitual hyperthermia (usually young women with low-grade fever but no organic disease)
   (i) thermoregulatory disorders (rare—abnormal temperature-regulating mechanism)
   (j) cyclic neutropenia
   (k) factitious fever

HIV = human immunodeficiency virus.

---

3. Ask about contact with domestic or wild animals or birds (e.g. psittacosis, brucellosis, Q fever, histoplasmosis, leptospirosis, toxoplasmosis).
4. Ask about close contact with persons who have tuberculosis.
5. Inquire about occupation and hobbies—veterinary surgeon, farming (fungal infection, raw milk ingestion, hypersensitivity pneumonitis), intravenous drug use (contaminants e.g. quinine).
6. Inquire about sexual practices (e.g. risk of human immunodeficiency virus [HIV] infection, sexually transmitted disease, pelvic inflammatory disease).
7. Ask about evidence of immunocompromised host (e.g. cytomegalovirus, *Pneumocystis carinii*).
8. Ask about medication used—drug fever (antibiotic allergy e.g. sulfonylureas, penicillin), arsenicals, iodides, thiouracils, antihistamines, non-steroidal anti-inflammatory drugs (NSAIDs), antihypertensives (methyldopa, hydralazine), antiarrhythmics (procainamide, quinidine).
9. Ask about anticoagulant use (accumulation of old blood in a closed space, e.g. retroperitoneal, perisplenic).

10. Ask about iatrogenic infection (e.g. catheter, arteriovenous fistula, prosthetic heart valve).
11. Ask about factitious fever from injection of contaminated material or tampering with thermometer readings—suspect the former diagnosis if there is an excessively high temperature, or the latter in the absence of tachycardia, chills or sweats; this is more common in medical or paramedical personnel.

The examination

Look at the temperature chart if available to see whether the fever pattern is characteristic. The temperature tends to fall to normal each day in pyogenic infections, tuberculosis and lymphoma, while in malaria the temperature can return to normal for days before rising again. Inspect the patient: note whether he or she appears ill or not, whether there is cachexia (suggesting a chronic disease process) and any skin rash (e.g. erythema multiforme, erythema nodosum).

Pick up the hands and look for stigmata of infective endocarditis or any vasculitic changes and for finger clubbing. Inspect the arms for injection sites (intravenous drug abuse). Palpate for epitrochlear and axillary lymphadenopathy (e.g. lymphoma, solid tumour spread, focal infections).

Examine the eyes for iritis or conjunctivitis (e.g. connective tissue disease, sarcoidosis) or jaundice (e.g. cholangitis, liver abscess). Look in the fundi for choroidal tubercles (miliary tuberculosis), Roth's spots (infective endocarditis), retinal haemorrhages or infiltrates (e.g. leukaemia). Note any facial rash (e.g. SLE). Feel the temporal arteries (temporal arteritis). Examine the mouth for ulcers and gum disease, and the teeth and tonsils for infection. Feel the parotids for parotitis and the sinuses for sinusitis. Palpate the cervical lymph nodes. Also examine for thyroid enlargement and tenderness (subacute thyroiditis).

Examine the chest. Palpate for bony tenderness over the sternum and shoulders. Carefully examine the respiratory system (e.g. for signs of tuberculosis, abscess, empyema, carcinoma) and the heart for murmurs (e.g. infective endocarditis, atrial myxoma) or prosthetic heart sounds or rubs (e.g. pericarditis).

Examine the abdomen. Inspect for skin rash (e.g. the rose-coloured spots of typhoid [an uncommon long case]). Palpate for tenderness (e.g. abscess), hepatomegaly (e.g. granulomatous hepatitis, hepatoma, cirrhosis, metastatic deposits), splenomegaly (e.g. haemopoietic malignancy, infective endocarditis, malaria), renal enlargement (e.g. obstruction, renal cell carcinoma). Feel the testes for enlargement (e.g. seminoma, tuberculosis). Feel for inguinal adenopathy.

Always ask for the results of the rectal examination (e.g. prostatic abscess, rectal cancer, Crohn's disease) and pelvic examination (pelvic pus). Look at the penis and scrotum for a discharge or rash.

Finally examine the nervous system for signs of meningism (chronic meningitis) or focal neurological signs (e.g. brain abscess, mononeuritis multiplex in polyarteritis nodosa). Check the results of the urine analysis.

Investigations

Determine how many blood cultures have been obtained and the results. Ask to review the blood count and smear (e.g. for neutropenia, eosinophilia, atypical lymphocytes), liver function tests, electrolytes and creatinine. Look at the chest X-ray. Rule out urinary tract disease if suspected. Selected serological tests may be helpful depending on the clinical setting (e.g. fungal, HIV, Q fever). An autoimmune screen—antinuclear antibodies (ANA), extractable nuclear antigen (ENA), erythrocyte sedimentation rate (ESR), C-reactive protein (CRP), an electrophoretogram (EPG) and complement levels—should be assessed if a connective tissue disease is suspected. However, remember that malignancy and infection can also cause an increase in acute phase reactants and a low-titre ANA. Check the purified protein derivative (PPD) for tuberculosis exposure. If abdominal disease is suspected or other tests have not provided a clue, obtain a computed tomography (CT) scan.

Biopsy of involved tissue (e.g. bone marrow, liver, lymph node, skin, muscle) may lead to a definitive diagnosis. The clinical setting determines what should be biopsied.

Exploratory laparotomy when all other tests are negative and in the absence of any evidence of abdominal disease is usually unproductive.

Treatment

Therapy directed at the underlying disease should be the goal of assessment. Therapeutic trials in the absence of a diagnosis (e.g. antibiotics, antituberculosis therapy, NSAIDs, steroids) may result in resistant bacterial infection or drug toxicity and may make accurate diagnosis difficult.

HIV/AIDS

The patient with human immunodeficiency virus (HIV) infection or the acquired immunodeficiency syndrome (AIDS) has become increasingly available for the long cases. Remember that the diagnosis of AIDS can be made when someone infected with HIV has a CD4$^+$ cell count of <200 cells/μL or an HIV-associated disease. These patients present numerous diagnostic and management problems. The candidate will be expected to display a logical approach to the case and, of course, show a sympathetic attitude to the patient with this chronic disease. There needs to be a strong emphasis in the discussion on the psychological and social effects of the illness. Public health implications may also have to be addressed. Candidates should have an approach to pretest counselling for patients being tested for HIV.

The history

1. Ask about the presenting symptoms. As usual for long cases, the candidate must find out what symptoms or complications are currently affecting the patient. These must be assessed in the context of possible longstanding disease affecting many systems of the body.
2. Inquire when the virus was acquired. This is especially important in helping predict the likely level of immunosuppression. Find out about symptoms of a possible seroconversion illness in the past (Table 6.76). Approximately 50% of people have a seroconversion illness. It occurs 3–6 weeks after infection and often resembles glandular fever. Remember that, without treatment, the development of AIDS takes roughly 7–10 years from the time of seroconversion. The occurrence of a seroconversion illness does not seem to be associated with a worse prognosis.

   Note from the history any of the conditions likely to occur during the period of mild-to-moderate immunosuppression that precedes the development of AIDS, and those related to severe immunosuppression that define the development of AIDS (Table 6.77).
3. Ask about the mode of acquisition of infection. Comorbidity differs between subgroups, so specific questions about risk factors are essential. For example, Kaposi's sarcoma is often found in the homosexual subgroup, while viral hepatitis, endocarditis, heroin nephropathy and other disorders related to drug abuse may complicate the disease in the intravenous drug-using group; many haemophilia A patients acquired HIV from pooled blood products.
4. Ask about sexual contacts. Contact tracing must be mentioned and the possibility of infection of sexual partners without their knowledge addressed. Ask the patient whether family and friends are aware of the diagnosis.

Table 6.76   Features of the seroconversion illness

A seroconversion illness occurs in more than 50% of cases. There is usually some combination of the following symptoms:
- Fever
- Lymphadenopathy
- Maculopapular rash
- Arthralgia
- Myalgia
- Pharyngitis
- Nausea
- Vomiting
- Diarrhoea
- Headache
- Meningism
- Weight loss
- Oral candidiasis

Table 6.77   HIV-related conditions with severe immunosuppression

Pneumocystis carinii pneumonia

Kaposi's sarcoma

Non-Hodgkin's lymphoma

Disseminated *Mycobacterium avium complex* infection

Cytomegalovirus infection

Cerebral toxoplasmosis

Oesophageal candidiasis

AIDS dementia complex

Note: This is a representative rather than an exhaustive list.

5. Ask about general constitutional symptoms. Symptoms of fever, lethargy and weight loss may indicate the AIDS-related complex, or suggest an underlying opportunistic infection or malignancy.
6. Inquire about specific symptoms:
   (a) respiratory—cough, dyspnoea, sputum—these may result from *Pneumocystis carinii* pneumonia, lymphoid interstitial pneumonitis, tuberculosis, bacterial pneumonia or fungal pneumonia
   (b) gastrointestinal—diarrhoea or weight loss as a result of cryptosporidiosis, microsporidiosis, mycobacterial infection or cytomegalovirus (CMV) colitis; odynophagia, as a result of oesophageal candidiasis, herpes simplex, or CMV ulceration; vomiting and abdominal pain owing to biliary tract disease; drug side-effects (e.g. didanosine-induced pancreatitis);—diarrhoea is usual when patients are treated with protease inhibitors

(c) neurological—meningism, caused by cryptococcal meningitis, focal neurological symptoms or seizures as a result of space-occupying lesions, toxoplasmosis or non-Hodgkin's lymphoma; cognitive decline as a result of HIV dementia or multifocal leukoencephalopathy; peripheral nervous system disease owing to peripheral neuropathy, CMV radiculopathy, or myopathy

(d) renal—nephrotic syndrome from HIV-associated nephropathy; renal failure owing to sepsis or drug side-effects

(e) ocular—deteriorating vision, which usually suggests advanced CMV retinitis

(f) dermatological—rashes may be caused by drug reactions, viral infection (e.g. herpes zoster virus [HZV] or herpes simplex virus [HSV]), or fungal infection; itch may be caused by scabies or drug reaction, and nodules can be caused by Kaposi's sarcoma or bacillary angiomatosis

(g) mouth—ulcers (aphthous or viral), gingivitis, periodontal disease, hairy leukoplakia or candidiasis

(h) cardiac—dyspnoea, chest pain or palpitations owing to myocarditis or pericarditis

(i) haematological—anaemia (bone marrow suppression or infiltration, treatment with zidovudine); thrombocytopenia and neutropenia are less common.

7. Ask about previous treatment. Find out about antiretroviral drug and antibiotic treatment and about any adverse effects of these. Inquire about specific side-effects (Table 6.78).

8. Ask about previous investigations. The HIV patient may be able to give much helpful information on previous investigations, including viral load results, T cell CD4$^+$ counts, magnetic resonance imaging (MRI) scans, CT scans, lumbar punctures, bone marrow biopsies and endoscopy.

9. Inquire about social, drug and alcohol history. The examiners will expect quite detailed knowledge of the patient's social, economic and family circumstances.

The examination

Note especially:

1. temperature
2. nutritional state (wasting is common in advanced disease)
3. skin (e.g. rashes, pigmentation and the lesions of Kaposi's sarcoma)
4. mouth (e.g. hairy leukoplakia, Kaposi's sarcoma lesions, periodontal disease, HSV mouth ulcers)
5. eyes—acuity, visual fields and fundoscopy (e.g. CMV retinal lesions)
6. cognition, gait and coordination (e.g. AIDS dementia)
7. chest—cough, sputum, crackles (e.g. opportunistic chest infection)
8. heart—cardiac failure, pericardial disease (e.g. AIDS cardiomyopathy)
9. abdomen—rectal examination, perianal disease (especially warts and HSV)
10. haematological system—lymph nodes and spleen.

Investigations

The patient is likely to have had many tests. The standard screening test for HIV is an ELISA or enzyme immunoassay (EIA) test. It usually tests against antigens of both HIV1 and HIV2 (very rare in Australia). It has a sensitivity of over 99%. Its specificity in low-risk populations is only about 90%. False positives can occur related to recent vaccinations, other viral infections and autoimmune diseases. The western blot test is more specific and a negative western blot means a positive EIA test is a false positive. Other tests are used to assess the severity of the illness and immunocompromisation and to look for associated conditions (e.g. syphilis) and complications. The currently relevant ones will depend on the clinical presentation. Certain tests are essential for all patients, either as a baseline or for monitoring.

Table 6.78 Side-effects of selected antiretroviral drugs

Drug	Side-effects
A. Nucleoside reverse transcriptase inhibitors	
Zidovudine (AZT)	Headache, nausea, myopathy, bone marrow suppression
Didanosine (Ddi)	Diarrhoea, pancreatitis, peripheral neuropathy
Zalcitabine (ddc)	Mouth and oesophageal ulcers, pancreatitis, peripheral neuropathy
Lamivudine (3TC)	Side-effects uncommon
Stavudine (d4t)	Peripheral neuropathy, nausea
Abacavir	Hypersensitivity syndrome (3%)
B. Non-nucleoside reverse transcriptase inhibitors	
Nevirapine	Rash, hepatitis
Efavirenz	Dizziness, cognitive disturbance, insomnia, fatigue, rash
Delavirdine	Rash
C. Protease inhibitors	
Indinavir	Nausea, diarrhoea, lipodystrophy, insulin resistance, hepatitis, renal calculi, hair and nail changes
Saquinavir	Diarrhoea, lipodystrophy, insulin resistance, hepatitis
Nelfinavir	As for saquinavir
Amprenavir	Diarrhoea, nausea, perioral paraesthesia, lipodystrophy, insulin resistance
Ritonavir	Nausea, diarrhoea, taste disturbance, perioral paraesthesia, lipodystrophy, insulin resistance

Baseline

Immune function needs to be established at this point with a full blood count, $CD4^+$ level (levels >200 cells/µL are associated with opportunistic infections) and HIV plasma serum viral load. A delayed-type hypersensitivity skin test will help define cellular immune function. The lower the $CD4^+$ (T helper cell) level and higher the HIV viral load, the more advanced the infection. $CD4^+$ levels may fall progressively to undetectable levels. Aggressive treatment of infections may allow continued survival of patients despite these low $CD4^+$ levels. Antiviral treatment may slow $CD4^+$ depletion or stabilise it for many years. About 5% of infected patients do not develop a reduction in $CD4^+$ counts even after more than 10 years without treatment. These patients are called 'non-progressors'.

It should also be established whether the patients have concurrent sexually transmitted diseases (syphilis serology, hepatitis B serology), tuberculosis (tuberculin test), and whether they are at risk of activation of latent infection (CMV, toxoplasma serology). Renal and liver function should be checked prior to commencing antiviral drugs.

Monitoring

The key investigations for monitoring progress are the HIV plasma viral load and the CD4$^+$ T cell count. Serial full blood counts and biochemistry will help assess any complications of disease or therapy.

Treatment

Candidates will be expected to know the clinical features and general treatment options for common complications of HIV infection, especially opportunistic infection and malignancy. This list would include *P. carinii* pneumonia, Kaposi's sarcoma, cerebral toxoplasmosis, CMV infection, *Mycobacterium avium* complex (MAC) infection, diarrhoeal syndromes and cryptococcal meningitis.

Prophylaxis for *P. carinii* with cotrimoxazole or pentamidine and MAC with azithromycin is an important consideration. Pneumococcal vaccination is routine even when the CD4$^+$ count remains >300 cells/μL. Herpes simplex prophylaxis with acyclovir and *Candida* prophylaxis with fluconazole or ketoconazole are appropriate for prevention after one episode has occurred.

Multiple antiretroviral agents are now available for the treatment of HIV (see Table 6.78). Known as HAART (highly active antiretroviral therapy), these drugs have dramatically improved quality of life and life expectancy in HIV disease. Some doubt remains as to the optimal time to commence therapy. It is clear that an increasing viral load (>20,000 copies/mL), falling CD4$^+$ count (<500 cells/μL) or clinical progression are definite indications, but many clinicians prefer to commence treatment before this. Drugs should be used only in combination to prevent emergence of resistance, and most regimens contain three or more drugs. Children and pregnant women should also be treated in this way. Treatment is not curative and must be continued indefinitely. Regimens can be changed if there is evidence of disease progression. HAART reduces the risk of vertical transmission and probably also the risk of seroconversion following occupational exposure (e.g. needlestick injury), if given promptly.

The short case

You see, but you do not observe.

Sir Arthur Conan Doyle (1859–1930)

The short case is a test of a candidate's ability to examine a patient smoothly, confidently and accurately. There is rarely the opportunity to go back and repeat the examination. It takes a long time to get used to being watched critically while examining. This is why it is important to have done short cases of every conceivable type so that the physical examination is performed automatically the correct way. While proceeding, the candidate should be consciously synthesising the results, not trying to remember what to do next.

Listen carefully to the introduction given. These introductions are now standardised. Each group of examiners gives the same introduction to all the candidates they examine. The wording is agreed by them after they have examined the patient themselves, and is usually written on a card. This is to make the case fairer. The introduction may well give a hint, so be attentive. Usually a short history will be given (e.g. 'This patient presented with chest pain') to indicate the problem, followed by an instruction to examine a particular system or organ (e.g. the cardiovascular system). These specific instructions must be followed. For example, if asked to examine a patient's gait, it is vital to get the patient to walk first. This may appear obvious but many candidates have failed because they have not followed their examiner's instructions. Time is a major factor here—it is limited and you do not want to run out of time before having got to the problem the examiners have raised.

The time allowed for each short case is 15 minutes. This means that time should be available for both examination and discussion. Patients are not included just as quick 'spot diagnosis' cases, but if you do 'spot the diagnosis' it will be a golden opportunity to demonstrate systematically the associated signs in full. With the current marking system, a candidate can fail a short case and still pass the examination. The commonest short cases are cardiovascular and neurological problems. Abdominal examinations are probably next in importance. We suggest that candidates aim to examine each short case proficiently within 8 minutes.

It is a good idea, when introduced to the patient, to step over and shake his or her hand firmly. This may endear you to the patient (and exclude dystrophia myotonica). Always position the patient properly (e.g. at 45 degrees for the cardiovascular examination or flat for the abdominal examination) and make sure that the appropriate parts are undressed.

Do not ask the patient any questions, with few exceptions. It is prudent to say 'Let me know if I hurt you' and, when examining the abdomen directly, to ask 'Are you tender anywhere?'. This is a test of bedside manner (and may give you a clue!). Always try to make the patient comfortable and avoid totally exposing him or her, or exposing parts that are not being examined.

It is always worthwhile taking a moment to stand back and look at the whole patient. This may prevent you missing an obvious spot diagnosis, such as myxoedema, a thymectomy scar in a patient with muscle weakness (myasthenia), a psoriatic rash in a patient with arthropathy or a cushingoid appearance in a hypertension examination. Practice really does help improve the ability to see clinical associations. A candidate will almost always fail the case if a major sign is missed.

Do remember that you are, in fact, demonstrating the signs (particularly in the case of a neurological short case) to the examiners. It is important to perform each manoeuvre accurately and deliberately. Be seen to be smooth and confident, as if you have done the examination a thousand times before. Also try to be confident of each sign before moving on to another area (e.g. on finding an abdominal mass, concentrate on excluding the various possibilities and coming to a firm conclusion), and don't worry too much about the time it takes. Practice will facilitate formation of conclusions accurately and quickly.

The examiners will very occasionally pull a candidate away in the middle of the examination. This is why it is important to be synthesising the data as you go. Do not get flustered—this usually means enough of the examination has been completed for you to have discovered the important signs. Examiners no longer require the interpretation of a particular sign in isolation (e.g. the collapsing carotid pulse in aortic regurgitation, or the double apex beat in hypertrophic cardiomyopathy).

Usually there is no interruption until the examination is almost finished. We suggest that candidates just keep on examining until told to stop and then list all the other things they would like to have done and why (e.g. urine analysis, rectal examination).

Before presenting the findings, listen closely to the examiners' instructions. A candidate will often be asked 'What did you find?', when he or she is expected to describe the relevant signs first and then comment on possible causes. Sometimes candidates will be asked 'What is your diagnosis?', when they are expected to give a diagnosis or differential diagnosis first and then list the signs supporting the contention.

One useful method of presentation is to first repeat the examiners' introduction, then give the provisional diagnosis and relevant findings, for example, 'I was asked to examine Mr Jones, a 60-year-old man who presented with dyspnoea. On examination of his cardiovascular system, I found . . .'. When describing the signs it is probably easiest to present them in the order that they were looked for (e.g. for the cardiovascular system—pulse rate, then blood pressure, then jugular venous pressure). It is important to state all the positive signs and the important negative ones. Be definite about each sign mentioned or do not mention the sign at all. There is no place for expressions such as 'slightly asymmetrical', 'minor', 'early clubbing', etc. Never use the phrase 'I think'; it will always be interpreted as uncertainty.

Alternatively, you may talk as you go. This is usually acceptable to the examiners but we recommend such an approach only in special cases in adult medicine because the processing of information is more difficult for candidates (see Chapter 8).

Confidence is critical to success in the short cases. Do not lose confidence if you make an error, just go on—the examiner may not even have noticed. If the examiner detects hyperventilation, tremor or other signs of extreme anxiety, he or she may wonder, perhaps unfairly, whether the candidate is capable of handling other stresses (e.g. during a cardiac arrest).

A short differential diagnosis is usually expected even if the diagnosis is obvious, for example, a patient with fasciculation, plus upper and lower motor neurone signs in the legs and no sensory loss, almost certainly has motor neurone disease, but a non-metastatic manifestation of carcinoma must be considered. Always mention common before rare diseases, and always consider the patient's age and sex. Never reel off any old list; the differential diagnosis must be tailored to the particular patient seen. Sometimes patients will have signs of two different problems. This shouldn't be ignored. For example, a patient with proximal muscle weakness as a result of polymyositis may have unrelated Dupuytren's contractures.

After presentation of the signs, several minutes or more are set aside for discussion. The examiners are not encouraged to take the candidate back for a second look at a sign but this does happen and presents a genuine second chance. If a candidate has done well in a case and there are a few minutes left for extra questions, the score can only go up, not down. Relevant X-rays or an electrocardiograph (ECG) may be shown to the candidate. Some diagnostic and therapeutic aspects may be discussed in the short case.

The College has moved away from the traditional 'spot' short case (e.g. acromegaly) and now concentrates more on 'realistic' cases (e.g. heart murmurs, abdominal masses). However, all types still crop up—the candidate must try to prepare for most possibilities. It is also true that the more straightforward the case, the higher the standard of examination that will be expected, and vice versa. Trick cases are deliberately avoided.

The value of some traditional clinical signs is now being questioned as *evidence-based* approaches to clinical examination help establish the reliability and validity of signs. There is much work still to be done in this area but an understanding of the value of signs is increasingly important. Some useful references that might assist the candidate are listed at the end of the book. A tactful approach may be needed with the examiners to prevent any resentment at the candidate's failing to look for a traditional sign that is a particular favourite of theirs.

There are four golden rules worth remembering:

1. Do *everything* properly when you examine—*never* take short cuts.
2. *Think* and *synthesise* as you examine the patient—be alert.
3. *Never* make up signs, and *never* ignore signs because they don't fit neatly together.
4. Don't say *anything* wrong when presenting—it is better to say that you don't know.

8

CHAPTER

Common short cases

The trouble with doctors is not that they don't know enough, but that they don't see enough.

Corrigan (1802–1880)

You may be asked to examine a system or a particular part of the patient. Now that 15 minutes is available for each case, 'spot' diagnoses alone are not likely to be asked for by the examiners. In the following pages a system for examining major short-case possibilities is outlined. Use these to help develop your own system. Many useful lists are also included in this section.

In all cases, before beginning a specific examination, you should stand back for a moment and carefully observe the patient. It is still important to look for an associated 'spot' diagnosis, such as peripheral neuropathy in a myxoedematous patient or aortic regurgitation in a patient with Marfan's syndrome.

The patient will normally be positioned and undressed for you. However, if either positioning or undressing is unsatisfactory, you must insist on having this corrected.

Cardiovascular system

Cardiovascular examination

This man presents with dyspnoea on exertion and orthopnoea. Please examine his cardiovascular system.

Method (Fig 8.1)

Figure 8.1 Cardiovascular system examination.

1. GENERAL INSPECTION (lying at 45°)
   Marfan's, Turner's, Down syndrome
   Rheumatological disorders—
   ankylosing spondylitis (aortic regurgitation)

   Acromegaly, etc.
   Dyspnoea

2. HANDS
   Radial pulses—right and left
   Radiofemoral delay

Clubbing
Signs of infective endocarditis—
  splinter haemorrhages, Osler's
  nodes, etc.
Peripheral cyanosis
Xanthomata

3. BLOOD PRESSURE

4. FACE
  Eyes
    Cornea: arcus cornea
    Sclerae: pallor, jaundice
    Pupils: Argyll Robertson (aortic
    regurgitation)
    Xanthelasma
  Malar flush (mitral stenosis,
    pulmonary stenosis)
  Mouth
    Cyanosis
    Palate (high arched—Marfan's)
    Dentition

5. NECK
  Jugular venous pressure
    Central venous pressure height
    Wave form (especially large *v*
    waves)
  Carotids
    Pulse character

6. PRAECORDIUM
  Inspect
    Scars—whole chest, back
    Deformity
    Apex beat—position, character
    Abnormal pulsations
  Palpate
    Apex beat—position, character
  Thrills
  Abnormal impulses
  Note: Beware of dextrocardia
  Auscultate
    Heart sounds

Murmurs
  Position patient left lateral
  position sitting forward (forced
  expiratory apnoea)
  Note: Palpate for thrills again on
  positioning.
Dynamic auscultation
  Respiratory phases
  Valsalva
  Exercise (isometric,
  e.g. handgrip)

7. BACK (sitting forward)
  Scars, deformity
  Sacral oedema
  Pleural effusion (percuss)
  Left ventricular failure
    (auscultate)

8. ABDOMEN (lying flat—1 pillow
  only)
  Palpate liver (pulsatile, etc.),
    spleen, aorta
  Percuss for ascites (right heart
    failure)
  Femoral arteries—palpate,
    auscultate)

9. LEGS
  Clubbing toes
  Cyanosis, cold limbs, trophic
    changes, ulceration (peripheral
    vascular disease)
  All peripheral pulses
  Oedema
  Xanthomata
  Calf tenderness

10. OTHER
  Urine analysis (infective
    endocarditis)
  Fundi (endocarditis)
  Temperature chart (endocarditis)

Position the patient at 45 degrees and make sure the chest and neck are fully exposed. For a woman, the requirements of modesty dictate that you cover her breasts with a towel or loose garment.

Inspect while standing back for the appearance of Marfan's, Turner's or Down syndromes. Also look for dyspnoea and cyanosis.

Pick up the patient's hand. While feeling the radial pulse, ask whether you may take the blood pressure. The examiners will usually supply you with the reading. Make sure you remember this value. Inspect the hands then for clubbing. Also look for the peripheral stigmata of infective endocarditis—splinter haemorrhages are common (and are also caused by trauma), while Osler's nodes and Janeway lesions are rare. Look quickly, but carefully, at each nail bed, otherwise it is easy to miss key signs. Note the presence of an intravenous cannula and, if an infusion is running, look at the bag to see what it is. There will usually be a peripheral or central line in situ if the patient is being treated for infective endocarditis. Note any tendon xanthomata (type II hyper-lipidaemia.

The pulse at the wrist should be timed for rate and rhythm. Pulse character is poorly assessed here. This is also the time to feel for radiofemoral delay (which occurs in coarctation of the aorta) and radial–radial inequality.

Next inspect the face. Look at the eyes briefly for jaundice (valve haemolysis) and xanthelasma (type II or III hyperlipidaemia). You may also notice the classic 'mitral facies' (owing to dilation of malar capillaries associated with severe mitral stenosis and caused by pulmonary hypertension and a low cardiac output). Then inspect the mouth using a torch for a high-arched palate (Marfan's syndrome and the possibility of aortic regurgitation and mitral valve prolapse), petechiae and the state of dentition (endocarditis). Look at the tongue or lips for central cyanosis.

The neck is very important, so take time to examine here. The jugular venous pressure (JVP) must be assessed for height and character (Table 8.1 and Fig 8.2). Use the right internal jugular vein to assess this. Look for a change with inspiration (Kussmaul's sign).

Now feel each carotid pulse separately (never together!). Assess the pulse character (Table 8.2).

Table 8.1   Jugular venous pressure

1. Wave form
   (a) Causes of dominant *a* wave:
       (i)   tricuspid stenosis (also causes a slow *y* descent)
       (ii) pulmonary stenosis
       (iii) pulmonary hypertension
   (b) Causes of dominant *v* wave:
       (i)   tricuspid regurgitation
   (c) Causes of cannon *a* waves:
       (i)   complete heart block
       (ii) paroxysmal nodal tachycardia with retrograde atrial conduction
       (iii) ventricular tachycardia with retrograde atrial conduction or atrioventricular dissociation
2. Causes of an elevated central venous pressure:
   (a) right ventricular failure
   (b) tricuspid stenosis or regurgitation
   (c) pericardial effusion or constrictive pericarditis
   (d) superior vena caval obstruction
   (e) fluid overload
   (f) hyperdynamic circulation (e.g. fever, anaemia, thyrotoxicosis, arteriovenous fistula, pregnancy, exercise, beri beri, hypoxia, hypercapnia)

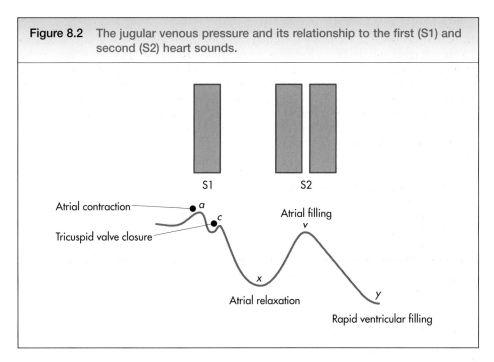

Figure 8.2 The jugular venous pressure and its relationship to the first (S1) and second (S2) heart sounds.

Proceed to the praecordium. Always begin by inspecting for scars, deformity, site of the apex beat and visible pulsations. Don't forget about pacemaker and cardioverter-defibrillator boxes. Mitral valvotomy scars (under the left or right breast) can be quite lateral and easily missed (with ghastly repercussions in the test).

Table 8.2	Arterial pulse character
Anacrotic	Small volume, slow upstroke, plus *a* wave on the upstroke. Cause: aortic stenosis.
Plateau	Slow upstroke. Cause: aortic stenosis.
Bisferiens	Anacrotic plus collapsing. Cause: aortic stenosis plus aortic regurgitation.
Collapsing	Causes: aortic regurgitation, hyperdynamic circulation, arteriosclerotic aorta (elderly patients particularly), patent ductus arteriosus, peripheral arteriovenous aneurysm.
Small volume	Causes: aortic stenosis, pericardial effusion.
Alternans	Alternating strong and weak beats. Cause: left ventricular failure.

Palpate for the apex beat position. Be seen to count down the correct number of intercostal spaces. The normal position is the fifth intercostal space, 1 cm medial to the midclavicular line. The character of the apex beat is important. There are a number of types. A *pressure-loaded* (hyperdynamic, systolic overloaded) apex beat is a forceful and sustained impulse (e.g. in aortic stenosis, hypertension). A *volume-loaded* (hyperkinetic, diastolic overloaded) apex beat is a forceful but unsustained impulse (e.g. in aortic regurgitation, mitral regurgitation). Don't miss the tapping apex beat of mitral stenosis (a palpable first heart sound) or the dyskinetic apex beat caused by a previous large myocardial infarction. The double or triple apical impulse in hypertrophic cardiomyopathy is very important too. Feel also for an apical thrill and time it.

Then palpate with the heel of your hand for a left parasternal impulse, which indicates right ventricular hypertrophy or left atrial enlargement. Now feel at the base of the heart for a palpable pulmonary component of the second heart sound (P2) and aortic thrills. Percussion is usually unnecessary.

Auscultation begins with listening in the mitral area with both the bell and the diaphragm. Spend most time here. Listen for each component of the cardiac cycle separately. Identify the first and second heart sounds (Table 8.3) and decide whether they are of normal intensity and whether they are split. Now listen for extra heart or prosthetic heart sounds (Tables 8.3 and 8.4) and for murmurs (Table 8.5). Do not be satisfied at having identified one abnormality—it is more common to get complex rather than simple lesions in the examination.

Repeat the approach at the left sternal edge and then at the base of the heart (aortic and pulmonary areas). Time each part of the cycle with the carotid pulse. Listen below the left clavicle for a patent ductus arteriosus murmur, which may be audible here and nowhere else.

It is now time to reposition the patient, first in the left lateral position. Again feel the apex beat for character (particularly tapping). Auscultate carefully for mitral stenosis with the bell. Next sit the patient forward and feel for thrills (with the patient in full expiration) at the left sternal edge and base. Then listen in those areas, particularly for aortic regurgitation.

Dynamic auscultation should always be done if there is any doubt about the diagnosis. The Valsalva manoeuvre should be performed whenever there is a pure systolic murmur. Hypertrophic cardiomyopathy is easily missed otherwise (p 241). The patient who seems familiar with the Valsalva manoeuvre may well have a murmur affected by it.

The patient is now sitting up. Percuss the back quickly to exclude a pleural effusion (e.g. due to left ventricular failure) and auscultate for inspiratory crackles (left ventricular failure). If there is radiofemoral delay, also listen for a coarctation murmur here. Feel for sacral oedema and note any back deformity (e.g. ankylosing spondylitis [p 283] with aortic regurgitation).

Next lay the patient flat and examine the abdomen properly (p 254) for hepatomegaly (e.g. as a result of right ventricular failure) and a pulsatile liver (tricuspid regurgitation). Feel for splenomegaly (endocarditis) and an aortic aneurysm. Palpate both femoral arteries. Then examine all the peripheral pulses. Look particularly for peripheral oedema, clubbing of the toes, Achilles tendon xanthomata, signs of peripheral vascular disease, and the stigmata of infective endocarditis.

At the end, ask the examiners for the results of the urine analysis (haematuria in endocarditis) and a temperature chart (fever in endocarditis) and examine the fundi (for Roth's spots in endocarditis and for hypertensive changes).

It is fairly unlikely that you will have time to complete all aspects of your examination. If you are stopped, mention the list of things you would still like to do that are particularly relevant.

If you have auscultated and there is nothing obvious at first, consider the following and exclude them:

Table 8.3   **Heart sounds**

First heart sound (S1)
Loud—mitral stenosis, tricuspid stenosis, tachycardia, hyperdynamic circulation
Soft—mitral regurgitation, calcified mitral valve, left bundle branch block,
    first-degree heart block

Second heart sound (S2)
Aortic (A2)
Loud—congenital aortic stenosis, systemic hypertension
Soft—calcified aortic valve, aortic regurgitation (when the leaflets cannot
    coapt)

Pulmonary (P2)
Loud—pulmonary hypertension
Soft—pulmonary stenosis

Increased normal splitting (wider on inspiration)
Right bundle branch block, pulmonary stenosis, ventricular septal defect, mitral
    regurgitation (earlier A2)

Fixed splitting
Atrial septal defect

Reversed splitting (P2 first)
Left bundle branch block, aortic stenosis (severe), coarctation of aorta, patent
    ductus arteriosus (large)

Third heart sound (S3)
Mechanism: possibly tautening of the mitral or tricuspid cusps at the end of rapid
    diastolic filling

Causes:
Left ventricular third heart sound (S3) (louder at apex and on expiration)
Physiological (under 40 years of age or during pregnancy), left ventricular failure,
    aortic regurgitation, mitral regurgitation, ventricular septal defect, patent ductus
    arteriosus

Right ventricular third heart sound (S3) (louder at left sternal edge and on inspiration)
Right ventricular failure, constrictive pericarditis

Fourth heart sound (S4)
Mechanism: a high atrial pressure wave is probably reflected back from a poorly
    compliant ventricle; is always abnormal.

Causes:
Left ventricular fourth heart sound
Aortic stenosis, acute mitral regurgitation, systemic hypertension, ischaemic heart
    disease, hypertrophic cardiomyopathy

Right ventricular fourth heart sound
Pulmonary hypertension, pulmonary stenosis

<table>
<tr><td colspan="3">Table 8.4   Prosthetic heart valves: physical signs</td></tr>
</table>

Type	Mitral	Aortic
Ball valve (e.g. Starr-Edwards)*	Sharp opening sound after S2; sharp closing sound at S1; 'rattles' in diastole; systolic ejection murmur	Sharp opening sound after S1; sharp closing sound at S2; 'rattles' in systole; systolic ejection murmur
Tilting disc (e.g. Bjork-Shiley)*	Soft opening sound after S2; sharp closing sound at S1; no murmur	Soft opening sound after S1; sharp closing sound at S2; systolic ejection murmur
Xenograft[†]	Systolic ejection murmur	Systolic ejection murmur

*Severe prosthetic dysfunction causes absence of the opening or closing sounds. Ball and cage valves cause more haemolysis than other types, and tilting disc valves are more thrombogenic.

[†]Biprosthetic obstruction or patient prosthetic mismatch causes diastolic rumbling.
Modified with permission from Stein JH (ed.) 1987 Internal medicine, 2nd edn. Little Brown, Boston, p 486.

1. mitral stenosis (see Fig 9.3) (position and exercise if necessary)
2. atrial septal defect (listen carefully for fixed splitting)
3. mitral valve prolapse (perform a Valsalva manoeuvre)
4. pulmonary hypertension
5. constrictive pericarditis.

Notes on valve diseases

After you have made a diagnosis of a valve lesion, the following are the types of facts you should know. An assessment of the lesion's severity is usually required.

Candidates should be able to make some recommendation as to appropriate follow-up. Most patients with valve abnormalities should be reviewed regularly and have repeat echocardiograms. For patients with mild abnormalities about every 3–4 years is sufficient but for more severe ones annual review is usually recommended. Patients who are not symptomatic but have severe disease may need 6-monthly review, usually with a repeat echocardiogram. Patients should be advised to return for earlier review if symptoms (e.g. dyspnoea, chest pain or exertional dizziness) occur.

Mitral stenosis

Valve area: normal, 4–6 cm^2; severe mitral stenosis, <1 cm^2.

Causes
1. Rheumatic (in women more often than men).
2. Congenital very rarely (e.g. parachute valve, with all chordae inserting into one papillary muscle).

Table 8.5	Differential diagnosis of murmurs
Pansystolic	Mitral regurgitation, tricuspid regurgitation, ventricular septal defect, aortopulmonary shunts
Midsystolic	Aortic stenosis, pulmonary stenosis, hypertrophic cardiomyopathy, pulmonary flow murmur of an atrial septal defect
Early systolic	Ventricular septal defect (either very small, or large plus pulmonary hypertension), acute mitral regurgitation, tricuspid regurgitation
Late systolic	Mitral valve prolapse, papillary muscle dysfunction (e.g. hypertrophic cardiomyopathy)
Early diastolic	Aortic regurgitation, pulmonary regurgitation
Mid-diastolic	Mitral stenosis, tricuspid stenosis, atrial myxoma, Austin Flint murmur of aortic regurgitation, Carey-Coombs murmur of acute rheumatic fever
Presystolic	Mitral stenosis, tricuspid stenosis, atrial myxoma

Continuous*
1. Patent ductus arteriosus
2. Arteriovenous fistula (coronary artery, pulmonary, systemic)
3. Venous hum (situated over the right supraclavicular fossa and abolished by ipsilateral compression of the internal jugular vein)
4. Rupture of a sinus of Valsalva into the right atrium or ventricle
5. Aortopulmonary connection (e.g. Blalock shunt)
6. 'Mammary souffle' (in late pregnancy or early postpartum period)

*Aortic stenosis and aortic regurgitation or mitral stenosis and mitral regurgitation may be confused with a continuous murmur.

Clinical signs of severity
1. Small pulse pressure.
2. Early opening snap (owing to raised left atrial pressure).
3. Length of the mid-diastolic rumbling murmur (persists as long as there is a gradient).
4. Diastolic thrill at the apex (rare).
5. Presence of pulmonary hypertension, the signs of which are:
   (a) prominent *a* wave in the JVP
   (b) right ventricular impulse
   (c) loud pulmonary component of the second heart sound (P2)
   (d) pulmonary regurgitation
   (e) tricuspid regurgitation.

Results of investigations
1. Electrocardiogram (ECG):
   (a) *P* mitrale in sinus rhythm

    (b)   atrial fibrillation (a sign of chronicity)
    (c)   right ventricular systolic overload (severe disease)
    (d)   right axis deviation (severe disease).
2. Chest X-ray film (see Fig 9.3):
    (a)   mitral valve calcification
    (b)   big left atrium:
        (i)   double left atrial shadow
        (ii)   displaced left main bronchus
        (iii) big left atrial appendage
    (c)   signs of pulmonary hypertension:
        (i)   large central pulmonary arteries
        (ii)   pruned peripheral arterial tree
    (d)   signs of cardiac failure.

Note: If the investigations suggest that left ventricular dilatation is present in the presence of a mitral stenosis murmur, consider these other possibilities:

1. associated mitral regurgitation
2. associated aortic valve disease
3. associated hypertension
4. associated ischaemic heart disease.

Echocardiograph (M mode, 2D Doppler and colour flow mapping)

The posterior mitral leaflet maintains its anterior position in diastole, and this is pathognomonic. A delayed mitral closure with decreased ejection fraction slope (an M mode index of mitral valve opening) is not pathognomonic but is very suggestive. There may be heavy echoes from thickened or calcified mitral leaflets. On two-dimensional (2D) scanning the valve can be seen doming in diastole. The mitral valve area can be quite accurately determined by 2D echocardiography and Doppler measurements. The valve area is estimated using the pressure half-time measurement. This analysis of Doppler left ventricular inflow is performed routinely when mitral stenosis is suspected. Colour flow mapping makes finding the inflow jet easier and is very sensitive for the detection of any associated mitral regurgitation.

Indications for surgery

These include progressive dyspnoea, pulmonary oedema or major haemoptysis that has failed to respond to medical therapy. This usually occurs when the valve area falls to about 1 cm^2.

    Remember: A declaration that the apex beat is 'tapping' in quality tells the examiner that you have made the diagnosis of mitral (or very rarely of tricuspid) stenosis. It is unwise to allow the word tapping to escape your lips unless you are happy that this is the diagnosis.

Mitral regurgitation

Causes—chronic

1. Degenerative disease.
2. Mitral valve prolapse.
3. Rheumatic (men more often than women)—rarely is mitral regurgitation the only murmur present.
4. Papillary muscle dysfunction:
    (a)   left ventricular failure
    (b)   ischaemia.
5. Connective tissue disease—rheumatoid arthritis, ankylosing spondylitis.
6. Congenital—endocardial cushion defect (including primum atrial septal defect [ASD] and cleft mitral leaflet), parachute valve, corrected transposition.

Causes—acute

1. Infective endocarditis (perforation of anterior leaflet), rupture of a myxomatous cord.
2. Myocardial infarction (chordae rupture or papillary muscle dysfunction).
3. Surgery.
4. Trauma.

Clinical signs of severity

1. Enlarged left ventricle.
2. Pulmonary hypertension (a late sign).
3. Third heart sound (not always reliable).
4. Early diastolic rumble.
5. Soft first heart sound.
6. Aortic component of second heart sound (A2) is earlier.
7. Small-volume pulse (very severe).
8. Left ventricular failure.

Results of investigations

1. ECG:
   (a) *P* mitrale
   (b) atrial fibrillation
   (c) left ventricular diastolic overload
   (d) right axis deviation.
2. Chest X-ray film:
   (a) large (sometimes gigantic) left atrium
   (b) increased left ventricular size
   (c) mitral annular calcification
   (d) pulmonary hypertension (much less common).
3. Echocardiography (Fig 8.3)—this will give information about the possible aetiology, the severity and any associated valve or structural abnormalities (*Note*: The valve leaflets may not appear abnormal.):
   (a) thickened leaflets—rheumatic aetiology
   (b) prolapsing leaflet(s)
   (c) left atrial size (a sign of chronicity and severity)
   (d) left ventricular size and function
   (e) Doppler detection of the regurgitant jet in the left atrium; colour mapping of jet size and detection of reversal of flow in the pulmonary veins
   (f) other abnormalities (e.g. aortic valve disease as a result of rheumatic carditis or an ASD associated with mitral valve prolapse)
   (g) calcification of the mitral annulus—common in elderly people.

Indications for surgery

In chronic mitral regurgitation, consider surgery if there are class III or IV symptoms or if there is left ventricular dysfunction or the left ventricular dimensions have increased progressively. In acute mitral regurgitation, operate if there is haemodynamic collapse (there usually is). Repair of a prolapsing posterior leaflet is now undertaken earlier than valve replacement. The short- and long-term results (1% recurrence per year) are so good that the operation should be recommended for even mild symptoms or once left ventricular dilatation occurs. Mitral valve replacement is usually with a mechanical valve. Tissue valves in the mitral position have a relatively short life (sometimes only 5–7 years).

Mitral valve prolapse (systolic click–murmur syndrome)

This is the commonest heart lesion in the community (3% of adults), and is more common in women. It is more likely to progress to cause significant regurgitation when it occurs in men.

Figure 8.3   Echocardiography report in a patient with mitral regurgitation and mitral valve prolapse.

Echocardiography Report

Reason for study
Middle and late systolic murmur ?MVP

Study quality	<u>Good</u>	Satisfactory	Poor

RV _____ 18 _____ (mm) (N 10–26)

Sept. ___ 8 ___ (mm) (N 7–11)

LVEDD 63 _____ (mm) (N 36–56)

LVESD 28 _____ (mm) (N 20–40)

LVPW ___ 10 _____ (mm) (N 7–11)

Aorta ___ 22 _____ (mm) (N 20–35)

LA _____ 46 _____ (mm) (N 24–40)

FS _____ 55 _____ % (N 27–40)

EF _____ 85 _____ % (N 55–70)

Valves

> **Mitral** MR, prolapse posterior MV leaflet
>
> **Tricus.** Trivial TR
>
> **Aortic** Thickened, not stenosed
>
> **Pulm.** Appears normal

Doppler–2D
The left ventricle is dilated. LV systolic function is preserved. LA is dilated. Severe prolapse of posterior MV leaflet. Possible flail segment.

Doppler—colour flow mapping
There is a large jet of mitral regurgitation extending into the left atrium.

Conclusions
Severe MR, possible flail mitral valve segment, severe MVP.

Comment
The echocardiography criteria for mitral valve prolapse have been tightened over the last several years. Redundancy of one or both of the mitral valve leaflets is common and probably represents a variation of normal in many cases. Bowing of the leaflet into the left atrium of at least 1 cm must be present before the diagnosis of mitral valve prolapse can be made. In this case, the posterior leaflet appears very abnormal and appears to move into the left atrium in an unrestrained fashion. This suggests its chordal attachment may have been severed. The chords may be involved in the abnormality of the mitral leaflets in patients with prolapse and are at risk of rupture.

The left ventricle is dilated, suggesting that the mitral regurgitation is of haemodynamic significance. Left ventricular ejection remains high in cases of mitral regurgitation until late in the illness. This is because the left ventricular afterload is low. Part of the left ventricular ejection is into the left atrium, which is a low-resistance chamber.

> The left atrial enlargement, present here, suggests that some mitral regurgitation has been present for some time. A large left atrium pleases the cardiac surgeons who have trouble getting their hands into the mitral valve through a normal-sized atrium.

Key

EF = ejection fraction; FS = fractional shortening; LA = left atrium; LV = left ventricle; LVEDD = left ventricular end-diastolic dimension; LVESD = left ventricular end-systolic dimension, LVPW = left ventricular posterior wall; MR = mitral regurgitation; MV = mitral valve; MVP = mitral valve prolapse; Pulm. = pulmonary; RV = right ventricle; Sept. = septal thickness; TR = tricuspid regurgitation; Tricus. = tricuspid.

Dynamic auscultation

The click murmur is affected by the:
1. Valsalva manoeuvre (decreases preload)—murmur longer, click earlier
2. handgrip (increases afterload) or squatting (increases preload)—murmur shorter.

Echocardiography

There is now thought to be a considerable variation in the normal range of the appearance of the mitral leaflets on echocardiography. Some redundancy of one or both leaflets is seen commonly in normal people. Prolapse of a leaflet of 1 cm or more into the left atrium behind the attachment point of the valve is considered abnormal. Antibiotic prophylaxis, however, is not necessary for these patients unless mitral regurgitation is detected on Doppler interrogation.

Associations

1. Marfan's syndrome.
2. ASD (secundum).
3. Anorexia nervosa (disproportion between normal-sized valve ring and small left ventricle).

Complications (more common for men with mitral value prolapse)

1. Mitral regurgitation.
2. Infective endocarditis (rare).
   Arrhythmias, embolism and sudden death are probably not complications of mitral valve prolapse.

Aortic regurgitation

Causes of chronic aortic regurgitation

Valvular

1. Rheumatic (rarely the only murmur in this case).
2. Congenital (e.g. bicuspid valve; ventricular septal defect—an associated prolapse of the aortic cusp is not uncommon).
3. Seronegative arthropathy, especially ankylosing spondylitis.

Aortic root (murmur may be maximal at the right sternal border)

1. Marfan's syndrome.
2. Aortitis (e.g. seronegative arthropathies, rheumatoid arthritis, tertiary syphilis).
3. Dissecting aneurysm.
4. Old age.

Causes of acute aortic regurgitation
Note: Murmur may be soft because of increased left ventricular end-diastolic pressure.
1. Valvular—infective endocarditis.
2. Aortic root—Marfan's syndrome, hypertension, dissecting aneurysm.

Clinical signs of severity in chronic aortic regurgitation
1. Collapsing pulse.
2. Wide pulse pressure.
3. Length of the *decrescendo* diastolic murmur.
4. Third heart sound (left ventricular).
5. Soft aortic component of the second heart sound (A2).
6. Austin Flint murmur (a diastolic rumble caused by limitation to mitral inflow by the regurgitation jet).
7. Left ventricular failure.

Note: A loud systolic murmur, rarely with a thrill, may be present in patients with severe aortic regurgitation without any organic aortic stenosis being associated. The peripheral signs of aortic regurgitation are the clue that this is the real lesion in this situation.

Results of investigations
1. ECG:
   (a) left ventricular hypertrophy (diastolic overload).
2. Chest X-ray film:
   (a) left ventricular dilation
   (b) valve calcification.
3. Echocardiography:
   (a) left ventricular dimensions and function
   (b) Doppler estimation of size of regurgitant jet
   (c) vegetations (endocarditis can be a cause of acute aortic regurgitation)
   (d) aortic root dimensions
   (e) valve cusp thickening or prolapse.

Indications for surgery
1. Symptoms—dyspnoea on exertion.
2. Worsening left ventricular function, such as low ejection fraction (in aortic regurgitation this is increased until late, severe disease intervenes) measured on a gated blood pool scan.
3. Progressive left ventricular dilatation on serial echocardiograms. Left ventricular end-systolic dimension of >5.5 cm.

Aortic stenosis

Valve area: 1.5–2.0 cm^2. Significant stenosis at <1 cm^2. In critical aortic stenosis, less than 0.7 cm^2/m^2 or a valve gradient >70 mmHg.

Causes
1. Degenerative senile calcific aortic stenosis (commonest cause in the elderly).
2. Rheumatic (rarely isolated).
3. Calcific bicuspid valve.

Clinical signs of severity
1. Plateau pulse.
2. Aortic thrill (very important sign of severe stenosis).
3. Length, harshness and lateness of the peak of the systolic murmur.
4. Fourth heart sound (S4).

5. Paradoxical splitting of the second heart sound (delayed left ventricular ejection and aortic valve closure).
6. Left ventricular failure (a late sign—right ventricular failure is preterminal).

Results of investigations

1. ECG:
   (a) left ventricular hypertrophy (systolic overload).
2. Chest X-ray film:
   (a) left ventricular hypertrophy
   (b) valve calcification.
3. Echocardiography (Fig 8.4):
   (a) Doppler estimation of gradient (*Note*: Doppler estimation of peak gradient usually overestimates the value compared with cardiac catheterisation.)
   (b) valve cusp mobility
   (c) left ventricular hypertrophy
   (d) left ventricular dysfunction.

Figure 8.4 Echocardiography report in a patient with aortic stenosis.

Echocardiography Report

Reason for study
Systolic ejection murmur ?AS

Study quality: Good   Satisfactory   Poor

RV	13	(mm) (N 10–26)
Sept.	13	(mm) (N 7–11)
LVEDD	53	(mm) (N 36–56)
LVESD	25	(mm) (N 20–40)
LVPW	12	(mm) (N 7–11)
Aorta	22	(mm) (N 20–35)
LA	38	(mm) (N 24–40)
FS	53	% (N 27–40)
EF	83	% (N 55–70)

Valves

Mitral	Trivial MR
Tricus.	Mild TR
Aortic	Thickened, calcified, reduced cusp movement.
Pulm.	Appears normal

Doppler—2D
There is mild symmetrical LV hypertrophy.
   The aortic valve is thickened and heavily calcified, it appears trileaflet. The mitral valve appears normal.

Doppler—colour flow mapping
The aortic outflow velocity is 4.6 m/s. The calculated peak aortic gradient is 85 mmHg. The mean gradient is 60 mmHg. Mild aortic regurgitation was detected. Mild MR is present. Mild TR. RV pressure = 24 mmHg.

Figure 8.4 Echocardiography report for a patient with aortic stenosis (cont.).

Conclusions

Severe calcific aortic stenosis and mild LVH.

Comments

This echocardiography report gives considerable information about the patient's murmur. The candidate who had not diagnosed AS would be in some difficulty.

In AS the aortic valve is usually thickened and calcified unless the patient is young and has congenital AS. Stenosed aortic valves are often congenitally bicuspid and so the echocardiographer will often report the number of valve leaflets. Sometimes there is a comment about reduction in valve cusp movement. An almost immobile valve is more likely to be severely stenosed.

Left ventricular hypertrophy is common when AS is significant. This LVH is mild; dimensions of 14 mm or more indicate severe LVH. Left ventricular dilatation and reduced fractional shortening are late signs.

Doppler measurement of the velocity of blood in the ascending aorta in systole allows calculation of the peak pressure difference across the valve (usually almost 0). This gradient tends to be higher than the gradient measured at cardiac catheterisation. The mean gradient is often closer to the catheter gradient.

Some AR is very often detected in the presence of significant AS. It is unlikely this mild AR would be audible and its presence on the report should not lead the candidate to panic.

Key

AR = aortic regurgitation; AS = aortic stenosis; EF = ejection fraction; FS = fractional shortening; LA = left atrium; LV = left ventricular; LVEDD = left ventricular end-diastolic dimension; LVESD = left ventricular end-systolic dimension; LVH = left ventricular hypertrophy; LVPW = left ventricular posterior wall; MR = mitral regurgitation; Pulm. = pulmonary; RV = right ventricle; Sept. = septal thickness; TR = tricuspid regurgitation; Tricus. = tricuspid.

Indications for surgery

1. Symptoms—exertional angina, exertional dyspnoea, exertional syncope (urgent).
2. Critical obstruction (based on catheterisation data) and severe left ventricular hypertrophy even if asymptomatic.

Choice of valve

Tissue (bovine pericardial or porcine or occasionally homograft valve) are usually offered to patients over the age of about 65 or to younger patients who wish to avoid warfarin. Their life expectancy before failing is up to 15 years or more.

Tricuspid regurgitation

Look for the following signs:

1. the jugular venous pressure—large v waves: the jugular venous pressure is elevated if right ventricular failure has occurred
2. palpation—right ventricular heave
3. auscultation—a pansystolic murmur, maximal at the lower end of the sternum and on inspiration, may be present, but the diagnosis can be made on the basis of the peripheral signs alone
4. abdomen—a pulsatile, large and tender liver is usually present; ascites and oedema with pleural effusions may also occur.

Causes

1. Functional (no disease of the valve leaflets)—right ventricular failure.
2. Rheumatic—only very rarely does tricuspid regurgitation occur alone; usually mitral valve disease is also present.
3. Infective endocarditis (right-sided endocarditis in intravenous drug abusers).
4. Congenital—Ebstein's anomaly.
5. Tricuspid valve prolapse (rare).
6. Right ventricular papillary muscle infarction.
7. Trauma (usually a steering-wheel injury to the sternum).

Results of investigations

Echocardiography enables detection of structural valve abnormality and estimation of the size of the regurgitant jet in the right atrium. Measurement of the velocity of this jet allows estimation of the pressure gradient across the valve. As right atrial pressure is usually 5–10 mmHg, the right ventricular pressure can be estimated in any patient with tricuspid regurgitation by adding 5 to this pressure gradient. Trivial tricuspid regurgitation is a common and normal Doppler echocardiogram finding.

Pulmonary stenosis (in adults)

Look for the following signs:

1. general signs—peripheral cyanosis because of a low cardiac output
2. the pulse—normal or reduced because of a low cardiac output
3. the JVP—giant *a* waves because of right atrial hypertrophy; the JVP may be elevated
4. palpation—right ventricular heave; thrill over the pulmonary area (common)
5. auscultation—the murmur may be preceded by an ejection click; a harsh ejection systolic murmur maximal in the pulmonary area and on inspiration is present; S4 may be present (owing to right atrial hypertrophy)
6. abdomen—presystolic pulsation of the liver may be present
7. signs of severe pulmonary stenosis—an ejection systolic murmur peaking late in systole; absence of an ejection click (also absent when the pulmonary stenosis is infundibular, i.e. below the valve level); presence of S4; signs of right ventricular failure.

Causes

1. Congenital.
2. Carcinoid syndrome.

Chronic constrictive pericarditis

This diagnosis must not be missed. The patient may appear cachectic. Look for the following signs:

1. pulse and blood pressure—a low blood pressure and pulsus paradoxus are typical
2. JVP—this is raised; Kussmaul's sign is rare; the *x* and *y* descents are prominent
3. apex beat—impalpable
4. heart sounds—these are distant; there may be an early third heart sound and an early pericardial knock (as rapid ventricular filling is abruptly halted)
5. hepatosplenomegaly, ascites and oedema provide important clues
6. underlying aetiology (e.g. radiation, tumour, tuberculosis, connective tissue disease, chronic renal failure, trauma).

Hypertrophic cardiomyopathy

It is always important to consider this diagnosis—it is a popular 'trap'! The classical signs are as follows.

1. Pulse: this is typically sharp, rising and jerky, owing to rapid ejection by a hyper-trophied ventricle early in systole, followed then by obstruction. It is not like the pulse of aortic stenosis.
2. Jugular venous pressure: there is a prominent *a* wave owing to forceful atrial contraction against a non-compliant ventricle.
3. Apex beat: there is typically a double or triple impulse owing to presystolic ventric-ular expansion following atrial contraction.
4. Auscultation:
    (a) late systolic ejection murmur (left sternal edge)
    (b) pansystolic murmur (apex) from mitral regurgitation
    (c) fourth heart sound.
    Note: There are no diastolic murmurs.
5. Dynamic manoeuvres: the murmur is louder with the Valsalva manoeuvre, standing and isotonic exercise (e.g. jogging—not usually possible under examination condi-tions). The murmur is softer with squatting, raising the legs and isometric exercise (e.g. forceful handgrip).

Results of investigations
1. ECG:
    (a) left ventricular hypertrophy and lateral ST segment and T wave changes
    (b) deep Q waves
    (c) conduction defects.
2. Chest X-ray film:
    (a) left ventricle enlarged with a hump along the border
    (b) no valve calcification.
3. Echocardiogram (Fig 8.5):
    (a) asymmetrical hypertrophy of the ventricular septum (ASH)
    (b) systolic anterior motion of the anterior mitral valve leaflet (SAM)
    (c) midsystolic closure of the aortic valve
    (d) Doppler detection of mitral regurgitation
    (e) Doppler estimation of the gradient in the left ventricular outflow tract.

Non-cyanotic congenital heart disease

These are difficult examination cases that not infrequently crop up in the test.

Atrial septal defect
There are two types (sinus venosus defects are not often seen in adults)—ostium secundum and ostium primum.

Ostium secundum

This is the commonest and presents in adult life with:

1. fixed splitting of the second heart sound (*Note:* Unfortunately, an ASD is still a possible diagnosis when some variation in splitting is detectable during the respiratory cycle.)
2. pulmonary systolic ejection murmur (increasing on inspiration)
3. pulmonary hypertension (late).

Results of investigations
1. ECG:
    (a) right axis deviation
    (b) right bundle branch block pattern
    (c) right ventricular hypertrophy (systolic overload).
2. Chest X-ray film (see Fig 9.4):
    (a) increased pulmonary vasculature

Figure 8.5 Echocardiography report in a patient with hypertrophic cardiomyopathy.

Echocardiography Report

Reason for study

Systolic murmur, family history of hypertrophic cardiomyopathy

Study quality   <u>Good</u>   Satisfactory   Poor

RV _____ 13 _____ (mm) (N 10–26)

Sept. _____ 18 _____ (mm) (N 7–11)

LVEDD 54 _____ (mm) (N 36–56)

LVESD 30 _____ (mm) (N 20–40)

LVPW 10 _____ (mm) (N 7–11)

Aorta _____ 22 _____ (mm) (N 20–35)

LA _____ 40 _____ (mm) (N 24–40)

FS _____ 44 _____ % (N 27–40)

EF _____ 75 _____ % (N 55–70)

Valves

    Mitral   Mild-to-moderate MR, SAM

    Tricus.   Appears normal

    Aortic   Appears normal

    Pulm.   Appears normal

Doppler — 2D

There is asymmetrical septal hypertrophy. LV systolic function appears normal. LA upper limit of normal size.

Doppler — colour flow mapping

There is a gradient in the left ventricular outflow tract of 80 mmHg. Moderate MR jet – ½ LA.

Conclusions

Hypertrophic cardiomyopathy with LVOT gradient of 80 mmHg. Systolic anterior motion of anterior mitral valve leaflet. Moderate MR.

Comment

The typical echocardiograph findings in this condition are seen here. The septum is thicker than 11 mm and there is abnormal anterior movement of the anterior mitral valve leaflet in systole—SAM. This movement is, in part, responsible for any LVOT gradient. The LVOT gradient only correlates roughly with symptoms and prognosis in this condition. In some cases of hypertrophic cardiomyopathy there may be no LVOT gradient.

Key

EF = ejection fraction; FS = fractional shortening; LA = left atrium; LV = left ventricle; LVEDD = left ventricular end-diastolic dimension; LVESD = left ventricular end-systolic dimension, LVOT = left ventricular outflow tract; LVPW = left ventricular posterior wall; MR = mitral regurgitation; Pulm. = pulmonary; RV = right ventricle; SAM = systolic anterior motion; Sept. = septal thickness; Tricus. = tricuspid.

    (b)   enlarged right atrium and ventricle
    (c)   dilated main pulmonary artery
    (d)   small aortic knob.
3. Echocardiogram:
    (a)   paradoxical septal motion, right ventricular dilation
    (b)   echo dropout in atrial septum
    (c)   Doppler detection of a shunt at the atrial level
    (d)   shunt (bubble) study using agitated saline.

Indication for surgery

Almost all need to be surgically closed when the left-to-right shunt is measured to be at least 1.5 to 1 (unless there is reversal of the shunt). A nuclear cardiac shunt study may help estimation of the size of the shunt.

Ostium primum

This is an endocardial cushion defect adjacent to the atrioventricular valves.

The signs are the same as for ostium secundum but associated mitral regurgitation, tricuspid regurgitation or ventricular septal defect is common. The ECG is particularly helpful as there is left axis deviation and right bundle branch block (and sometimes a prolonged P–R interval).

Look also for the presence of Down syndrome and skeletal upper limb defects (Holt–Oram syndrome).

Ventricular septal defect (VSD)

The clues to the diagnosis of VSD are a thrill and a harsh pansystolic murmur confined to the left sternal edge. Sometimes mitral regurgitation is also present. Down syndrome is associated.

The ECG and chest X-ray film may show left ventricular hypertrophy. The chest X-ray film may also show increased pulmonary vasculature and an enlarged right ventricle. The echocardiogram will show the defect and detect the shunt. Estimation of the pressure gradient between the ventricles will allow detection of right ventricular hypertension. As right ventricular pressure rises, the gradient across the defect falls (right ventricular pressure is closer to left ventricular)—a sign that the shunt is causing trouble.

Indication for surgery

Closure is indicated when the left-to-right shunt is moderate to large, with the pulmonary-to-systemic flow being >1.5 to 1.

Patent ductus arteriosus (PDA)

In this condition there is a vessel from the bifurcation of the pulmonary artery to the aorta. The shunt is usually from the aorta to the pulmonary artery. Reversal of the shunt leads to differential cyanosis and clubbing (toes, *not* fingers). Often a continuous murmur is heard. Confusion with aortic stenosis and regurgitation commonly occurs when candidates examine these patients.

The ECG may show left ventricular hypertrophy (diastolic overload).

The chest X-ray film may show increased pulmonary vasculature, calcification of the duct (trumpet-shaped calcification) and an enlarged left ventricle.

Doppler echocardiography will demonstrate continuous flow in the main pulmonary artery. Left atrial size will be increased.

The indication for surgery or use of a closure device (surgery for this condition in adults is difficult and is now largely replaced by the use of percutaneous catheter closure devices) is the diagnosis of PDA with more than a trivial shunt (unless there is pulmonary hypertension). (*Note*: The detection of a trivial shunt at echocardiography in a patient without a significant murmur or any symptoms is not an indication for closure.)

Coarctation of the aorta

The commonest site for this lesion is just distal to the origin of the left subclavian artery.

Look for a better developed upper body, radiofemoral delay, hypertension in the arms only, chest collateral vessels, a midsystolic murmur over the praecordium and back, and changes of hypertension in the fundi. Turner's syndrome may be associated in some cases.

Results of investigations

1. The ECG may show left ventricular hypertrophy (systolic overload).
2. The chest X-ray film may show (see Fig 9.7):
   (a) enlarged left ventricle
   (b) enlarged left subclavian artery
   (c) dilated ascending aorta
   (d) aortic indentation
   (e) aortic prestenotic and poststenotic dilation
   (f) rib notching—second to sixth ribs on the inferior border.
3. The echocardiogram may show:
   (a) left ventricular hypertrophy
   (b) coarctation shelf in the descending aorta
   (c) abnormal flow patterns in the same area.

Cyanotic congenital heart disease

This is a very difficult area. You will probably not be expected to identify the lesion exactly. A cardiac cause should be suspected if the patient is clubbed and cyanosed.

The common causes of the problem in adults are:

1. Eisenmenger's syndrome—pulmonary hypertension plus a large communication between the left and right circulations (e.g. VSD, PDA, ASD)
2. tetralogy of Fallot
3. complex lesions—univentricular heart, Ebstein's anomaly (if there is an associated atrial septal defect with a right-to-left shunt).

You must decide while examining the patient whether pulmonary hypertension is present as this distinguishes Eisenmenger's syndrome from the tetralogy of Fallot.

Eisenmenger's syndrome

This syndrome may be found in older adults who had right-to-left shunting before the availability of open-heart surgery. The physical signs may include cyanosis, clubbing and polycythaemia. The jugular venous pressure pattern may have a dominant *a* wave and sometimes a prominent *v* wave. A right ventricular heave and a palpable pulmonary component of the second heart sound (P2) may be found. On auscultation there may be a loud P2, a fourth heart sound, a pulmonary ejection click, pulmonary regurgitation and sometimes tricuspid regurgitation (but there may be no murmurs).

The signs all add up to pulmonary hypertension in a cyanosed patient.

To work out the level of the shunt, pay close attention to the second heart sound:

1. wide fixed split—ASD
2. single second sound—VSD
3. normal second sound or reversed splitting—PDA (look for differential cyanosis).

Results of investigations

1. The ECG may show:
   (a) right ventricular hypertrophy
   (b) *P* pulmonale.

2. The chest X-ray film may show (see Fig 9.4):
    (a) right ventricular and right atrial enlargement
    (b) pulmonary artery prominence
    (c) increased hilar vascular markings but attenuated peripheral vessels
    (d) a heart *not* boot-shaped.
3. The echocardiogram will define the anatomy and enable measurement of pulmonary pressures.

Tetralogy of Fallot

There are four features:

1. ventricular septal defect
2. right ventricular outflow obstruction (which determines severity)
3. overriding aorta
4. right ventricular hypertrophy.

The physical signs may include cyanosis, clubbing, polycythaemia, a right ventricular heave and a thrill at the left sternal edge, but not cardiomegaly. On auscultation there may be a single second heart sound (A2) and a short pulmonary ejection murmur.

Results of investigations

1. The ECG may show:
    (a) right ventricular hypertrophy
    (b) right axis deviation.
2. The chest X-ray film may show (see Fig 9.5):
    (a) a normal-sized heart with a boot shape (i.e. a left concavity where the pulmonary artery is normally situated plus a prominent elevated apex)
    (b) right ventricular enlargement
    (c) decreased vascularity of lung vessels
    (d) right-sided aortic knob, arch and descending aorta (25%).
3. The echocardiogram will demonstrate the anatomical abnormalities.

Hypertensive examination

This man has hypertension. Please examine him.

Method

Stand back and inspect. Look for evidence of Cushing's syndrome, acromegaly, polycythaemia and uraemia (Table 8.6). If one of these is present, modify your examination appropriately.

Next, confirm that the blood pressure is elevated. Ask to measure it in both arms and both lying and standing. Measurement in the legs in a young patient may be important.

Feel the radial pulse and very carefully feel for radiofemoral delay. Palpate for radial–radial asymmetry and inspect both hands for vasculitic changes.

Now look at the face. Inspect the conjunctivae for injection (polycythaemia), then examine the fundi for hypertensive changes (Table 8.7). Describe what you see when presenting rather than just giving a grade.

Examine the rest of the cardiovascular system, looking especially for left ventricular failure and coarctation of the aorta. Usually a fourth heart sound is present in severe hypertension.

The abdomen should be examined for renal masses, adrenal masses and an abdominal aneurysm. Auscultate for renal bruits (as a result of fibromuscular dysplasia or atheroma). These may have a diastolic component. Listen first just to the right or left of the midline

Table 8.6   Causes of hypertension

Essential (>95%) *Secondary* (<5%)	
Renal disease	Renovascular disease (renal artery atherosclerosis, fibromuscular disease, aneurysm, vasculitis) Diffuse renal disease
Endocrine	Cushing's syndrome (especially steroid treatment) 17- and 11-beta-hydroxylase defects Conn's syndrome (primary aldosteronism) Phaeochromocytoma Acromegaly Myxoedema Contraceptive pill
Coarctation of the aorta	
Other	Polycythaemia rubra vera Toxaemia of pregnancy Neurogenic (increased intracranial pressure, lead poisoning, acute intermittent porphyria) Hypercalcaemia Alcohol Sleep apnoea

Note: Alcohol consumption and obesity are associated with essential hypertension.

Table 8.7   Fundoscopy changes in hypertension

Grade	Changes
Grade I	Silver wiring
Grade II	Above change plus arteriovenous nipping
Grade III	Above changes plus haemorrhages (characteristically flame-shaped) and exudates: soft exudates, also called cotton wool spots, owing to ischaemia; hard exudates owing to lipid residues from leaky vessels
Grade IV	Above changes plus papilloedema

above the umbilicus. Then sit the patient up and listen in the flanks (a systolic–diastolic bruit in the costovertebral area suggests a renal arteriovenous fistula). Ask at the end for the results of urine analysis (signs of renal disease). Also remember that cerebrovascular accidents, secondary to hypertension, may cause other physical signs.

Marfan's syndrome

This man has a heart murmur. Please examine him.

Method

Fortunately, you notice a marfanoid habitus. While performing your normal cardio-vascular examination look also for the following signs.

- *Hands and arms.* Look for arachnodactyly (spider fingers) and joint hypermobility as well as long, thin limbs.
- *Face.* You may notice a long and narrow face. Look for lens dislocation or lens replace-ment. The sclerae may be blue. Look in the mouth for a high-arched palate.
- *Chest.* Note any pectus carinatum or excavatum.
- *Heart.* Auscultate for aortic regurgitation and mitral valve prolapse. Also look for the signs of dissecting aneurysm or coarctation of the aorta.
- *Back.* Look for kyphoscoliosis and hypermobility.

Always ask at the end to measure the arm span, which will exceed the height. The upper segment to lower segment ratio will be less than 0.85 (the upper segment is from the crown to the symphysis pubis, while the lower segment is from the symphysis pubis to the ground).

Investigations

Many of these patients will have had serial echocardiograms in the hope that progres-sive aortic root dilation will warn of an increased risk of dissection before this occurs.

A slit-lamp examination may be required to diagnose lens dislocation.

Oedema

This man has oedema. Please assess him.

Method

First stand back and look. Note whether the oedema is localised or generalised and whether it is gravitational or not.

Assess nutrition quickly (as hypoalbuminaemia and also beri beri owing to vitamin B_1 deficiency can cause oedema). Also look for any obvious signs of myxoedema (p 266) must never be missed.

Undress the patient and further define the areas affected. Palpate for pitting. Proceed, depending on your findings (Table 8.8).

Table 8.8 **Causes of oedema**

1. Cardiac—congestive cardiac failure, constrictive pericarditis
2. Hepatic—cirrhosis
3. Renal—nephrotic syndrome (Table 6.71)
4. Drugs—calcium antagonists
5. Malabsorption or starvation
6. Protein-losing enteropathy
7. Beri beri ('wet')
8. Myxoedema
9. Cyclical oedema

Pitting lower limb oedema

Define the extent of the oedema. Look for signs of deep venous thrombosis (≥2 cm difference in calf swelling, prominent superficial veins and increased warmth have minor diagnostic value; Homan's test is unhelpful). Note the presence of varicose veins (a common cause of mild peripheral oedema) and the presence of vein-harvesting scars (for coronary artery surgery). Feel the inguinal nodes. Go to the abdomen and look for abdominal wall oedema, prominent abdominal wall veins (inferior vena caval obstruction), ascites, any abdominal masses and evidence of liver disease. A pulsatile liver (tricuspid regurgitation) or malignant involvement should be particularly looked for. Examine next the JVP. Then examine for signs of right ventricular failure and constrictive pericarditis. Feel all the node groups. Finally examine for delayed ankle jerks (to exclude hypothyroidism) and look at the urine analysis.

Remember that vasodilating drugs used for hypertension or angina are very common causes of oedema.

Non-pitting lower limb oedema

Consider the various causes, including lymphoedema (from malignant infiltration, congenital disease, filariasis, Milroy's disease) and myxoedema.

Superior vena caval obstruction (Table 8.9)

The patient may appear cushingoid, from either a tumour or treatment with steroids. Note the plethoric cyanosed face with periorbital oedema. There may be exophthalmos and conjunctival injection. Examine the pupils: a mass in the chest may have caused Horner's syndrome. Examine the fundi for venous dilation. Examine the neck, which is enlarged. The jugular venous pressure is raised, but the vein is not pulsatile. Decide whether the thyroid gland is enlarged). Feel for supraclavicular lymphadenopathy and listen over the trachea for inspiratory stridor. Examine the chest carefully for distended venous collaterals. One or both arms may be oedematous. Look for all the peripheral manifestations of lung carcinoma.

Table 8.9   **Causes of superior vena caval obstruction**

1. Lung carcinoma (90%)
2. Retrosternal tumours—lymphoma, thymoma, dermoid
3. Retrosternal goitre
4. Massive mediastinal lymphadenopathy
5. Aortic aneurysm

Respiratory system

Respiratory examination

This patient presented with breathlessness. Please examine him.

Method (Fig 8.6)

Undress the patient to the waist and sit him over the side of the bed. While standing back to make your usual inspection, ask whether sputum is available for you to look at. A large volume of purulent sputum is an important clue to bronchiectasis. Haemoptysis suggests lung carcinoma or pulmonary infection. Look for evidence of

---

Figure 8.6   Respiratory system examination.

Sitting up

1. **GENERAL INSPECTION**
   Sputum mug contents (blood, pus, etc.)
   Type of cough
   Rate and depth of respiration
   Accessory muscles of respiration

2. **HANDS**
   Clubbing
   Cyanosis (peripheral)
   Nicotine staining
   Wasting, weakness—finger abduction
   Wrist tenderness (HPO)
   Pulse (tachycardia; pulsus paradoxus)
   Flapping tremor (CO_2 narcosis)

3. **FACE**
   Eyes—Horner's syndrome (apical tumour), jaundice, anaemia
   Mouth—central cyanosis
   Voice—hoarseness (recurrent laryngeal nerve palsy)

4. **TRACHEA**

5. **FORCED EXPIRATORY TIME**

6. **CHEST POSTERIORLY**
   Inspect
     Shape of chest and spine
     Scars
     Radiotherapy marks
     Prominent veins (determine direction of flow)
   Palpate
     Cervical lymph nodes

   Expansion
   Vocal fremitus
   Percuss
     Supraclavicular region
     Back
     Axillae
     Tidal percussion (diaphragm)
   Auscultate
     Breath sounds
     Adventitial sounds
     Vocal resonance

7. **CHEST ANTERIORLY**
   Inspect
   Palpate
     Supraclavicular nodes
     Vocal fremitus
     Axillary nodes
   Percuss
   Auscultate
   Pemberton's sign (SVC obstruction)

8. **CARDIOVASCULAR SYSTEM (lying at 45°)**
   Jugular venous pressure (SVC obstruction, etc.)
   Apex beat
   Pulmonary hypertension
   Cor pulmonale

9. **OTHER**
   Temperature chart (infection)
   Fundi (CO_2 narcosis)
   Evidence of malignancy or pleural effusion: examine breasts, abdomen, rectal examination, lymph nodes, etc.

HPO = hypertrophic pulmonary osteoarthropathy; SVC = superior vena cava.

---

dyspnoea at rest and count the respiratory rate. Note the use of the accessory muscles of respiration and any intercostal indrawing of the lower ribs anteriorly (a sign of emphysema). General cachexia should also be noted.

Pick up the hands. Note clubbing (Table 8.10), peripheral cyanosis, nicotine (actually, tar) staining and anaemia, and look for wasting of the small muscles of the hands and weakness of finger abduction (which may be caused by a lower trunk brachial plexus lesion from apical lung carcinoma involvement). Palpate the wrists for tenderness if there is clubbing (hypertrophic pulmonary osteoarthropathy [HPO]). While holding the hand, palpate the radial pulse for tachycardia or obvious pulsus paradoxus.

Table 8.10 Causes of clubbing

1. Respiratory:
   (a) lung carcinoma (usually *not* small cell carcinoma)
   (b) chronic pulmonary suppuration (e.g. bronchiectasis, lung abscess, empyema)
   (c) idiopathic pulmonary fibrosis, asbestosis
   (d) cystic fibrosis
   (e) pleural fibroma or mesothelioma
   (f) mediastinal disease (e.g. thymoma, lymphoma, carcinoma)
2. Cardiovascular:
   (a) infective endocarditis
   (b) cyanotic congenital heart disease
3. Other:
   (a) inflammatory bowel disease
   (b) cirrhosis
   (c) coeliac disease
   (d) thyrotoxicosis
   (e) brachial arteriovenous aneurysm or arterial graft sepsis (unilateral)
   (f) neurogenic diaphragmatic tumours
   (g) familial (usually before puberty) or idiopathic
   (h) hemiplegic stroke (unilateral)

Note: Clubbing does *not* occur with chronic obstructive pulmonary disease, sarcoidosis, extrinsic allergic alveolitis, coal worker's pneumoconiosis or silicosis. With this important sign decide whether it is definitely present or absent. Don't call it 'early' if in doubt.

Go on to the face. Look closely at the eyes for ptosis and constriction of the pupils (Horner's syndrome, p 287). Inspect the tongue for central cyanosis.

Palpate the position of the trachea. This is a most important sign, so spend time on it. If the trachea is displaced, you must concentrate on the upper lobes for physical signs. Also note the presence of a tracheal tug, which indicates gross overexpansion of the chest with airflow obstruction. Now ask the patient to cough and note whether this is a loose cough, a dry cough or, because of recurrent laryngeal nerve palsy, a bovine cough. Next measure the forced expiratory time (FET). Tell the patient to take a maximal inspiration and blow out as rapidly and completely as possible. Note audible wheeze. Prolongation of expiration beyond 3 seconds is evidence of chronic airflow limitation.

The next step is to examine the chest. You may wish to examine this anteriorly first, or go around to the back initially. The advantage of the latter is that there are usually more signs there, unless the trachea is obviously displaced.

Inspect the back. Look for kyphoscoliosis. Don't miss ankylosing spondylitis (p 283), which causes decreased chest expansion and upper lobe fibrosis. Look for thoracotomy scars and prominent veins. Also note any skin changes from radiotherapy.

Palpate first the cervical nodes from behind. Then examine for expansion. First, upper lobe expansion is best seen by looking over the patient's shoulders at clavicular movement during moderate respiration. The affected side will show a delay or decreased movement. Then examine lower lobe expansion by palpation. Note asymmetry and reduction of movement.

Now ask the patient to bring his elbows together in front of him to move the scapulae out of the way. Examine for vocal fremitus. Then percuss the back of the chest and include both axillae. Do not miss a pleural effusion (Table 8.11).

Table 8.11	Pleural effusion

Causes
1. Transudate (protein <30 g/L, pleural:serum protein <0.5, lactate dehydrogenase [LDH] <200 U/L, pleural:serum LDH <0.6):
   (a) cardiac failure
   (b) nephrotic syndrome
   (c) liver failure
   (d) Meigs' syndrome (ovarian fibroma and effusion)
   (e) hypothyroidism (but classically an exudate)
2. Exudate (protein ≥30 g/L, pleural/serum protein >0.5, LDH >200 U/L, pleural:serum LDH >0.6):
   (a) pneumonia
   (b) neoplasm—lung carcinoma, metastatic carcinoma, mesothelioma
   (c) tuberculosis, sarcoidosis
   (d) pulmonary infarction
   (e) subphrenic abscess
   (f) pancreatitis
   (g) connective tissue disease—rheumatoid arthritis, systemic lupus erythematosus
   (h) drugs—nitrofurantoin (acute), methysergide (chronic), drugs causing lupus, chemotherapeutic agents, bromocriptine
   (i) radiation

Pleural fluid analysis: differential diagnosis

pH <7.2	Empyema, tuberculosis, neoplasm, rheumatoid arthritis, oesophageal rupture
Glucose <3.33 mmol/L	Infection, carcinoma, mesothelioma, rheumatoid arthritis
Red blood cells >5000/μL	Pulmonary infarction, neoplasm, trauma, asbestosis, tuberculosis, pancreatitis
Amylase >2000 U/L	Pancreatitis, abdominal viscera rupture, oesophageal rupture
Complement decreased	Rheumatoid arthritis, systemic lupus erythematosus
Chylous	Tumour (usually lymphoma), thoracic duct trauma, tuberculosis, tuberous sclerosis

Auscultate the chest. Note breath sounds (whether bronchial or vesicular) and their intensity (normal or reduced) (Table 8.12). Listen for adventitial sounds (crackles and wheezes) (Table 8.13). Finally examine for vocal resonance. If a localised abnormality is found, try to determine the abnormal lobe and segment.

Return to the front of the chest. Inspect again for chest deformity, symmetry of chest wall movement, distended veins, radiotherapy changes and scars. Palpate the supraclavicular nodes carefully. Palpate the apex beat and measure chest expansion. Then test for vocal fremitus and proceed with percussion and auscultation as before. Listen high up in the axillae too. Before leaving the chest, feel the axillary nodes and breasts.

Lay the patient down at 45 degrees and visually measure the jugular venous pressure. Then examine the praecordium for signs of pulmonary hypertension and cor pulmonale. Finally examine the liver and look for peripheral oedema. Check for Pemberton's sign (p 266).

Before leaving the patient, ask whether you may see the temperature chart.

Table 8.12   **Breath sounds**

1. *Vesicular.* Normal, likened to wind rustling in the leaves.
2. *Bronchial.* The expiratory phase is prolonged and has a blowing quality. The breath sounds heard over the trachea and right and left main bronchi are sometimes rather bronchial in quality.

Causes:
- (a) lobar pneumonia (common)
- (b) localised fibrosis or collapse
- (c) above a pleural effusion
- (d) large lung cavity

3. *Reduced.* Use this term rather than 'air entry'.

Causes:
- (a) emphysema
- (b) large lung mass
- (c) collapse, fibrosis or pneumonia
- (d) effusion
- (e) pneumothorax

Table 8.13   **Added sounds**

1. Wheezes (rhonchi)
   Inspiratory wheezes—characteristic of asthma or upper airway extrathoracic obstruction
   Expiratory wheezes—occur in asthma and chronic obstructive pulmonary disease
   Fixed inspiratory wheeze (monophonic—does not change with respiration)—an important sign of fixed bronchial obstruction, usually due to a carcinoma
2. Crackles (crepitations)
   Late or pan inspiratory crackles:
   - fine—caused by fibrosis—dry crackles
   - medium—caused by left ventricular failure
   - coarse—caused by bronchiectasis or retained secretions
   Early inspiratory crackles: coarse—caused by chronic obstructive pulmonary disease

Chest X-ray films

Hints on how to read a chest X-ray

This is a very valuable investigation and some even consider a chest X-ray an extension of the physical examination. It is essential to be familiar with the various radiographic appearances (see Chapter 9). As a physician, one should feel personally responsible for viewing all the patient's radiographs.

When first viewing the chest radiograph, check:

1. film date
2. type of film—posteroanterior (PA) or anteroposterior (AP) film; the latter (which may be labelled 'portable') magnifies heart size, making assessment of cardiac diameter difficult
3. correct orientation—the left side is most reliably determined by the position of stomach gas
4. film 'centring'—the medial ends of each clavicle should be equidistant from the spines of the vertebrae. Rotation affects mediastinal and hilar shadows, causing undue prominence on the side opposite that to which the patient was turned.

Next, systematically examine the PA film, comparing right and left sides carefully for abnormalities of:

1. soft tissues (e.g. mastectomy, subcutaneous emphysema) and bony skeleton (e.g. rib fractures, malignant deposits)
2. tracheal displacement, paratracheal masses
3. heart size, borders and retrocardiac density
4. aorta and upper mediastinum (count ribs, look for mediastinal shift)
5. diaphragm (right higher than left by 1–3 cm normally), cardiophrenic and costophrenic angles
6. lung hila (left normally above right by up to 3 cm, usually no larger than an average thumb)
7. lung fields—upper zone (to lower border of second rib), midzone (from upper zone to lower border of fourth rib) and lower zone (from midzone to diaphragm)
8. pleura
9. gastric bubble (normally there should be no opacity >0.5 cm above the air bubble)
10. the presence of monitoring leads, a permanent or temporary pacemaker, central lines or other 'hardware'.

Learn to do all this rapidly and accurately.

Finally, always ask to look at a lateral film. Examine it just as carefully. The lateral film is used to help decide the exact anatomical site of an abnormality. Candidates must learn the normal position of the fissures (the horizontal fissure, seen sometimes on the PA and lateral film, is a fine horizontal line at the level of the fourth costal cartilage, whereas the oblique fissure is only seen sometimes on the lateral, beginning at the level of the fifth thoracic vertebra and running downwards to the diaphragm at the junction of its anterior and middle thirds). The lung segments must also be memorised (Fig 8.7). Remember, abnormalities in the lung fields are described by terms such as 'mottling', 'opacity' or 'shadow'—it is usually unwise to attempt to make a precise diagnosis of the underlying pathology in your initial assessment of the chest X-ray (Table 9.1).

Some common radiological abnormalities

In Chapter 9, Figures 9.2 to 9.17, selected films of important conditions are presented. Practise looking at films—it will pay handsome dividends!

Gastrointestinal system

Abdominal examination

Please examine this patient's abdomen.

Figure 8.7 The lung segments.

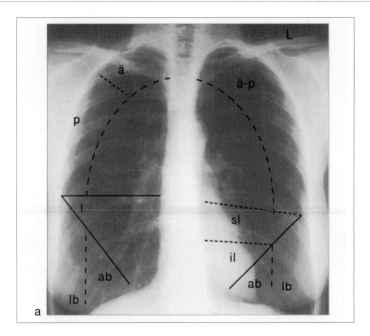

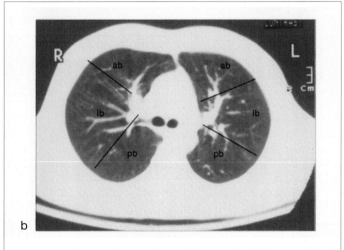

(a) Postero-anterior view. (b) CT scan through lung bases. (c) Left lateral view. (d) Right lateral view.

Right upper lobe: ä = apical segment; a = anterior segment; p = posterior segment. **Left upper lobe**: ä-p = apico-posterior segment; a = anterior segment; sl = superior lingular segment; il = inferior lingular segment. **Right lower lobe**: äl = apical segment; mb = medial basal segment; lb = lateral basal segment; ab = anterior basal segment; pb = posterior basal segment. **Left lower lobe**: äl = apical segment; lb = lateral basal segment; ab = anterior basal segment; pb = posterior basal segment.

Figure 8.7 The lung segments (cont.).

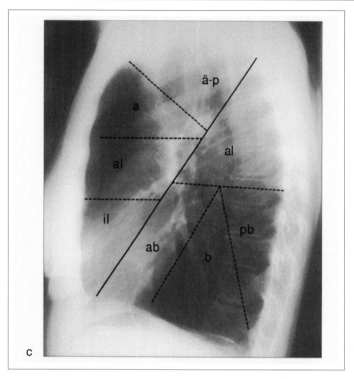

c

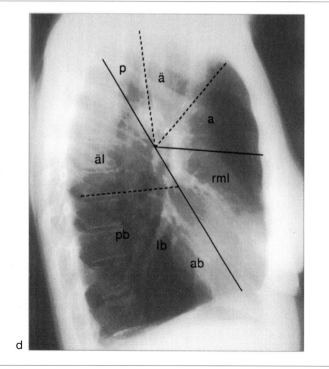

d

Method (Fig 8.8)

Figure 8.8 Gastrointestinal system examination.

Lying flat (1 pillow)

1. **GENERAL INSPECTION**
   Jaundice (liver disease, etc.)
   Pigmentation (e.g. haemochromatosis)
   Xanthomata (e.g. primary biliary cirrhosis, chronic biliary tract obstruction)
   Mental state (encephalopathy)

2. **HANDS**
   Nails—Clubbing
      —Leuconychia (white nails)
   Palmar erythema
   Dupuytren's contractures (alcohol)
   Arthropathy
   Hepatic flap

3. **ARMS**
   Spider naevi
   Bruising
   Wasting
   Scratch marks (chronic cholestasis)

4. **FACE**
   Eyes—Sclera: jaundice, anaemia, iritis
      —Cornea: Kayser-Fleischer rings (Wilson's disease)
   Parotids (alcohol)
   Mouth—Breath: fetor hepaticus
      —Lips: stomatitis, leucoplakia, ulceration, localised pigmentation (Peutz-Jeghers syndrome), telangiectasia (hereditary haemorrhagic telangiectasia)
      —Gums: gingivitis, bleeding, hypertrophy, pigmentation, *Candida*
      —Tongue: atrophic glossitis, leucoplakia, ulceration

5. **CERVICAL/AXILLARY LYMPH NODES**

6. **CHEST**
   Gynaecomastia
   Spider naevi

7. **ABDOMEN**
   Inspect
      Scars
      Distension
      Prominent veins—determine direction of flow (caput medusae; inferior vena caval obstruction)
      Striae
      Bruising
      Localised masses
      Visible peristalsis
   Palpate
      Superficial palpation—tenderness, rigidity, outline of any mass
      Deep palpation—organomegaly (liver, gallbladder, spleen, kidney), abnormal masses
   Roll on to right side (spleen)
   Percuss
      Viscera outline
      Ascites—shifting dullness
   Auscultate
      Bowel sounds
      Bruits, hums
      Rubs

8. **GROIN**
   Genitalia
   Lymph nodes
   Hernial orifices (standing up and coughing)

9. **LEGS**
   Bruising
   Oedema
   Neurological signs (alcohol)

10. **OTHER**
   Rectal examination—inspect (fistulae, tags, blood on glove, etc.), palpate (masses)
   Urine analysis (bile, etc.)
   Blood pressure (renal disease)
   Cardiovascular system (cardiomyopathy)
   Neurological system (Wernicke's encephalopathy, etc.)
   Temperature chart (infection)

Position the patient correctly, with one pillow for the head and complete exposure of the abdomen.

Briefly look at the patient's general appearance and inspect particularly for signs of chronic liver disease and renal disease.

Inspect the abdomen now from the side, squatting to the patient's level. Large masses may be visible. Ask the patient to take slow, deep breaths. Now stand up and look for scars, distension, prominent veins, striae, bruising and pigmentation.

Palpate lightly in each quadrant for masses (Tables 8.14 to 8.19). Ask first if any particular area is tender (to avoid causing pain and also to obtain a clue to the site of possible pathology). Next palpate more deeply in each quadrant and then feel specifically for hepatomegaly and splenomegaly. A palpable liver may be a result of enlargement or ptosis. If there is hepatomegaly (Table 8.14), confirm with percussion and estimate the span (normal span is approximately 12.5 cm). The same procedure is followed for splenomegaly (use a two-handed technique) (Table 8.18). Percussion is useful to exclude splenomegaly (over the lowest intercostal space in the left anterior axillary line: if dull in full inspiration, suspect splenomegaly and palpate again). Always roll the patient on to the right side and palpate again if no spleen is palpable.

Carefully feel for the kidneys bimanually. Remember that any left-sided mass may arise from a number of sites. Always consider, if you have found hepatosplenomegaly, the possibility of associated polycystic kidneys (a common trap for young players in the test).

The usual distinguishing features of a spleen as opposed to a kidney are as follows:

1. The spleen has no palpable upper border.
2. The spleen has a notch.
3. The spleen moves inferomedially on respiration.
4. There is usually no resonance over a splenic mass.
5. The spleen is not bimanually palpable (i.e. not 'ballottable').
6. A friction rub may occasionally be heard over the spleen.

Percuss for ascites as a routine. If the abdomen is resonant out to the flanks on percussion, do not roll the patient over. Otherwise, look for shifting dullness. The technique is usually performed by percussing away from your side of the bed until you reach a dull note, then rolling the patient towards you and waiting at least a short time before percussing again for resonance.

Always auscultate briefly over the liver, spleen and renal areas. Listen for bruits, rubs and a venous hum. Note the presence of bowel sounds. An arterial systolic bruit over the liver is usually caused by either hepatocellular carcinoma or acute alcoholic hepatitis. A friction rub over the liver may be caused by tumour, recent liver biopsy, infarction or gonococcal perihepatitis; splenic rubs indicate infarction. A venous hum occurs uncommonly in portal hypertension.

Examine the groins next. Palpate for inguinal lymphadenopathy. Always ask if you may palpate the testes.

If you now suspect liver disease, you must go on and look for the peripheral stigmata of chronic liver disease. In this instance, it is probably better to proceed from the abdomen to the chest wall. Look for gynaecomastia, spider naevi, hair loss (in men) and breast atrophy (in women). Examine the breasts if you suspect intra-abdominal malignant disease.

Sit the patient at 45 degrees and visually measure the jugular venous pressure so as not to miss constrictive pericarditis as a cause of cirrhosis. Palpate anteriorly for supraclavicular nodes, then sit the patient forwards and feel posteriorly for the other cervical nodes. Look at the back for sacral oedema and spider naevi. If ascites is present, examine the chest for pleural effusions.

Look at the face next. Note any scleral abnormality (jaundice, anaemia or iritis) and look at the corneas for Kayser-Fleischer rings. Xanthelasma are common in patients with

Table 8.14   Differential diagnosis in liver palpation

Hepatomegaly
1. Massive
   (a) metastases
   (b) alcoholic liver disease with fatty infiltration
   (c) myeloproliferative disease
   (d) right heart failure
   (e) hepatoma
2. Moderate
   (a) the above causes
   (b) haemochromatosis
   (c) haematological disease—chronic myeloid leukaemia, lymphoma
   (d) fatty liver—obesity, diabetes mellitus, toxins
3. Mild
   (a) the above causes
   (b) hepatitis (viral, drugs)
   (c) cirrhosis
   (d) biliary obstruction
   (e) granulomatous disorders
   (f) hydatid disease
   (g) amyloid and other infiltrative diseases
   (h) HIV infection
   (i) ischaemia

Firm and irregular liver
1. Cirrhosis
2. Metastatic disease
3. Hydatid disease, granuloma, amyloid, cysts, lipoidoses

Tender liver
1. Hepatitis
2. Rapid liver enlargement—right heart failure, Budd-Chiari syndrome
3. Hepatoma

Pulsatile liver
1. Tricuspid regurgitation
2. Hepatoma
3. Vascular abnormalities

HIV = human immunodeficiency virus.

advanced primary biliary cirrhosis. Feel for parotid enlargement, which may be present soon after an acute alcoholic binge. Inspect the mouth with a torch and spatula for angular stomatitis, ulceration and atrophic glossitis. Smell the breath for fetor hepaticus.

Look at the arms for bruising and spider naevi. Next examine the hands. Ask the patient to extend his arms and hands and look for evidence of hepatic flap. Look also at the nails for clubbing and white nails (leuconychia), and note any palmar erythema and Dupuytren's contractures (the latter are associated with alcohol or trauma). The arthropathy of haemochromatosis may also be present (a degenerative arthritis that particularly involves the second and third metacarpophalangeal joints).

Next examine the legs for oedema and bruising. Look for the nervous system signs of alcoholism—namely, peripheral neuropathy, proximal myopathy, cerebellar syndrome, Wernicke's encephalopathy (bilateral VI nerve palsies) and Korsakoff's psychosis.

Table 8.15   Causes of renal masses

Bilateral
1. Polycystic kidneys (Table 8.16)
2. Hydronephrosis or pyonephrosis (bilateral)
3. Hypernephroma (bilateral renal cell carcinoma)
4. Acute renal vein thrombosis (bilateral)
5. Amyloid, lymphoma and other infiltrative diseases
6. Acromegaly

Unilateral
1. Renal cell carcinoma
2. Hydronephrosis or pyonephrosis
3. Polycystic kidney (asymmetrical enlargement)
4. Acute renal vein thrombosis
5. Normal right kidney or a solitary kidney (uncommon)

Note: In very thin patients, bilateral renal enlargement owing to early diabetic nephropathy or nephrotic syndrome is occasionally detectable.

Table 8.16   Adult polycystic kidneys

If you find polycystic kidneys, remember these very important points:
1. Take the blood pressure (75% have hypertension).
2. Examine the urine for haematuria (owing to haemorrhage into a cyst) and proteinuria (usually less than 2 g/day when measured).
3. Look for evidence of anaemia (as a result of chronic renal failure) or polycythaemia (owing to high erythropoietin levels). *Note*: The haemoglobin level is higher than expected for the degree of renal failure.
4. Note the presence of hepatic (30%) and splenic cysts (rare). These may cause confusion when examining the abdomen.

Note: Subarachnoid haemorrhage occurs in 3% of patients as a result of intracranial aneurysm. As this is an autosomal dominant condition, all family members of patients with polycystic kidney disease should be assessed for kidney disease. Cerebral aneurysms can be screened for in patients with kidney disease by MRI, in the absence of a previous history of subarachnoid haemorrhage.

Candidates are almost always stopped well before this stage. Don't forget to ask to perform a rectal examination and urine analysis. Also ask to look at the temperature chart. Examine for hernias by asking the patient to stand and cough.

If, on the other hand, you have found signs consistent with a haematological problem, proceed as described in that section.

If you find a pulsatile liver, examine the cardiovascular system and particularly note any signs of tricuspid regurgitation.

If an enlarged kidney is present (Table 8.15), ask to check the blood pressure and the urine. If malignant disease is suspected, examine all the node groups, the lungs and the breasts after a thorough abdominal examination. Non-haematological malignant disease which causes hepatomegaly rarely leads to splenomegaly unless the portal vein is directly involved.

Table 8.17   **Some other causes of abdominal masses**

Right iliac fossa
Appendiceal abscess
Carcinoma of the caecum
Crohn's disease
Pelvic kidney
Ovarian tumour or cyst
Carcinoid tumour
Amoebiasis
Psoas abscess
Ileocaecal tuberculosis

Left iliac fossa
Faeces (*Note*: Can be indented.)
Carcinoma of sigmoid or descending colon
Diverticular disease
Ovarian tumour or cyst
Psoas abscess

Upper abdomen
Retroperitoneal lymphadenopathy (e.g. lymphoma, teratoma)
Abdominal aortic aneurysm (pulsatile)
Carcinoma of stomach
Pancreatic pseudocyst or tumour
Pyloric stenosis
Carcinoma of transverse colon

Haemochromatosis, an autosomal recessive disorder, is an important cause of liver disease and is common in the examination. Consider this diagnosis if any of the following signs are present:
1. pigmentation (bronze)
2. arthropathy (typically degenerative arthritis of the metacarpophalangeal joints of the index and middle finger, but may involve any other joint; pseudogout may occur)
3. testicular atrophy (owing to iron deposition in the pituitary gland)
4. dilated cardiomyopathy
5. glycosuria (as a result of diabetes mellitus).
Note: If you are asked to examine the 'gastrointestinal system' rather than the 'abdomen', begin by examining the hands and go on to the arms, face, chest, abdomen and legs as described (see Fig 8.8).

Haematological system

Haemopoietic examination

Please examine this man's haemopoietic system.

Method (Fig 8.9)

Position the patient as for a gastrointestinal examination. Make sure he is fully undressed. Look for bruising, pigmentation, cyanosis, jaundice, scratch marks (owing

---

Table 8.18   Causes of splenomegaly

---

1. Massive
   (a) chronic myeloid leukaemia
   (b) myelofibrosis
   (c) primary lymphoma of spleen, hairy cell disease, malaria, kala-azar (all rare)
2. Moderate
   (a) the above causes
   (b) portal hypertension
   (c) lymphoma
   (d) leukaemia (chronic or acute)
   (e) thalassaemia
   (f) storage diseases (e.g. Gaucher's disease)
3. Small
   (a) the above causes
   (b) other myeloproliferative disorders—polycythaemia rubra vera, essential thrombocythaemia
   (c) haemolytic anaemia
   (d) megaloblastic anaemia (rarely)
   (e) infection—viral (infectious mononucleosis [glandular fever], hepatitis), bacterial (infective endocarditis)
   (f) connective tissue disease or vasculitis—rheumatoid arthritis, systemic lupus erythematosus, polyarteritis nodosa
   (g) infiltration—amyloidosis, sarcoidosis

Note: Secondary carcinomatosis is a rare cause of splenomegaly.

Table 8.19   Causes of hepatosplenomegaly

---

1. Chronic liver disease with portal hypertension
2. Haematological disease—myeloproliferative disease, lymphoma, leukaemia, pernicious anaemia, sickle cell anaemia
3. Infection—acute viral hepatitis, glandular fever, cytomegalovirus
4. Infiltration—amyloid, sarcoid
5. Connective tissue disease—systemic lupus erythematosus
6. Acromegaly
7. Thyrotoxicosis

---

to myeloproliferative disease or lymphoma) and leg ulceration (see below). Also note the presence of frontal bossing and the racial origin of the patient (thalassaemia is more common in people of Asian or Greek background).

Pick up the patient's hands. Look at the nails for koilonychia (spoon-shaped nails, which are rarely seen today and which indicate iron deficiency) and the changes of vasculitis. Pale palmar creases indicate anaemia (usually the haemoglobin level is >90 g/L). Evidence of arthropathy may be important, for example, rheumatoid

---

Figure 8.9 Haematological system examination.

Lying flat (1 pillow)

1. **GENERAL INSPECTION**
   Bruising (thrombocytopenia,
      scurvy, etc.)
   —Petechiae (pinhead bleeding)
   —Ecchymoses (large bruises)
   Pigmentation (lymphoma)
   Rashes and infiltrative lesions
      (lymphoma)
   Ulceration (neutropenia)
   Cyanosis (polycythaemia)
   Plethora (polycythaemia)
   Jaundice (haemolysis)
   Scratch marks (myeloproliferative
      disease)
   Racial origin

2. **HANDS**
   Nails—koilonychia
   Palmar crease pallor (anaemia)
   Arthropathy (haemophilia;
   secondary
      gout; drug treatment, etc.)
   Pulse

3. **ARMS**
   Epitrochlear nodes (non-Hodgkin's
   lymphoma, chronic lymphocytic
      leukaemia, intravenous drug
      use, sarcoid)
   Axillary nodes

4. **FACE**
   Sclera—jaundice, pallor, conjunctival
      suffusion (polycythaemia)
   Mouth—gum hypertrophy
      (monocytic leukaemia),
      ulceration,

infection, haemorrhage (marrow
   aplasia, etc.); atrophic glossitis,
   angular stomatitis (iron, vitamin
   deficiencies)
Tonsils—enlarged (lymphoma)

5. **CERVICAL NODES** (sitting up)
   Palpate from behind

6. **BONY TENDERNESS**
   Sternum
   Clavicles
   Shoulders
   Spine

7. **ABDOMEN** (lying flat) and
   GENITALIA
   Detailed examination

8. **INGUINAL NODES**

9. **LEGS**
   Vasculitis (Henoch-Schönlein
      purpura—buttocks, thighs)
   Bruising
   Pigmentation
   Ulceration
   Neurological signs (subacute
      combined degeneration,
      peripheral neuropathy)

10. **OTHER**
    Fundi (hyperviscosity,
       haemorrhages, infection, etc.)
    Temperature chart (infection)
    Urine analysis (haematuria, bile,
       etc.)
    Rectal examination (blood loss)
    Hess test

---

arthritis and Felty's syndrome, recurrent haemarthroses in bleeding disorders or secondary gout in myeloproliferative disorders.

Examine the epitrochlear nodes. Do this by placing your palm under the patient's elbow—your thumb will be placed over the appropriate area (proximal and slightly anterior to the medial epicondyle). A palpable node is usually pathological and may indicate non-Hodgkin's lymphoma. Note any arm bruising. Remember petechiae are pinhead haemorrhages, whereas ecchymoses are larger bruises. Palpable purpura suggests vasculitis, dysglobulinaemia or bacteraemia.

Go to the axillae and palpate the axillary nodes. Do this by raising the patient's arm and placing your fingers as high as possible. Then position the patient's forearm comfortably over your own forearm. Use your left hand for the patient's right axilla and vice versa. There are four main areas: central, lateral (above and lateral), pectoral (most medial), and subscapular (most inferior).

Look at the face. Inspecting the eyes, note jaundice, pallor or haemorrhage of the sclera, or the injected sclera of polycythaemia. Examine the mouth. Note gum hypertrophy (differential diagnosis includes acute monocytic leukaemia and scurvy), ulceration, infection (e.g. *Candida*), haemorrhage, atrophic glossitis (secondary to iron, vitamin B_{12} or folate deficiency) and angular stomatitis. Look for tonsillar and adenoid enlargement (Waldeyer's ring).

Sit the patient up. Examine the cervical nodes from behind. There are seven groups: submental, submandibular, jugular chain, posterior triangle, postauricular, preauricular and occipital. Then feel the supraclavicular area from the front. Tap the spine with your fist for bony tenderness (which can be caused by an enlarging marrow—e.g. in myeloma, carcinoma). Also gently press the sternum, clavicles and shoulders for bony tenderness.

Lay the patient flat again. Examine the abdomen, particularly for splenomegaly (see Table 8.18) and hepatomegaly (see Tables 8.14 and 8.19). Spring the hips for pelvic tenderness. Palpate the inguinal nodes. There are two groups—along the inguinal ligament and along the femoral vessels. Don't forget to feel the testes, and ask to do a rectal examination (e.g. for melaena).

Examine the legs. Note particularly leg ulcers, which may occur with hereditary spherocytosis, sickle cell syndromes, thalassaemia, macroglobulinaemia and Felty's syndrome. Ask to examine the legs from a neurological aspect for evidence of vitamin B_{12} deficiency. Remember, hypothyroidism and lead poisoning can cause anaemia and peripheral neuropathy. Do not miss Henoch-Schönlein purpura over the buttocks and legs.

Finally, ask to examine the fundi (engorged retinal vessels, papilloedema, haemorrhages, etc.) and look at the temperature chart. Also ask whether you can perform a Hess test if you suspect thrombocytopenia or capillary fragility. Be able to describe the Hess test—inflate the blood pressure cuff to 10 mmHg above diastolic blood pressure. After 5 minutes, deflate the cuff, then wait another 5 minutes and count the number of petechiae; more than $20/cm^2$ is definitely abnormal. Causes of generalised lymphadenopathy are presented in Table 8.20.

Table 8.20   **Causes of generalised lymphadenopathy**

1. Lymphoma (rubbery and firm)
2. Leukaemia (chronic lymphocytic leukaemia, acute lymphoblastic leukaemia particularly)
3. Malignant disease (metastases or reactive changes causing usually asymmetrical, very firm nodes)
4. Infections—viral (e.g. cytomegalovirus, HIV, infectious mononucleosis [glandular fever]), bacterial (e.g. tuberculosis, brucellosis), protozoal (e.g. toxoplasmosis)
5. Connective tissue diseases—rheumatoid arthritis, systemic lupus erythematosus
6. Infiltrations—sarcoidosis
7. Drugs—phenytoin (pseudolymphoma)

HIV = human immunodeficiency virus.

Endocrine system

The thyroid gland

Please examine this woman's neck.

Method (Fig 8.10)

> **Figure 8.10 Neck examination.**
>
> **Sitting up**
>
> 1. **GENERAL INSPECTION**
>   Face—thyrotoxicosis, myxoedema,
>   other diagnostic facies (Table 8.28)
>
> 2. NECK
>   Inspection
>   Scars
>   Swelling
>   Prominent veins
>   Swallowing (a glass of water)
>   Palpation (from behind with neck
>   flexed)
>   Thyroid enlargement—note size,
>   shape, consistency, borders,
>   mobility
>   Thyroid tenderness
>   Thyroid thrill
>   Cervical nodes
>   Palpation (from in front)
>   Thyroid (as above)
>   Carotid arteries
>
> Supraclavicular nodes
> Trachea position
> Sternomastoid function
> Percuss
>   Upper manubrium
> Auscultate
>   Thyroid bruit
>   Carotid bruit
> Pemberton's sign
>
> 3. OTHER
> Signs of thyrotoxicosis/myxoedema
>   elsewhere
> Thyroidectomy scar—test for
>   hypoparathyroidism (Chvostek's
>   and Trousseau's signs)
> Jugular venous pressure—superior
>   vena cava obstruction
> Causes of localised cervical gland
>   enlargement—chest, abdomen,
>   head and neck examination

The most likely problem is thyroid disease but you should also consider in the neck examination the possibilities of superior vena caval obstruction, cervical lymphadenopathy, carotid aneurysm or bruit, jugular venous pressure abnormalities and tracheal deviation.

Glance first at the face for signs of thyrotoxicosis or myxoedema (see below).

Inspect the neck for scars, swelling and prominent veins with the patient sitting up and the neck fully exposed. Look at the front and the sides. Next ask the patient to swallow a sip of water and look for thyroid enlargement. The thyroid moves up with swallowing.

First palpate gently from behind, with the neck flexed, feeling for any thyroid mass (Table 8.21). Note the shape, consistency and distribution of the thyroid enlargement. If a nodule is palpable, determine whether this is single or part of a multinodular goitre. Ask the patient whether the gland is tender (a clue to subacute thyroiditis) and note any hoarseness of the voice (which may be caused by recurrent laryngeal nerve palsy). Decide whether you can palpate the lower border of the gland (to exclude retrosternal extension) and whether there is a thrill. Feel for cervical lymphadenopathy from behind. Palpate each carotid artery (absence possibly indicating malignant infiltration). Test the sternomastoid function, as malignant disease may infiltrate this muscle. Finally, palpate the gland from in front and note the tracheal position.

Table 8.21 Causes of a diffuse goitre

1. Idiopathic (majority)
2. Puberty, pregnancy and postpartum
3. Graves' disease
4. Thyroiditis—Hashimoto's thyroiditis, subacute thyroiditis (tender), chronic fibrosing (Riedel's) thyroiditis (rare)
5. Simple goitre (iodine deficiency)
6. Goitrogens—iodine excess, drugs (e.g. lithium, phenylbutazone)
7. Inborn errors of thyroid hormone synthesis—Pendred's syndrome, an autosomal recessive condition associated with nerve deafness

---

Percuss over the upper part of the manubrium from one side to the other right across the bone and note any change from resonant to dull (a sign of retrosternal extension).

Auscultate over the thyroid gland for bruits (a sign of active thyrotoxicosis) and also over the carotid arteries.

Remember Pemberton's sign. Ask the patient to lift her arms over her head. Look for suffusion of the face, elevation of the jugular venous pressure and inspiratory stridor. Any retrosternal mass may cause these changes.

If there is evidence of a goitre and obvious eye disease (indicating the presence of *thyrotoxicosis*, Table 8.22), proceed to the face. Examine the eyes for exophthalmos by noting the presence of sclera below the cornea when the patient is looking straight ahead. Note lid retraction by looking for the presence of sclera above the cornea. Then test for lid lag by asking the patient to follow your finger descending at a moderate rate. Now examine the conjunctiva for chemosis. Test eye movements for ophthalmoplegia. The inferior oblique muscle power is lost first, then convergence is affected, followed by the other muscles in thyrotoxicosis. Examine the fundi because optic atrophy can occur late. Then look from behind, over the patient's forehead, when she is looking forward, for proptosis.

Examine the outstretched hands for tremor. It is worthwhile placing a sheet of paper over the dorsal aspects of the fingers. Look at the nails for onycholysis (Plummer's nails)—distal separation of the nail from its bed—and thyroid acropachy (this looks like clubbing and is clubbing but is not called clubbing). Note any palmar erythema. Feel for warmth and sweating. Feel the radial pulse for sinus tachycardia, atrial fibrillation or a collapsing pulse.

Test for proximal myopathy in the arms and tap the arm reflexes for briskness.

If there is time, proceed to the legs and look for skin manifestations: pretibial myxoedema—bilateral firm, elevated dermal nodules and plaques which can be pink, brown, or skin-coloured and which are caused by mucopolysaccharide accumulation—and vitiligo. Test for proximal myopathy and hyperreflexia in the legs.

Ask to examine the chest for evidence of gynaecomastia in men, and the heart for an ejection systolic murmur and signs of congestive cardiac failure. Although rarely of importance, there may also be signs of mild splenomegaly and hepatomegaly on abdominal examination, as well as generalised lymphadenopathy.

If a thyroidectomy scar is present, ask to look for the *signs of hypocalcaemia* (i.e. Chvostek's and Trousseau's signs). Chvostek's sign may be present in normal patients. It is tested by tapping over the facial nerve 3–5 cm below and in front of the ear. The facial muscle twitches briefly in the presence of hypocalcaemia. Trousseau's sign is tested by pumping up a sphygmomanometer cuff above systolic blood pressure and looking for *main d'accoucheur* (a strongly adducted thumb with fingers extended except at the metacarpophalangeal joints) that occurs within 2 minutes.

Table 8.22 Causes of thyrotoxicosis

Primary
1. Graves' disease
2. Toxic adenoma or multinodular goitre
3. Hashimoto's thyroiditis (early in its course), subacute thyroiditis (transient) and painful (granulomatous) or painless (lymphatic)
4. Iodine-induced (after previous iodine deficiency)—termed the Jod-Basedow phenomenon
5. Excess thyroid hormone replacement
6. Postpartum thyroiditis (non-tender)
7. Drugs—amiodarone (via Jod-Basedow), lithium (rare)

Secondary
1. Pituitary or ectopic thyroid-stimulating hormone hypersecretion (very rare)
2. Hydatidiform mole or choriocarcinoma (hCG secretion—rare)
3. Struma ovarii (rare)
4. Factitious

Note: The three components of Graves' disease—viz. eye signs, hyperthyroidism with goitre, and pretibial myxoedema—run independent courses.

hCG = human chorionic gonadotrophin.

If there is a suspicion of *hypothyroidism* (when goitre is unusual) (Table 8.23), proceed as follows. Examine the hands. Note peripheral cyanosis, swelling and dry, cold skin. Look at the palmar creases for anaemia (Table 8.24). Feel the pulse for bradycardia and a small volume. Test for carpal tunnel syndrome. Ask the patient to flex both wrists for 30 seconds—paraesthesiae will often be precipitated in the affected hand if the syndrome is present (Phalen's wrist flexion test).

Test for delayed relaxation of the biceps jerk. Examine for proximal myopathy, which is rare.

Proceed to the face. Note here any general swelling and periorbital oedema. Look for loss of the outer one-third of the eyebrows and periorbital xanthelasma. Note whether the skin is dry, fine and smooth. There may be signs of carotenaemia, alopecia or vitiligo. Look at the tongue, which may be swollen, then ask the patient to tell you her name and address and note any hoarseness or slowness of speech. Test for nerve deafness, which may be bilateral.

Go to the legs next. Examine them neurologically, starting with the ankle jerks, noting particularly any evidence of slow relaxation, which is best seen with the patient kneeling on a chair. Then examine for peripheral neuropathy and look for other uncommon neurological abnormalities (Table 8.25).

Finally ask to examine the chest for pleural and pericardial effusions. There may be dry, rough 'sandpaper-like' skin over the chest.

Panhypopituitarism

This man has lost his libido. Please assess him.

Method

You cleverly note that this man looks 'panhypopituitary' (Table 8.26). Proceed as follows. Ask him to stand and make sure he is fully undressed. Note the pale skin and

---

Table 8.23   Causes of hypothyroidism

Primary
Without a goitre (decreased or absent thyroid tissue)
Idiopathic atrophy
Treatment (e.g. iodine-131, surgery)
Agenesis or a lingual thyroid
Unresponsiveness to thyroid-stimulating hormone
With a goitre (decreased synthesis)
Chronic thyroiditis (e.g. late Hashimoto's disease, Riedel's thyroiditis)
Drugs (e.g. lithium, amiodarone)
Endemic iodine deficiency
Iodine-induced hypothyroidism
Inborn errors (enzyme deficiency)

Secondary
Pituitary lesions

Tertiary
Hypothalamic lesions

Transient
Thyroid hormone treatment withdrawn
Subacute thyroiditis
Postpartum thyroiditis

Table 8.24   Causes of anaemia in patients with hypothyroidism

1. Chronic disease (direct or erythropoietin-mediated depressive effect on bone marrow)
2. Folate deficiency secondary to bacterial overgrowth
3. Pernicious anaemia associated with myxoedema
4. Iron deficiency in women owing to menorrhagia
5. Haemolysis secondary to hypercholesterolaemia-induced spur-cell anaemia

---

the lack of hair. The patient may have short stature (failure of growth hormone secretion before growth is complete) and no secondary sexual characteristics (gonadotrophin failure before puberty).

Look at the face more closely. Multiple fine skin wrinkles around the eyes and mouth are characteristic of growth hormone deficiency. Look closely for a hypophysectomy scar on the forehead near the inner canthus of the eye. Examine the eyes for signs of a pituitary tumour (visual fields, especially for bitemporal hemianopia, fundi for optic atrophy) and assess cranial nerves III, IV and VI, as well as the first division of V (affected by tumour extension into the cavernous sinus). Feel the facial hair over the beard area in men.

Go to the chest and look for decreased body hair, pale skin and gynaecomastia. Lay the patient down and look for loss of pubic hair and testicular atrophy (testes are small and soft—the normal size is 15–25 mL in volume).

Table 8.25   **Neurological associations of hypothyroidism**

Common
1. Entrapment (e.g. carpal tunnel, tarsal tunnel)
2. Delayed relaxation phase of ankle jerks
3. Nerve deafness

Uncommon
1. Peripheral neuropathy
2. Proximal myopathy (with normal creatine kinase levels)
3. Hypokalaemic periodic paralysis
4. Eaton-Lambert syndrome or deterioration or unmasking of myasthenia gravis
5. Cerebellar syndrome
6. Psychosis
7. Coma
8. Cerebrovascular disease
9. High cerebrospinal fluid protein
10. Muscle cramps

Table 8.26   **Causes of panhypopituitarism**

1. Chromophobe adenoma (commonest cause in males)
2. Other space-occupying lesion (craniopharyngioma, metastatic carcinoma, granuloma)
3. Iatrogenic (surgery, radiation)
4. Sheehan's syndrome (postpartum necrosis)
5. Head injury
6. Idiopathic

Note: Loss of function (in order)
60% pituitary loss: growth hormone, FSH and LH
80% pituitary loss: TSH
100% pituitary loss: ACTH
ACTH = adrenocorticotrophic hormone; FSH = follicle-stimulating hormone;
LH = luteinising hormone; TSH = thyroid-stimulating hormone.

Test the ankle jerks (for slow relaxation in hypothyroidism—there is no myxoede-matous appearance) and ask to check the blood pressure lying and standing (hypotension with adrenocorticotrophic hormone [ACTH] deficiency).

Cushing's syndrome

This patient has noted weight gain. Please examine him.

Method (Fig 8.11)

This type of introduction may mean Cushing's syndrome in the clinical examination. Make sure that the patient is undressed to his underpants and ask him to stand. Look at him from the front, sides and behind.

Figure 8.11 Cushing's syndrome examination.

Standing

1. GENERAL INSPECTION
   Central obesity and thin limbs
   Skin bruising, atrophy
   Pigmentation (ACTH tumour—
      rare—or bilateral adrenalectomy)
   Poor wound healing

2. ARMS
   Purple striae (proximally)
   Proximal myopathy

Sitting

1. FACE
   Plethora, hirsutism, acne,
      telangiectasia
   Moon shape
   Eyes—visual fields (pituitary tumour),
      fundi (atrophy, papilloedema, signs
      of hypertension or diabetes)
   Mouth—thrush
   Neck—supraclavicular fat pads,
      acanthosis nigricans

2. BACK
   Buffalo hump (interscapular fat pad)
   Kyphoscoliosis (osteoporosis)

Tenderness of vertebrae (osteoporotic
   fractures)

3. LEGS
   Squat (proximal myopathy)
   Striae (thighs)
   Bruising, oedema

4. MENTAL STATE
   Depression
   Psychosis
   Irritability

Lying flat

1. ABDOMEN
   Purple striae
   Adrenal masses, adrenalectomy
      scars
   Liver (tumour deposits)

2. OTHER
   Urine analysis (glycosuria, evidence
      of renal stone disease)
   Blood pressure (hypertension)
   Signs of ectopic tumour (e.g. lung
      small cell carcinoma or
      carcinoid)—rare

Note central obesity with peripheral sparing, and the skin for bruising, atrophy and pigmentation of extensor areas. Hyperpigmentation suggests an ectopic ACTH-secreting tumour, or it may indicate an ACTH-secreting pituitary adenoma in a patient who has had a bilateral adrenalectomy (Nelson's syndrome).

Test for proximal myopathy of the arms and also of the legs (initially by getting the patient to squat). Examine the back for a buffalo hump and feel it. Look for kyphoscoliosis and tap the spine for bony tenderness as a result of osteoporotic vertebral crush fractures.

Then sit the patient on the side of the bed. Look at the face for plethora, hirsutism, acne, telangiectasia and a moon shape.

Test the eyes for visual field defects (which are uncommon) and look in the fundi for papilloedema (caused by benign intracranial hypertension or a pituitary tumour) and optic atrophy, as well as hypertensive or diabetic changes (see Tables 8.7 and 8.36). Then look at the neck for supraclavicular fat pads and acanthosis nigricans.

Ask the patient to lie down. Examine the abdomen (p 254) for adrenalectomy scars, pigmentation, striae and adrenal masses. Look at the genitalia. Virilisation in women or gynaecomastia in men suggests that adrenal carcinoma is more likely. Next look at the legs for oedema, bruising and poor wound healing.

Don't forget to ask for the results of urine analysis (glucose) and take the blood pressure (hypertension). Diagnostic tests are summarised in Table 8.27.

Table 8.27   Diagnosis of Cushing's syndrome*

Screening tests
1. Cortisol levels morning and evening (serum or salivary): loss of diurnal rhythm (evening cortisol level should be less than half the morning value) of little diagnostic value.
2. 24-hour urine collection for urinary free cortisol determination (an indirect assessment of cortisol production).
3. Overnight dexamethasone suppression test (1 mg dexamethasone at midnight causes suppression of cortisol in normal subjects at 9.00 a.m.). No suppression is found in Cushing's syndrome, but this may also occur with alcoholism, induction of hepatic enzymes (e.g. phenytoin), depression, in patients taking the contraceptive pill and in some obese patients.
4. Blood count (secondary polycythaemia, neutrophil leucocytosis, eosinopenia).
5. Electrolyte levels (hypokalaemic alkalosis, particularly with ectopic ACTH-producing tumours).
6. Blood sugar level (hyperglycaemia).

Definitive tests
1. 2 mg dexamethasone suppression tests (0.5 mg 6-hourly for 48 hours). No suppression of plasma cortisol or urinary free cortisol occurs in Cushing's syndrome, but usually suppression does occur in normal subjects, obese patients and depressed patients.
2. 8 mg dexamethasone suppression test (2 mg 6-hourly for 48 hours). Suppression occurs in Cushing's disease, but no suppression is usually found in adrenal adenoma or carcinoma or in the presence of ectopic ACTH production. False-positive results can occur in patients taking anticonvulsants (which accelerate dexamethasone metabolism).
3. Corticotropin-releasing hormone (CRH) stimulation test[†]—CRH stimulates the release of ACTH normally; in Cushing's disease an intravenous injection of ovine CRH increases plasma ACTH, but this does not occur with ectopic ACTH production or adrenal neoplasms.
4. ACTH level—high in ectopic ACTH production, low with adrenal adenoma or carcinoma, high or normal in Cushing's disease. Ectopic secretion of CRH by tumours is a very rare cause of Cushing's syndrome.
5. Petrosal sinus ACTH sampling—a central-to-peripheral venous cortisol ratio of >2:1 is diagnostic of Cushing's disease; lateralisation of ACTH production helps the neurosurgeon plan trans-sphenoidal exploration of the sella.

* Cushing's disease is specifically pituitary ACTH overproduction.
[†] Not available in Australia.

Note: If Cushing's disease is present, pituitary assessment is necessary. If adrenal disease is suspected, CT scanning is useful to assess the anatomy. Remember, ectopic ACTH production by a tumour (e.g. small cell carcinoma of lung, carcinoid of lung or thymus, pancreatic islet cell carcinoma, ovarian carcinoma) does not usually cause cushingoid clinical features but may present with hyperpigmentation, hypokalaemic alkalosis and hypertension.

ACTH = adrenocorticotrophic hormone.

Acromegaly

This patient has noted some change in his facial appearance. Please examine him.

Method (Fig 8.12)

Figure 8.12 Acromegaly examination.

1. GENERAL INSPECTION
   Diagnostic facies

2. HANDS
   Shape
   Sweat
   Phalen's test (carpal tunnel)

3. ULNAR NERVE
   Thickened

4. PROXIMAL MYOPATHY

5. AXILLAE
   Skin tags
   Acanthosis nigricans
   Greasy skin

6. FACE
   Frontal bossing
   Hirsutism
   Macroglossia
   Prognathism
   Hoarseness

7. EYES
   Visual fields

Cranial nerves III, IV, VI, V
Fundi

8. NECK
   Thyroid gland (diffuse or nodular
   goitre)

9. HEART
   Cardiac failure

10. ABDOMEN
    Organomegaly

11. LOWER LIMBS
    Hips ⎫
    Knees ⎭ osteoarthritis, pseudogout
    Entrapment neuropathy
    Heel pad thickening

12. OTHER
    Urine analysis (glycosuria)
    Rectal examination—colonic
       polyps (correlate with skin
       tags)
    Blood pressure (hypertension)
    Sleep apnoea

Consider the possible diagnostic facies (Table 8.28). If the patient looks acromegalic, proceed as follows.

Have the patient stand or sit on the side of the bed. Look at the hands. Look for the coarse features and spade-like shape as well as increased sweating and warmth. Perform Phalen's wrist flexion test for the carpal tunnel syndrome (median nerve entrapment—more accurate than Tinel's sign). Feel the ulnar nerve for thickening at the elbow. Go to the arms and test for proximal myopathy. Also look in the axillae for skin tags (molluscum fibrosum), greasy skin and acanthosis nigricans (brown-to-black velvety elevation of the epidermis owing to multiple confluent papillomas).

Go on to the face. Look for frontal bossing as a result of a large supraorbital ridge (which may also occur in rickets, Paget's disease, hydrocephalus or achondroplasia). Note whether there is a large tongue (sometimes too big to fit into the mouth neatly). Enlargement of the lower jaw (called prognathism) and splaying of the teeth may be present. Notice any acne or hirsutism in women (see Table 8.37), and test the voice, which may be deep, husky and resonant.

Table 8.28   **Common diagnostic facies**

---

1. Acromegalic (p 272)
2. Thyrotoxic (p 266)
3. Myxoedematous (p 266)
4. Cushingoid (p 269)
5. Pagetic (p 185)
6. Myopathic (p 316)
7. Myotonic (p 317)
8. Parkinsonian (p 321)
9. Thalassaemic (p 133)
10. Marfanoid (p 248)
11. Mitral (p 232)

The eyes must be carefully examined. Visual fields should be checked—look particularly for bitemporal hemianopia, but many field defects are possible (Fig 8.16). Examine the fundi for optic atrophy, papilloedema and angioid streaks (red, brown or grey streaks 3–5 times the diameter of the retinal veins appearing to emanate from the optic disc and owing to degeneration of Bruch's membrane with resultant fibrosis, Table 8.29). There may also be diabetic or hypertensive changes.

Examine the thyroid gland for diffuse enlargement or a multinodular goitre (p 265).

Examine the cardiovascular system for signs of congestive cardiac failure, the abdomen for organomegaly—of liver, spleen and kidney—and for signs of hypogonadism (secondary to an enlarging pituitary adenoma). Examine the lower limbs for osteoarthritis and pseudogout. Also, look for foot drop (entrapment of common peroneal nerve) and heel pad thickening.

If there is time, look for evidence of hypothyroidism and adrenocortical insufficiency (from an enlarging pituitary adenoma).

Don't forget to ask for the results of a urine analysis to exclude glycosuria secondary to glucose intolerance, and take the blood pressure (hypertension is an association). Decide whether the acromegaly is active (Table 8.30). Ask if any photographs taken of the patient over the years are available for inspection (typically, manifestations begin in middle age). See Table 8.31 for the diagnostic evaluation.

Table 8.29   **Causes of angioid streaks (PASH)**

---

1. P—Paget's disease, pseudoxanthoma elasticum, poisoning (lead)
2. A—Acromegaly
3. S—Sickle cell anaemia
4. H—Hyperphosphataemia (familial)

Addison's disease

This patient has weakness, anorexia and weight loss. Please assess him.

Method

Fortunately, you suspect Addison's disease. Undress the patient and look for pigmentation (particularly in the palmar creases, elbows, gums and buccal mucosa, genital areas

---

Table 8.30   Evidence of activity in acromegaly

1. Skin tag number
2. Excessive sweating
3. Presence of glycosuria
4. Increasing visual field loss or development of cranial nerve palsies of III, IV, VI and V
5. Enlarging goitre
6. Hypertension
7. Symptoms of headache, or increasing ring size, shoe size or dentures

---

Table 8.31   The diagnosis of acromegaly

Anatomical (99% pituitary adenoma)
Skull X-ray film (enlarged sella, double floor)
CT or MRI scan

Biochemical
Insulin-like growth factor (IGF-1) (somatomedin C) level in plasma (elevated in active acromegaly)
Glucose tolerance test (no suppression or a paradoxical rise in growth hormone level)
Thyrotropin-releasing hormone test (abnormal release of growth hormone in 80%)
Evaluate pituitary function—static and dynamic tests

---

and scars) and vitiligo, owing to an autoimmune disease association. Ear lobe calcification occurs rarely.

Take the blood pressure and test for a postural drop. Ask for the results of a urine analysis, as diabetes is associated with Addison's disease. Remember that the rest of the autoimmune cluster may also be associated (Table 8.32), and the possible causes (Table 8.33). Diagnostic tests are summarised in Table 8.34.

Table 8.32   Autoimmune-associated disease

Addison's disease
Hypoparathyroidism
Mucocutaneous candidiasis
Diabetes mellitus (type 1)
Hashimoto's thyroiditis
Graves' disease
Primary ovarian failure
Pernicious anaemia
Vitiligo
Alopecia
Hypophysitis
Myasthenia gravis

Table 8.33   Causes of Addison's disease (chronic adrenal insufficiency)*

Iatrogenic
Primary
Autoimmune adrenal disease (>80% of all cases)
Polyglandular syndromes:
Type I: Addison's disease, hypoparathyroidism and mucocutaneous candidiasis (anti-IgA antibodies)
Type II: Addison's disease, type 1 diabetes mellitus and Hashimoto's thyroiditis or Graves' disease
Tuberculosis, histoplasmosis
Infiltration (e.g. amyloidosis, sarcoidosis)
Metastatic malignant disease
Demyelinating disease—adrenoleucodystrophy (asymmetrical cortical signs and
   Addison's disease), adrenomyeloneuropathy (spastic paraparesis and Addison's
   disease)
Drugs—heparin (bilateral adrenal haemorrhage), aminoglutethimide, ketoconazole,
   HIV infection

Secondary
Pituitary or hypothalamic disease (usually *no* mineralocorticoid deficiency)

* Acute adrenal insufficiency may follow any stress in a patient with chronic hypoadrenalism or
   abrupt cessation of prolonged high-dose steroid therapy.

HIV = human immunodeficiency virus.

Table 8.34   Diagnosis of Addison's disease

Screening tests
Electrolyte levels (hyponatraemia, hyperkalaemia, hyperchloraemic acidosis,
   hypercalcaemia)
Hypoglycaemia
Blood count (lymphocytosis, eosinophilia)
Chest X-ray film (tuberculosis, small heart)
Plain abdominal X-ray film (adrenal calcification)

Definitive tests
Short Synacthen test (0.25 mg synthetic ACTH given intramuscularly)
Long Synacthen test (8-hour intravenous infusion or depot administration) if
   subnormal response
Plasma ACTH level

Diabetes mellitus

Please examine this diabetic patient.

Method (Fig 8.13)

Figure 8.13 Diabetes mellitus examination.

Lying

1. GENERAL INSPECTION
   Weight—obesity
   Hydration
   Endocrine facies (Table 8.29)
   Pigmentation—haemochromatosis,
   etc.

2. LEGS
   Inspect
   Skin—necrobiosis, hair loss,
     infection, pigmented scars,
     atrophy, ulceration, injection sites
   Muscle wasting
   Palpate
     Temperature of feet (cold, blue
     owing to small or large vessel
     disease)
   Peripheral pulses
     Femoral (auscultate)
     Popliteal
     Posterior tibial
     Dorsalis pedis
   Oedema
   Neurological assessment
     Femoral nerve mononeuritis
     Peripheral neuropathy

3. ARMS
   Inspect
     Injection sites
     Skin lesions
   Pulse

4. EYES
   Fundi—cataracts, rubeosis, retinal
     disease, III nerve palsy, etc.

5. MOUTH AND EARS
   Infection

6. NECK
   Carotid arteries—palpate, auscultate

7. CHEST
   Signs of infection

8. ABDOMEN
   Liver—fat infiltration; rarely
     haemochromatosis
   Fat hypertrophy—insulin injection sites

9. OTHER
   Urine analysis—glycosuria, ketones,
     proteinuria
   Blood pressure and pulse—lying
     and standing

General inspection may reveal a characteristic facial appearance (e.g. Cushing's syndrome or acromegaly) or pigmentation (e.g. haemochromatosis), which will modify the examination approach. Otherwise, expose the patient's legs. This is the only case in which there is an advantage in starting at the legs.

Look for necrobiosis lipoidica over the shins (a central yellow scarred area with a surrounding red margin, if active, owing to atrophy of subcutaneous collagen—it is rare), pigmented scars, skin atrophy, small rounded plaques with raised borders lying in a linear fashion over the shins (diabetic dermopathy), ulceration and infection. Look at the thigh for injection sites, fat atrophy (owing to the use of impure insulin) or fat hypertrophy (owing to repeated injections into the same site, which leads to scarring and hypertrophy), and quadriceps wasting, from femoral nerve mononeuritis—called (inaccurately) diabetic amyotrophy.

Look for loss of hair, skin atrophy and blue, cool feet (small vessel vascular disease). Feel all the peripheral pulses and note capillary return. Feel for pitting oedema. Auscultate over the femoral artery for bruits.

Test proximal muscle power and test the reflexes. Assess for peripheral neuropathy, including dorsal column loss—called diabetic pseudotabes (p 315). Charcot's joints (owing to proprioceptive loss) may rarely be present. (*Note*: Neuropathic joint disease: sensory loss [e.g. from diabetes, tabes dorsalis, amyloid, leprosy, meningomyelocele] allows repeated joint trauma, producing bony overgrowth, synovial effusion and joint instability.)

Go to the upper limbs. Look at the nails for *Candida* infection. Feel the upper arm injection sites. Ask for the blood pressure and take the pulse lying and standing to detect autonomic neuropathy (Table 8.35).

Now examine the eyes for visual acuity. Remember, episodes of poor control cause lens abnormalities acutely. Look for Argyll Robertson pupils (which are rare). Remember, a diabetic third nerve palsy is usually pupil sparing—infarction affects the inner more than the outer fibres, whereas compressive lesions affect the outer fibres first and so involve the pupil early. Look in the fundi (Table 8.36). While performing

---

Table 8.35 Autonomic neuropathy

Clinical features
Postural hypotension (a blood pressure fall of >30/20 mmHg on standing upright from a supine position)
Loss of sinus arrhythmia
Valsalva manoeuvre causes no slowing of the pulse
Loss of sweating
Erectile dysfunction
Nocturnal diarrhoea
Urine retention, incontinence

Table 8.36 Features of diabetic retinopathy

Non-proliferative
Haemorrhages:
1. Dot-haemorrhage into the inner retinal areas
2. Blot-haemorrhage into more superficial nerve fibre layers
   Hard exudates (have straight edges)—leakage of protein and lipids from damaged capillaries
   Soft exudates (cotton wool spots) have a fluffy appearance owing to microinfarcts
   Microaneurysms
   Dilated veins

Proliferative
New vessels
Vitreous haemorrhage
Scar formation
Retinal detachment (opalescent sheet that balloons forward into the vitreous)
Laser scars (small brown or yellow spots)

fundoscopy, also note the presence of cataracts and any new blood vessel formation over the iris (rubeosis). Always test the III, IV and VI cranial nerves and remember that other cranial nerves may be affected. Periorbital and perinasal swelling with gangrene can occur with rhinocerebral mucormycosis, an opportunistic fungal infection. Look in the mouth for *Candida* and other infections. Look in the ears for infection (e.g. malignant otitis externa caused by *Pseudomonas aeruginosa*). Feel and auscultate the carotid arteries.

Examine for hepatomegaly as a result of fatty infiltration and then ask for the results of urine analysis with respect to glucose and protein. There may be signs of chronic renal failure with advanced disease. Ask whether you may weigh the patient.

Hirsutism

A diagnostic approach is summarised in Table 8.37.

Table 8.37 Hirsutism

Clinical approach:
General appearance—acromegaly, cushingoid
Skin changes of porphyria cutanea tarda

Hair distribution
Face
Midline (front and back)
Genital

Signs of virilisation
Receding hairline and increased oiliness of skin
Breast atrophy
Muscle bulk
Clitoromegaly

Abdomen
Adrenal masses (rarely palpable)
Polycystic ovaries or ovarian tumour (rarely palpable)

Blood pressure
Raised in C-11-hydroxylase deficiency

Causes of hirsutism
1. Constitutional (normal endocrinology)
2. Polycystic ovaries, ovarian tumour, idiopathic ovarian disease
3. Adrenal—Cushing's syndrome, congenital adrenal hyperplasia (21- and 11-hydroxylase deficiency), virilising adrenal tumour
4. Ovary (e.g. tumour)
5. Drugs (e.g. phenytoin, diazoxide, streptomycin, minoxidil, androgen, glucocorticoids)
6. Other (e.g. acromegaly, porphyria cutanea tarda)

Rheumatology

In this section only the common joints that are encountered in the examination are discussed.

The hands

Please examine this patient's hands.

Method (Fig 8.14)

Figure 8.14   Hand examination.

Sitting up (hands on a pillow)

1. **GENERAL INSPECTION**
   Cushingoid
   Weight
   Iritis, scleritis, etc.
   Obvious other joint disease

2. **FEEL AND MOVE PASSIVELY**
   Wrists
      Synovitis
      Effusions
      Range of movement
      Crepitus
      Ulnar styloid tenderness
   Metacarpophalangeal joints
      Synovitis
      Effusions
      Range of movement
      Crepitus
      Subluxation
   Proximal and distal interphalangeal
      joints
         As above
   Palmar tendon crepitus
   Carpal tunnel syndrome tests

3. **HAND FUNCTION**
   Grip strength
   Key grip
   Opposition strength
   Practical ability

4. **LOOK**
   Dorsal aspect

Wrists
   Skin—scars, redness, atrophy, rash
   Swelling—distribution
   Deformity
   Muscle wasting
Metacarpophalangeal joints
   Skin
   Swelling—distribution
   Deformity—ulnar deviation, volar subluxation, etc.
Proximal and distal
   interphalangeal joints
Skin
Swelling—distribution
Deformity–swan necking, boutonnière, Z, sausage-shaped, etc.
Nails
   Psoriatic changes—pitting, ridging, onycholysis, hyperkeratosis, discolouration
Palmar aspect
   Skin—scars, palmar erythema, palm creases (anaemia), discolouration
   Muscle wasting

5. **OTHER**
   Elbows—subcutaneous nodules, psoriatic rash
   Other joints
   Signs of systemic disease

When you are asked to examine the hands consider the possibilities of arthropathy, acromegaly, a peripheral nerve lesion, a myopathy or a neuropathy. If there is obvious joint disease, examine as follows.

First make the patient comfortable, expose as much of the hands and forearms as possible and place the patient's hands on a pillow, palms down. You may talk as you go. We believe this is the best way to proceed with a joint examination. However, also practise examining this sort of case by presenting at the end of the examination. Be gentle while examining—don't hurt the patient.

If the patient has arthropathy with an obvious rheumatoid distribution, start by stating that the patient has a symmetrical deforming polyarthropathy involving the wrists and hands. Then describe the forearms and wrists—look at the skin for erythema, ecchymoses or skin atrophy (this may indicate steroid use), scars and rashes (e.g. psoriasis). Then look for swelling and its distribution, wrist deformity and muscle wasting involving the forearms and interosseous muscles.

Go on to the metacarpophalangeal (MCP) joints. Mention, if present, any skin abnormalities, swelling and deformity, particularly ulnar deviation and volar subluxation.

Next describe the proximal (PIP) and distal interphalangeal (DIP) joints. Symmetrical wrist, MCP and proximal joint swellings suggest rheumatoid arthritis. Swelling in the PIP joints and DIP joints is suggestive of osteoarthritis. Again mention any skin changes that may be present, swelling over each joint if present, and deformity, particularly 'swan necking' and boutonnière deformity of the fingers, and 'Z' deformity of the thumb. Sausage-shaped phalanges occur in psoriatic arthropathy as well as ankylosing spondylitis and Reiter's disease. Look for telangiectasiae.

Next look at the nails and describe any psoriatic nail changes, namely pitting, onycholysis, hyperkeratosis, ridging and discolouration. Note the signs of vasculitis (splinter haemorrhages, or black to brown 1–2 mm skin infarcts usually in a periungual location) and mention this to the examiners.

Now ask the patient to open and close the hands. This will reveal tendon ruptures and fixed flexion deformities.

Next turn the wrists over and look at the palms for scars, palmar erythema and muscle wasting.

Now go on and palpate each joint, starting with the wrists. Feel for synovitis (boggy swelling) and effusions. Describe the range of passive movement of the joint. Also note any joint crepitus. Palpate the ulnar styloid for tenderness. When examining the MCP joints, also feel for subluxation. Test for palmar tendon crepitus (tenosynovitis).

Having examined each joint, assess the function of the hand. This is very important. Test grip strength, key grip and opposition strength (thumb and little finger), and ask the patient to perform a practical procedure, such as undoing a button.

A formal neurological examination of the hand is not required in assessing arthropathy. However, a ganglion or tenosynovitis may cause the carpal tunnel syndrome. Ask the patient to flex both wrists together for 30 seconds—paraesthesiae will often be precipitated in the affected hand if the carpal tunnel syndrome is present (Phalen's wrist flexion test). Tap over the carpal tunnel while the wrist is held in extension for Tinel's sign (paraesthesiae in the distribution of the median nerve). These tests have similar but limited specificity and sensitivity. After you have finished with the hands, feel at the elbows for rheumatoid nodules and look carefully for any psoriatic rash there also.

You should now have an idea of the pattern and severity of the deformity as well as the extent of the loss of function, and the activity of the disease.

Always consider the differential diagnosis of a deforming polyarthropathy:

1. rheumatoid arthritis
2. seronegative arthropathies—particularly psoriatic arthritis
3. polyarticular gout or pseudogout
4. primary generalised osteoarthritis (where DIP and PIP joint involvement is common).

Look carefully while doing your hand examination for any of these possibilities.

At the end, ask whether you may examine all the other joints that are likely to be involved and the other systems likely to be affected.

The knees

Examine this patient's knees.

Method

Expose both knees and thighs fully and have the patient lie on his or her back.

Look for quadriceps wasting and then over the knees for any skin abnormalities (scars or rashes), swelling and deformity. Synovial swelling is seen medial to the patella and in the suprapatellar area. Fixed flexion deformity must be assessed. This is looked for by inspecting the knee from the side (a space beneath the knee is seen).

Feel the quadriceps for wasting. Ask about tenderness and palpate for warmth and synovitis over the knee joint. Examine for effusions—the patella tap (ballottement) is used to confirm a large effusion. Here the fluid from the suprapatellar bursa is pushed by the hand into the joint space by squeezing the lower part of the quadriceps and then pushing the patella downwards with the fingers. The patella will be ballottable if fluid is present under it. Pressing over the lateral knee compartment may produce a noticeable medial bulge as a result of fluid displacement in patients with a smaller effusion.

Test flexion and extension passively and note the range of movement and the presence or absence of crepitus. Now examine for fixed flexion deformity by gently extending the knee. Test the ligaments next. The lateral and medial collateral ligaments are tested by having the knee slightly flexed, holding the leg with the right hand and arm, steadying the thigh with the left hand and moving the leg laterally and medially. Movements of more than 5–10 degrees are abnormal. The cruciate ligaments are tested by steadying the foot with your elbow and moving the leg anteriorly and posteriorly with the other hand. Again, laxity of more than 5–10 degrees is abnormal. Use McMurray's test for meniscal integrity. Hold the lower leg and foot, flex and extend the knee while internally and externally rotating the tibia. Pain or clicking is very suggestive of a meniscal tear.

Finally, ask the patient to stand up and examine for a Baker's cyst, which is felt in the popliteal fossa and is more obvious when the knee is extended.

Proceed then to examine other joints that may be involved.

The feet

Examine this patient's feet.

Method

Start by inspecting the ankles. Look at the skin (for scars and rashes) and look for swelling, deformity and muscle wasting. Examine the midfoot and forefoot similarly. Deformities affecting the forefoot include hallux valgus and clawing and crowding of the toes (in rheumatoid arthritis). Note any psoriatic nail changes. Look at the transverse and longitudinal arches. Look for callus over the metatarsal heads, which occurs in subluxation. Note any obvious painless deformities or Charcot's joint.

Palpate, starting with the ankle, feeling for synovitis and effusion. Passive movement of the talar joints (dorsiflexion and plantarflexion) and subtalar joints (inversion and eversion) must be assessed. The best way to examine the subtalar and midtarsal joints is to fix the os calcaneus and ankle joint with the left hand while inverting and everting the midfoot with the right. Tenderness on movement is more important than range of movement. The midfoot (midtarsal joint) allows rotation of the forefoot on a fixed hindfoot. Squeeze the metatarsophalangeal joints for tenderness. Examining the individual toes is useful in seronegative spondyloarthropathies and psoriatic arthritis, where a sausage-like swelling of the toe is characteristic.

Finally, feel the Achilles tendon for nodules and palpate the inferior aspect of the heel for tenderness (plantar fasciitis).

Go on to examine other joints as appropriate.

The back

Examine this man's back.

Method

The initial inspection suggests that this is a case of ankylosing spondylitis (Table 8.38). Ask the patient to undress to his underpants and stand up. Look for deformity, inspecting from both the back and the side, particularly for loss of kyphosis and lumbar lordosis. Palpate each vertebral body for tenderness and palpate for muscle spasm.

Table 8.38   The seronegative spondyloarthropathies

	HLA-B27
1. Ankylosing spondylitis	95%
2. Psoriatic spondylitis	50%
3. Reactive arthritis, including Reiter's syndrome	80%
4. Enteropathic arthritis	75%

HLA = human leucocyte antigen.

Test movement next. Measure the finger–floor distance (inability to touch the toes suggests early lumbar disease). Next look at extension, lateral flexion and rotation of the back. Ask whether you may perform a modified Schober's test. This involves identifying the level of the posterior iliac spine on the vertebral body (approximately at L5). Place a mark 5 cm below this point and another 10 cm above this point. The patient is asked to touch his toes. There should normally be an increase of 5 cm or more in the distance between the marks. In ankylosing spondylitis there will be little separation of the marks, as all the movement is taking place at the hips. Next test the occiput-to-wall distance. Ask the patient to place his heels and back against the wall and ask him to touch the wall with the back of his head without raising the chin above the carrying level; inability to touch the wall suggests cervical involvement, and the distance from occiput to wall is measured.

Ask the patient to go back to his bed and lie on his stomach.

A simple (and unreliable) test for sacroiliac disease is to push with the heel of the hand on the sacrum and note the presence of tenderness in either sacroiliac joint on springing. (*Note*: Usually there is bilateral disease in ankylosing spondylitis.)

Go to the heels and examine for Achilles tendonitis and plantar fasciitis, which are characteristic of the spondyloarthropathies. Evaluate the other large joints, particularly knees, hips and shoulders.

Next examine the chest for decreased lung expansion (chest expansion of less than 3 cm at the nipple line suggests early costovertebral involvement) and for signs of apical fibrosis. Examine the heart for aortic regurgitation, mitral valve prolapse and evidence of conduction defects, and the eyes for uveitis.

Examine the gastrointestinal system for evidence of inflammatory bowel disease (p 115) and for signs of amyloid deposition (e.g. hepatosplenomegaly, abnormal urine analysis results). Remember also to check for signs of psoriasis and Reiter's syndrome, which may cause spondylitis and unilateral sacroiliitis. Rarely patients with ankylosing spondylitis have a cauda equina compression (Table 8.39). X-ray changes are described in Table 8.40.

Table 8.39 **The cauda equina syndrome**

Back, buttock and leg pain

Saddle sensory loss

Lower limb weakness

Loss of sphincter control

Table 8.40 **X-ray changes in ankylosing spondylitis**

Sacroiliac joints
1. Cortical outline lost (early)
2. Juxta-articular osteosclerosis
3. Erosions
4. Joint ankylosis

Lumbar spine
1. Loss of lumbar lordosis
2. Squaring of vertebrae
3. Syndesmophytes (thoracolumbar region)
4. Bamboo spine (bony bridging of vertebrae) and osteoporosis
5. Apophyseal joint fusion

Nervous system

Cranial nerves

Examine this man's cranial nerves.

Method

Inspect the head and neck briefly first. Have the patient sit over the edge of the bed facing you and look for any craniotomy scars (often well disguised by hair), neurofibromata, Cushing's syndrome, acromegaly, Paget's disease, facial asymmetry and obvious ptosis, proptosis, skew deviation of the eyes or pupil inequality. Look for the characteristic facies of myasthenia gravis or myotonic dystrophy.

First nerve (p 288)
Ask the examiners whether they want you to test smell. They will rarely allow you to proceed as it is time-consuming and not usually fruitful in examinations. If you are required to test smell, a series of sample bottles will be provided by the examiners containing vanilla, coffee or other non-pungent substances. Remember to test each nostril separately (go to p 288 for the causes of anosmia).

Second nerve (p 288)

Test visual acuity (with the patient's spectacles on, as refractive errors are not cranial nerve abnormalities) using a visual acuity chart (p 27). Test each eye separately, covering the other eye with a small card.

Examine the visual fields by confrontation using a red-tipped hatpin (p 27), making sure your head is level with the patient's head. A red hatpin enables you to detect earlier peripheral field loss. Test each eye separately. If the patient has such poor acuity that a hatpin is difficult to use, map the fields with your fingers. When you are testing his right eye, he should look straight into your left eye. His head should be at arm's length and he should cover the eye not being tested with his hand. Bring the hatpin from the four main directions diagonally towards the centre of the field of vision.

Next map out the blind spot by asking about disappearance of the hatpin lateral to the centre of the field of vision of each eye. A gross enlargement may be detectable by comparison with your own blind spot.

Look into the fundi (p 286).

Third, fourth and sixth nerves (p 291–2)

Look at the pupils. Note the shape, relative sizes and any associated ptosis. Use your pocket torch and shine the light from the side to gauge the reaction to light on both sides. Don't bore the examiners by shining the light repeatedly into each eye—practise assessing the direct and consensual responses rapidly.

Look for the Marcus Gunn phenomenon (afferent pupillary defect) by moving the torch in an arc from pupil to pupil. The affected pupil will paradoxically dilate after a short time when the torch is moved from a normal eye to one with optic atrophy or very decreased visual acuity from other causes. Test accommodation by asking the patient to look into the distance and then at your red hatpin placed about 15 cm from his nose.

Assess eye movements with both eyes first. Ask the patient to look voluntarily and then follow the red hatpin in each direction—right and left lateral gaze, plus up and down in the lateral position. Look for failure of movement and nystagmus. Ask about diplopia (double vision) when the eyes are in each position. With complex lesions then assess each eye separately. Move the patient's head if the patient is unable to follow movements. Beware of strabismus.

Fifth nerve (p 294)

Ask permission first to test the corneal reflexes. Make sure you touch the cornea (not the conjunctiva) gently with a piece of cotton wool. Come in from the side and do this only once on each side. If the nerve pathways are intact, the patient will blink both eyes. Ask him whether he can actually feel the touch (V is the sensory component). *Note*: With an ipsilateral seventh nerve palsy, only the contralateral eye will blink—sensation is preserved (nerve VII is the motor component). Also with an ipsilateral seventh nerve palsy, the eye on the side of the lesion may roll superiorly with the corneal stimulus ('Bell's phenomenon').

Test facial sensation in the three divisions: ophthalmic, maxillary and mandibular. Use a pin first to assess pain. Map out any area of sensory loss from dull to sharp and check for any loss up on the posterior part of the head (C2) and neck (C3). Light touch must be tested also, as there may be some sensory dissociation. *Note*: A medullary or upper cervical lesion of the fifth nerve causes loss of pain and temperature sensation with preservation of light touch. A pontine lesion may cause loss of light touch with preservation of pain and temperature sensation.

Examine the motor division by asking the patient to clench his teeth (feeling the masseter muscles) and open his mouth; the pterygoid muscles will not allow you to force it closed if the nerve is intact. A unilateral lesion causes the jaw to deviate towards the weak (affected) side.

Always test the jaw jerk (with the mouth just open, the finger over the jaw is tapped with a tendon hammer). An increased jaw jerk occurs in pseudobulbar palsy.

Seventh nerve (p 295)

Look for facial asymmetry and then test the muscles of facial expression. Ask the patient to look up and wrinkle his forehead. Look for loss of wrinkling and feel the muscle strength by pushing down on each side. This is preserved in an upper motor neurone lesion because of bilateral cortical representation of these muscles.

Next ask the patient to shut his eyes tight—compare how deeply the eyelashes are buried on the two sides and then try to open each eye. Tell him to grin and compare the nasolabial grooves.

If a lower motor neurone lesion is detected, quickly check for ear and palatal vesicles of herpes zoster of the geniculate ganglion—the Ramsay Hunt syndrome. Examining for taste on the anterior two-thirds of the tongue is not usually required.

Eighth nerve (p 295)

Whisper a number softly about 0.5 m away from each ear and ask the patient to tell you the number. Perform Rinné's and Weber's tests with a 256 Hertz tuning fork (p 295). If indicated, ask for an auroscope (wax is the commonest cause of conductive deafness).

Ninth and tenth nerves (p 296)

Look at the palate and note any uvular displacement. Ask the patient to say 'aaah' and look for asymmetrical movement of the soft palate. With a unilateral tenth nerve lesion the uvula is drawn towards the unaffected (normal) side.

Testing the gag reflex is traditional but adds little to the examination. If the palate moves normally and the patient can feel the spatula, the same information is obtained (the ninth nerve is the sensory component and the tenth nerve the motor component): touch the back of the pharynx on each side. Remember to ask the patient if he feels the spatula each time. You may not attain top marks if the patient vomits all over the examiners. If the spatula is used correctly, the patient will gag only if the reflex is hyperactive.

Ask the patient to speak (to assess hoarseness) and to cough (listen for a bovine cough, which may occur with a recurrent laryngeal nerve lesion). *Note:* You will not usually be required to test taste on the posterior third of the tongue (i.e. ninth nerve).

Eleventh nerve

Ask the patient to shrug his shoulders and then feel the trapezius bulk and push the shoulders down. Then instruct the patient to turn his head against resistance (your hand) and also feel the muscle bulk of the sternomastoids.

Twelfth nerve (p 297)

While examining the mouth, inspect the tongue for wasting and fasciculation (best seen with the tongue not protruded and which may be unilateral or bilateral). Next ask the patient to protrude his tongue. With a unilateral lesion the tongue deviates towards the weaker (affected) side.

The way to finish your assessment depends entirely on your findings. For example, if you discover evidence of a particular syndrome (such as the lateral medullary syndrome), you should proceed to confirm your impressions by examining more peripherally, if allowed (especially for sensory long tract and cerebellar signs, see below). If you discovered multiple lower cranial nerve palsies, you would want to assess, among other features, the nasopharynx for signs of tumour.

Auscultating for carotid or cranial bruits (over the mastoids, temples and orbits), as well as taking the blood pressure and testing the urine for sugar, are often relevant.

Eyes

Examine this man's eyes.

Method (Fig 8.15)

Figure 8.15   Eye examination.

Sitting up

1. **GENERAL INSPECTION**
   Diagnostic facies (Table 8.29)

2. **CORNEA**
   Corneal arcus
   Band keratopathy
   Kayser-Fleischer rings

3. **SCLERA**
   Jaundice
   Pallor
   Injection

4. **PTOSIS**

5. **EXOPHTHALMOS**

6. **EYELIDS**
   Xanthelasma

7. **LID LAG**

8. **ORBITS**
   Palpate—tenderness—brow (for
      loss of sweating in Horner's
      syndrome)
   Listen for a bruit

9. **NEUROLOGICAL EXAMINATION**
   Acuity
      Eye chart—each eye separately
   Fields
      Red hatpin confrontation—each
   eye
      Central vision
   Fundi
      Cornea
      Lens
      Humor
      Colour of disc and state of cup
      Retina—vessels, exudates,
      haemorrhages, pigmentation, etc.
   Pupils
      Shape, size, symmetry
      Light reflex—direct and
        consensual
      Marcus Gunn phenomenon
      Accommodation
   Eye movements
      III, IV, VI nerves—movement,
      diplopia, nystagmus
      Gaze palsies (e.g. supranuclear
      lesions)
      Fatiguability (myasthenia)
   Corneal reflex (V)

10. **OTHER**
    Depends on findings—other cranial
       nerves, long tract signs, urine
       analysis (diabetes)

Always inspect the eyes first, with the patient sitting over the end of the bed facing you at eye level if possible.

First note any corneal abnormalities, such as band keratopathy (in hypercalcaemic states) or Kayser-Fleischer rings (Wilson's disease). Look at the sclerae for colour (e.g. jaundice, blue in osteogenesis imperfecta), pallor, injection and telangiectasia. Inspect carefully for subtle ptosis or strabismus.

Look for exophthalmos from behind and above the patient, as well as in front (p 266).

Proceed then as for the cranial nerve eye examination, testing acuity, fields and pupils and then performing fundoscopy.

Begin fundoscopy by examining the cornea and lens, and then the retina. Note any corneal, lens or humor abnormalities. Look for retinal changes of diabetes mellitus (see

Table 8.36) and hypertension (see Table 8.7). Also carefully inspect for optic atrophy, papilloedema, angioid streaks (see Table 8.29), retinal detachment, central vein or artery thrombosis and retinitis pigmentosa.

Test eye movements. Also look for fatiguability of eye muscles by asking your patient to look up at your hatpin for half a minute (myasthenia gravis, p 208). Test for lid lag if you suspect hyperthyroidism.

Test the corneal reflex.

Palpate the orbits for tenderness and auscultate the eyes with the bell of the stethoscope (the eye being tested is shut, the other is open and the patient is asked to stop breathing).

Don't forget that the patient may have a glass eye. Suspect this if visual acuity is zero in one eye and no pupillary reaction is apparent. Lengthy attempts to examine the fundus of a glass eye are embarrassing (and not uncommon).

One-and-a-half syndrome

This is rare but important to recognise. These patients have a horizontal gaze palsy when looking to one side (the 'one') plus impaired adduction on looking to the other side (the 'and-a-half'). Other features often include turning out (exotropia) of the eye opposite the side of the lesion (paralytic pontine exotropia). The one-and-a-half syndrome can be caused by a stroke (infarct), plaque of multiple sclerosis or tumour in the dorsal pons.

Horner's syndrome

If you find a partial ptosis and a constricted pupil (which reacts normally to light), Horner's syndrome is likely (Table 8.41). Proceed as follows.

Test for a difference in sweating over each brow with the back of your finger (even though your brow is usually more sweaty than the patient's); this occurs only when the lesion is proximal to the carotid bifurcation. Absence of sweating differences does not exclude the diagnosis of Horner's syndrome.

Examine the appropriate cranial nerves next to exclude the lateral medullary syndrome:

1. nystagmus (to the side of the lesion)
2. ipsilateral fifth (pain and temperature), ninth and tenth cranial nerve lesions
3. ipsilateral cerebellar signs
4. *contralateral* pain and temperature loss over the trunk and limbs.

Ask the patient to speak and note any hoarseness (which may be caused by recurrent laryngeal nerve palsy from a chest lesion or a cranial nerve lesion).

Look at the hands for clubbing. Test finger abduction to screen for a lower trunk brachial plexus (C8, T1) lesion.

Table 8.41 **Causes of Horner's syndrome**

1. Carcinoma of the lung apex (usually squamous cell carcinoma)
2. Neck—thyroid malignancy, trauma
3. Carotid arterial lesion—carotid aneurysm or dissection, pericarotid tumour, cluster headache
4. Brain stem lesions—vascular disease (especially the lateral medullary syndrome), syringobulbia, tumour
5. Retro-orbital lesions
6. Syringomyelia (rare)

If there are signs of hoarseness or a lower trunk brachial plexus lesion, proceed to a respiratory examination, concentrating on the apices for signs of lung carcinoma (p 249).

Examine the neck for lymphadenopathy, thyroid carcinoma and a carotid aneurysm or bruit (e.g. fibromuscular dysplasia causing dissection).

As syringomyelia may rarely cause this syndrome, finish off the assessment by examining for dissociated sensory loss. Remember, this lesion may cause a *bilateral* Horner's syndrome (a trap for the unwary).

Notes on the cranial nerves
First (olfactory) nerve (p 283)

Causes of anosmia

Bilateral
1. Upper respiratory tract infection (commonest)
2. Meningioma of the olfactory groove (late)
3. Ethmoid tumours
4. Head trauma (including cribriform plate fracture)
5. Meningitis
6. Hydrocephalus
7. Congenital—Kallmann's syndrome (hypogonadotrophic hypogonadism)

Unilateral
1. Meningioma of the olfactory groove (early)
2. Head trauma

Second (optic) nerve (p 284)

Light reflex
Constriction of the pupil in response to light is relayed via the optic nerve and tract, the superior quadrigeminal brachium, the Edinger-Westphal nucleus and its efferent parasympathetic fibres, which terminate in the ciliary ganglion. There is no cortical involvement.

Accommodation reflex
Constriction of the pupil with accommodation originates in the cortex (in association with convergence) and is relayed via parasympathetic fibres in the third nerve.

Causes of absent light reflex but intact accommodation reflex
1. Midbrain lesion (e.g. Argyll Robertson pupil)
2. Ciliary ganglion lesion (e.g. Adie's pupil)
3. Parinaud's syndrome (p 293)
4. Bilateral anterior visual pathway lesions (i.e. bilateral afferent pupil deficits)

Causes of absent convergence but intact light reflex
Cortical lesion (e.g. cortical blindness), midbrain lesions (rare).

Visual field defects (Fig 8.16)

Pupil abnormalities

Causes of constriction
1. Horner's syndrome.
2. Argyll Robertson pupil.
3. Pontine lesion (often bilateral but reactive to light).

Figure 8.16 Visual field defects associated with lesions of the visual system.

1. TUNNEL VISION: concentric diminution (glaucoma, papilloedema, syphilis)

2. ENLARGED BLIND SPOT: optic nerve head enlargement

3. CENTRAL SCOTOMATA: optic nerve head to chiasmal lesion (e.g. demyelination, toxic, vascular, nutritional)

4. UNILATERAL FIELD LOSS: optic nerve lesion (e.g. vascular, tumour)

5. BITEMPORAL HEMIANOPIA: optic chiasm lesion (e.g. pituitary tumour, sella meningioma)

6. HOMONYMOUS HEMIANOPIA: optic tract to occipital cortex, lesion at any point (e.g. vascular, tumour)
   Note: Incomplete lesion results in macular (central) vision sparing.

7. UPPER QUADRANT HOMONYMOUS HEMIANOPIA: temporal lobe lesion (e.g. vascular, tumour)

8. LOWER QUADRANT HOMONYMOUS HEMIANOPIA: parietal lobe lesion

---

4. Narcotics.
5. Pilocarpine drops.
6. Old age.

Causes of dilation
1. Mydriatics, atropine poisoning or cocaine.
2. Third nerve lesion.
3. Adie's pupil.
4. Iridectomy, lens implant, iritis.
5. Post-trauma, deep coma, cerebral death.
6. Congenital.

Holmes-Adie syndrome

Cause
Lesion in the efferent parasympathetic pathway.

Signs
1. Dilated pupil.
2. Decreased or absent reaction to light (direct and consensual).
3. Slow or incomplete reaction to accommodation with slow dilation afterwards.
4. Decreased tendon reflexes.
5. The patients are commonly young women.
6. Denervation supersensitivity to a weak (e.g. 0.125%) pilocarpine solution.

Argyll Robertson pupil

Cause
Lesion of the iridodilator fibres in the midbrain, as in:

1. syphilis
2. diabetes mellitus
3. alcoholic midbrain degeneration (rarely)
4. other midbrain lesions.

Signs
1. Small, irregular, unequal pupil.
2. No reaction to light.
3. Prompt reaction to accommodation.
4. If tabes associated, decreased reflexes.
5. Some mydriatics (e.g. atropine, cocaine) dilate slowly. Direct sympathetic agonists dilate promptly.

Papilloedema versus papillitis

Papilloedema	Papillitis
Optic disc swollen without venous pulsation	Optic disc swollen*
Acuity normal (early)	Acuity poor
Colour vision normal	Colour vision affected (particularly red desaturation)
Large blind spot	Large central scotoma
Peripheral constriction of visual fields	Pain on eye movement
Usually bilateral	Onset usually sudden and unilateral

*In retrobulbar neuritis and old papillitis the optic disc becomes pale.

Causes of papilloedema
1. Space-occupying lesion (causing raised intracranial pressure) or a retro-orbital mass.
2. Hydrocephalus (associated with large ventricles):
   (a) obstructive (block in the third ventricle, aqueduct or outlet to fourth ventricle—e.g. tumour)
   (b) communicating:
      (i) increased formation—choroid plexus papilloma
      (ii) decreased absorption—tumour causing venous compression, subarachnoid space obstruction from meningitis.
3. Benign intracranial hypertension (pseudotumour cerebri, associated with small ventricles):
   (a) idiopathic
   (b) the contraceptive pill
   (c) Addison's disease
   (d) drugs—nitrofurantoin, tetracycline, vitamin A, steroids
   (e) lateral sinus thrombosis
   (f) head trauma.
4. Hypertension (grade IV).
5. Central retinal vein thrombosis.

6. Cerebral venous sinus thrombosis.
7. High cerebrospinal fluid protein level—Guillain-Barré syndrome.

Causes of optic atrophy
1. Chronic papilloedema or optic neuritis.
2. Optic nerve pressure or division.
3. Glaucoma.
4. Ischaemia.
5. Familial—retinitis pigmentosa, Leber's disease, Friedreich's ataxia.

Causes of optic neuropathy
1. Multiple sclerosis.
2. Toxic—ethambutol, chloroquine, nicotine, alcohol.
3. Metabolic—vitamin B_{12} deficiency.
4. Ischaemia—diabetes mellitus, temporal arteritis, atheroma.
5. Familial—Leber's disease.
6. Infective—infectious mononucleosis (glandular fever).

Causes of cataract
1. Old age (senile cataract).
2. Endocrine—diabetes mellitus, steroids.
3. Hereditary or congenital—dystrophia myotonica, Refsum's disease.
4. Ocular disease—glaucoma.
5. Irradiation.
6. Trauma.

Causes of ptosis
1. With normal pupils:
   • myasthenia gravis
   • myotonic dystrophy
   • fascioscapulohumeral dystrophy
   • ocular myopathy
   • thyrotoxic myopathy
   • senile ptosis
   • botulism, snake bite
   • congenital
   • fatigue.
2. With constricted pupils:
   • Horner's syndrome
   • tabes dorsalis.
3. With dilated pupils:
   • third nerve lesion.

Third (oculomotor) nerve (p 284)

Clinical features of a third nerve palsy
1. Complete ptosis (partial ptosis may occur with an incomplete lesion).
2. Divergent strabismus (eye 'down and out').
3. Dilated pupil unreactive to direct or consensual light and unreactive to accommodation.

Note: Always exclude a fourth (trochlear) nerve lesion when a third nerve lesion is present. Do this by tilting the head to the same side as the lesion. The affected eye will intort if the fourth nerve is intact. Or ask the patient to look down and across to the opposite side from the lesion and look for intortion. Remember 'SIN': *s*uperior (oblique muscle), supplied by the IV nerve, *in*torts the eye.

Aetiology

Central
1. Vascular (e.g. brain stem infarction).
2. Tumour.
3. Demyelination (rare).
4. Trauma.
5. Idiopathic.

Peripheral
1. Compressive lesions:
    (a) aneurysm (usually on the posterior communicating artery)
    (b) tumour causing raised intracranial pressure (dilated pupil occurs early)
    (c) nasopharyngeal carcinoma
    (d) orbital lesions—Tolosa-Hunt syndrome (superior orbital fissure syndrome—painful lesion of the third, fourth, sixth and the first division of the fifth cranial nerves)
    (e) basal meningitis.
2. Infarction—diabetes mellitus, arteritis (pupil is usually spared).
3. Trauma.
4. Cavernous sinus lesions.

Sixth (abducens) nerve (p 284)

Clinical features of a sixth nerve palsy
1. Failure of lateral movement.
2. Affected eye is deviated inwards in severe lesions.
3. Diplopia—maximal on looking to the affected side. The images are horizontal and parallel to each other. The outermost image is from the affected eye and disappears on covering this eye (this image is also usually more blurred).

Aetiology

Bilateral
1. Trauma (head injury).
2. Wernicke's encephalopathy.
3. Raised intracranial pressure.
4. Mononeuritis multiplex.

Unilateral
1. Central:
    (a) vascular
    (b) tumour
    (c) Wernicke's encephalopathy
    (d) multiple sclerosis (rare).
2. Peripheral:
    (a) diabetes, other vascular lesions
    (b) trauma
    (c) idiopathic
    (d) raised intracranial pressure.

Eye movements

With the eye abducted: the elevator is the superior rectus (third nerve). The depressor is the inferior rectus (third nerve). With the eye adducted: the elevator is the inferior oblique (third nerve). The depressor is the superior oblique (fourth nerve).

Causes of nystagmus

Jerky
1. Horizontal:
   (a) vestibular lesion (*Note*: Chronic lesions cause nystagmus to the side of the lesion—fast component.)
   (b) cerebellar lesion (*Note*: Unilateral disease causes nystagmus to the side of the lesion.)
   (c) internuclear ophthalmoplegia (*Note*: Nystagmus is in the abducting eye, with failure of adduction on the affected side. This is a result of a medial longitudinal fasciculus lesion. The commonest cause in young adults with bilateral involvement is multiple sclerosis [p 205]; in the elderly, consider brain stem infarction. When the medial longitudinal fasciculus and the abducens nucleus on the same side are affected, the only horizontal movement the patient can make is abduction of the contralateral eye—*one-and-a-half syndrome*.)
2. Vertical:
   (a) brain stem lesion
       (i) upbeat nystagmus suggests a lesion in the floor of the fourth ventricle
       (ii) downbeat nystagmus suggests a foramen magnum lesion
   (b) toxic—phenytoin, alcohol (may also cause horizontal nystagmus).

Pendular
1. Retinal (decreased macular vision)—albinism.
2. Congenital.

Supranuclear palsy

Loss of vertical upward gaze and sometimes downward gaze. Clinical features (distinguishing from third, fourth and sixth nerve palsy):
1. both eyes affected
2. pupils often unequal
3. no diplopia
4. reflex eye movements (e.g. on flexing and extending the neck) intact.

Steele-Richardson-Olszewski syndrome (progressive supranuclear palsy)
1. Loss of vertical downward gaze first, later vertical upward gaze and finally horizontal gaze.
2. Associated with pseudobulbar palsy, long tract signs, extrapyramidal signs, dementia and neck rigidity.

Parinaud's syndrome
Loss of vertical upward gaze often associated with convergence–retraction nystagmus on attempted convergence and pseudo Argyll Robertson pupils.

Causes of Parinaud's syndrome
Central:

1. pinealoma
2. multiple sclerosis
3. vascular lesions.

Peripheral:

1. trauma
2. diabetes
3. other vascular lesions
4. idiopathic
5. raised intracranial pressure.

Fifth (trigeminal) nerve palsy (p 284) (Fig 8.17)

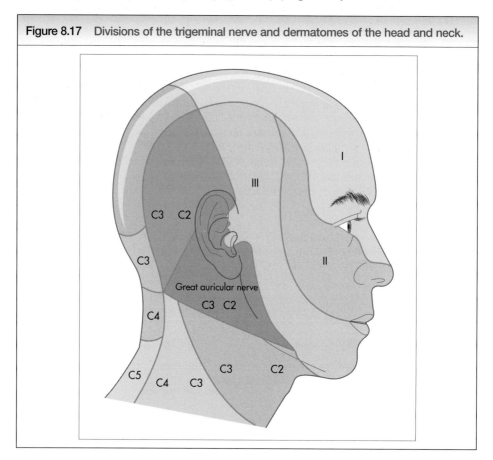

Figure 8.17 Divisions of the trigeminal nerve and dermatomes of the head and neck.

Aetiology

Central (pons, medulla and upper cervical cord)
1. Vascular.
2. Tumour.
3. Syringobulbia.
4. Multiple sclerosis.

Peripheral (posterior fossa)
1. Aneurysm.
2. Tumour (skull base, e.g. acoustic neuroma).
3. Chronic meningitis.

Trigeminal ganglion (petrous temporal bone)
1. Meningioma.
2. Fracture of the middle fossa.

Cavernous sinus (associated third, fourth and sixth nerve palsies)
1. Aneurysm.
2. Thrombosis.
3. Tumour.

Other

Sjögren's syndrome, systemic lupus erythematosus (SLE), toxins, idiopathic.
Remember, if there is:

1. loss of all sensation in all three divisions—consider a lesion at the ganglion or sensory root
2. total sensory loss in one division—consider a postganglionic lesion
3. loss of pain but preservation of touch—consider a brain stem or upper cervical cord lesion
4. loss of touch but pain sensation preserved—consider a pontine nucleus lesion.

Seventh (facial) nerve palsy (p 285)

Aetiology

Upper motor neurone lesion (supranuclear)
1. Vascular.
2. Tumour.

Lower motor neurone lesion
Pontine (often associated with nerves V, VI):

1. vascular
2. tumour
3. syringobulbia
4. multiple sclerosis.

Posterior fossa:

1. acoustic neuroma
2. meningioma.

Petrous temporal bone:

1. Bell's palsy
2. Ramsay Hunt syndrome
3. otitis media
4. fracture.

Parotid:

1. tumour
2. sarcoid.

Causes of bilateral lower motor neurone facial weakness:

1. Guillain-Barré syndrome
2. bilateral parotid disease (e.g. sarcoid)
3. mononeuritis multiplex (rare).

Note: Myopathy and neuromuscular junction defects can also cause bilateral facial weakness.

Eighth (acoustic) nerve (p 285)

To differentiate nerve deafness from conductive deafness, use the following tests.

Rinné's test

A 256-Hertz vibrating tuning fork is first placed on the mastoid process, behind the ear and, when the sound is no longer heard, it is placed in line with the external meatus.

Results
1. Normal—the note is audible at the external meatus.
2. Nerve deafness—the note is audible at the external meatus as air and bone conduction are reduced equally, so that air conduction is better (as is normal). Positive result.
3. Conduction (middle ear) deafness—no note is audible at the external meatus. Negative result.

Weber's test
A 256-Hertz tuning fork is placed on the centre of the forehead.

Results
1. Normal—the sound is heard in the centre of the forehead.
2. Nerve deafness—the sound is transmitted to the normal ear.
3. Conduction deafness—the sound is heard louder in the abnormal ear.

Note: Although of traditional importance, these tests are not very accurate and are now rarely used by neurologists.

Causes of deafness
Nerve (sensorineural) deafness:

1. degeneration (e.g. presbycusis)
2. trauma (e.g. high noise exposure, fracture of the petrous temporal bone)
3. toxic (e.g. aspirin, alcohol, streptomycin)
4. infection (e.g. congenital rubella syndrome, congenital syphilis)
5. tumour (e.g. acoustic neuroma)
6. brain stem lesions
7. vascular disease of the internal auditory artery.

Conductive deafness:

1. wax
2. otitis media
3. otosclerosis
4. Paget's disease of bone.

Ninth (glossopharyngeal) and tenth (vagus) nerve palsy (p 285)

Aetiology

Central
1. Vascular (e.g. lateral medullary infarction owing to vertebral or posterior inferior cerebellar artery disease).
2. Tumour.
3. Syringobulbia.
4. Motor neurone disease (vagus nerve only).

Peripheral—posterior fossa
1. Aneurysm.
2. Tumour.
3. Chronic meningitis.
4. Guillain-Barré syndrome (vagus nerve only).

Twelfth (hypoglossal) nerve palsy (p 285)

Aetiology

Upper motor neurone lesion

1. Vascular.
2. Motor neurone disease.
3. Tumour.
4. Multiple sclerosis (p 205).

Note: The syndrome of bilateral upper motor neurone lesions of the ninth, tenth and twelfth nerves is called pseudobulbar palsy.

Lower motor neurone lesion—unilateral

Note: It is difficult to detect unilateral lesions as the tongue muscles (except the genioglossus) are bilaterally innervated.

Central:

1. vascular—thrombosis of the vertebral artery
2. motor neurone disease
3. syringobulbia.

Peripheral (posterior fossa):

1. aneurysm
2. tumour
3. chronic meningitis
4. trauma
5. Arnold-Chiari malformation
6. fracture or tumour of the base of the skull.

Note: The Arnold-Chiari malformation is a protrusion of the cerebellar tonsils through the foramen magnum. The more severe types (II–IV) cause basilar compression with lower cranial nerve palsies, cerebellar limb signs (owing to tonsillar compression) and upper motor neurone signs in the legs.

Lower motor neurone lesion—bilateral

1. Motor neurone disease.
2. Arnold-Chiari malformation.
3. Guillain-Barré syndrome.
4. Polio.

Causes of multiple cranial nerve palsies

Think of *cancer* first.

1. Nasopharyngeal *carcinoma*.
2. Chronic meningitis (e.g. *carcinoma*, tuberculosis, sarcoidosis).
3. Guillain-Barré syndrome (spares nerves I, II and VIII), including the Miller-Fisher variant.
4. Brain stem lesions. These are usually as a result of vascular disease causing crossed sensory or motor paralysis (i.e. cranial nerve signs on one side and contralateral long tract signs). Patients with brain stem *gliomas* may have similar signs and may live for many years.
5. Arnold-Chiari malformation.
6. Trauma.
7. Lesion of the base of the skull (e.g. Paget's disease, large *meningioma*, *metastasis*).
8. Mononeuritis multiplex, rarely (e.g. diabetes mellitus).

Higher centres

Examine this man's higher centres.

Method (Fig 8.18)

Figure 8.18 Higher centres' examination.

Lying or sitting

1. GENERAL INSPECTION
   Diagnostic facies (Table 8.29)
   Obvious cranial nerve or limb
     lesions
   Ask patient about handedness, level
     of education
   Shake hands

2. ORIENTATION
   Time
   Place
   Person

3. SPEECH
   Name objects (nominal dysphasia)

4. PARIETAL LOBES
   Dominant (ALF or Gerstmann's
     syndrome)
     Acalculia—(mental arithmetic)
     Agraphia (write)
     Left–right disorientation
     Finger agnosia (name fingers)
   Non-dominant
     Dressing apraxia

Both
   Sensory inattention
   Visual inattention
   Cortical sensory loss (loss of
     graphaesthesia, two-point
     discrimination, joint position
     sense and stereognosis)
   Constructional apraxia

5. MEMORY (temporal lobe)
   Short-term (e.g. names of flowers)
   Long-term

6. FRONTAL LOBE
   Reflexes—grasp
            —pout
            —palmar mental
   Proverb interpretation
   Smell
   Fundi
   Gait

7. OTHER
   Visual fields
   Bruits
   Blood pressure, etc.

In this assessment especially, you must be guided by your findings. The introduction is important. For example, if you are told the patient also presents with right-sided weakness, you should concentrate on looking for dominant parietal lobe signs.

Shake the patient's hand, noting any obvious focal weakness, and introduce yourself. Tell him you will be asking him some questions.

First, ask if he is right- or left-handed. Then ask questions about orientation (person, place and time). Ask his name, the present location and the date.

This also allows you to test for speech abnormality. Assess any nominal dysphasia by asking the patient to name some objects, such as your watch or a pen (Table 8.42). Ask the patient to repeat a phrase or sentence, for example, 'The barrister's closing argument convinced him'. This allows you to assess the fluency of speech as well as comprehension and repetition. Next ask the patient to perform one- and two-step commands, such as 'point to the ceiling, but first take off your spectacles'. This assesses the patient's comprehension.

Table 8.42 Examination of dysphasia

Fluent speech (receptive, conductive or nominal dysphasia usually)
1. Naming of objects—patients with nominal, conductive or receptive aphasia all name objects poorly.
2. Repetition—conductive and receptive aphasics cannot repeat.
3. Comprehension—only receptive aphasic patients cannot follow commands (verbal or written).
4. Reading—conductive and receptive aphasic patients have difficulty.
5. Writing—conductive aphasic patients have impaired writing (dysgraphia), while receptive aphasic patients have abnormal content. Dysgraphia may also occur with dominant frontal lobe lesions.

Non-fluent speech (usually expressive aphasia)*
1. Naming of objects–poor (but may be better than spontaneous speech).
2. Repetition—may be possible with great effort. Phrase repetition (e.g. 'no ifs, ands or buts') is poor.
3. Comprehension—near normal (written and verbal commands are followed).
4. Writing—dysgraphia may be present.
5. Look for hemiparesis—arm more affected than leg.

* As the patient is aware of his deficit, he is often frustrated and depressed.

Assess the parietal lobes next. Begin with the dominant parietal lobe, as Gerstmann's syndrome is common in examinations. Examine for *acalculia* (test mental arithmetic), *agraphia* (test for an inability to write), *left–right disorientation* (e.g. by asking the patient to put his right palm on his left ear, then vice versa), and *finger agnosia* (inability to name individual fingers). This is caused by a left angular gyrus lesion in right-handed and about half of left-handed patients. (A mnemonic for Gerstmann's syndrome is ALF.)

Test general parietal functions (involving either lobe). Examine for sensory and visual inattention. Also test for agraphaesthesia (inability to appreciate numbers drawn on the palm) and astereognosis (inability to name objects placed in the hand). Assess constructional apraxia by asking the patient to draw a clock face and fill in the numbers.

The major specific non-dominant parietal dysfunction is dressing apraxia. This can be tested by turning the patient's pyjama top inside out and asking him to put it on correctly.

Assess memory, both short- and long-term. This is a medial temporal lobe function. Ask the patient to remember the name of three flowers (e.g. *r*ose, *o*rchid and *t*ulip—mnemonic *rot* for those candidates with a poor memory) and repeat them immediately. Then assess long-term memory, such as by asking when World War II finished. Ask the names of the flowers again at the end of your higher centres' examination.

Test frontal lobe problems, first by assessing the primitive reflexes, normally not present in adults. The grasp reflex, pout reflex, and palmar–mental reflex are usually all that need be tested. Then ask for interpretation of a common proverb, such as 'A rolling stone gathers no moss'. Test for anosmia (cranial nerve I) and gait apraxia (a frontal gait abnormality is marked by gross unsteadiness in walking—the feet typically behave as if glued to the floor, resulting in a hesitant shuffling gait with freezing). Look at the fundi to exclude the rare Foster Kennedy syndrome (optic atrophy on the side of the lesion and papilloedema in the opposite fundus) if there is evidence of a frontal lobe lesion.

Any abnormality of the parietal, temporal or occipital lobes may cause a characteristic visual field loss. This should be tested, if appropriate, at the conclusion of your examination. Other important signs to look for are carotid bruits, hypertension and relevant focal neurological signs.

Speech

Assess this man's speech.

Method

Immediately ask the patient to state his name, age and present location. Then ask him to say 'British Constitution'. By now you should have decided if the problem is dysphasia, dysarthria or dysphonia.

Dysphasia
If the speech is fluent but conveys information imperfectly, often with paraphasic errors (e.g. 'treen' for train—substitution of a word of similar sound), the main possibilities are nominal and receptive aphasia. Test for these by asking the patient to name objects, to repeat a statement after you and then follow commands. Then ask him to read and write if the above are abnormal (Table 8.42).

If the speech is slow and non-fluent (hesitant), exactly the same procedure is followed but an expressive aphasia is likely. At the end ask to assess for a hemiparesis (Table 8.42).

Remember, large lesions may cause global aphasia, with inability to comprehend or speak, plus hemiparesis (Table 8.43).

Table 8.43 The sites of lesions in aphasia

Receptive aphasia
Wernicke's area—posterior part of first temporal gyrus in the dominant lobe

Expressive aphasia
Broca's area—posterior part of the third frontal gyrus

Conductive aphasia
Arcuate fasciculus (temporal lobe)

Nominal aphasia
Angular gyrus (temporal lobe)—small localised lesion
Other causes: encephalopathies (metabolic, toxic), pressure effects from a distant space-occupying lesion
Recovery phase from any dysphasia

Dysarthria
This is a disorder of articulation with no disorder of the content of speech. Consider cerebellar disease and lower cranial nerve lesions particularly. Cerebellar speech is slurred or 'scanning' (i.e. irregular and staccato). Pseudobulbar palsy causes slow,

hesitant, hollow-sounding speech with a harsh, strained voice, while bulbar palsy causes nasal speech with imprecise articulation.

Ask the patient to say 'British Constitution', 'West Register Street', 'Me Me Me' and 'Lah Lah Lah'. If the speech is cerebellar, go on to this system (p 319). If palsy of a lower cranial nerve is likely, examine the lower cranial nerves carefully. Don't forget to elicit the jaw jerk. Look in the mouth too for ulceration or other local lesions.

Less common causes of dysarthria include extrapyramidal disease and myopathies (p 316).

Dysphonia

This is huskiness of the voice from a laryngeal disorder, recurrent laryngeal nerve palsy or focal dystonia. Assess the quality of the cough too.

Upper limbs

This man has noticed weakness in his arms. Please examine him.

Method (Fig 8.19)

> **Figure 8.19** Upper limb neurological examination.
>
> 1. **GENERAL INSPECTION**
>   Diagnostic facies (Table 8.29)
>   Scars
>   Skin (e.g. neurofibromata, café-au-lait)
>   Abnormal movements
>
> 2. **SHAKE HANDS**
>
> 3. **MOTOR SYSTEM**
>   Inspect arms, shoulder girdle—
>   extend both arms
>   Wasting
>   Fasciculation
>   Tremor
>   Drift
>   Palpate
>   Muscle bulk
>   Muscle tenderness
>   Tone
>   Wrist
>   Elbow
>   Power
>   Shoulder
>   Elbow
>   Wrist
>   Fingers
>
> Ulnar, median nerve function
> Reflexes
>   Biceps
>   Triceps
>   Supinator
>   Finger
> Coordination
>   Finger–nose test—intention tremor, past pointing
>   Dysdiadochokinesis
>   Rebound
>
> 4. **SENSORY SYSTEM**
>   Pain (pinprick)
>   Vibration (128 Hz tuning fork)
>   Proprioception—distal interphalangeal joint (each hand)
>   Light touch (cotton wool)
>
> 5. **OTHER**
>   Thickened nerves (wrist, elbow)
>   Axillae
>   Neck
>   Lower limbs
>   Cranial nerves
>   Urine analysis, etc.

Look at the whole patient briefly. Note particularly evidence of a myopathic face, parkinsonian features or stroke.

Shake the patient's hand firmly and introduce yourself. If he cannot let go, you have made the diagnosis (myotonia, usually caused by dystrophia myotonica). Ask him to sit over the side of the bed facing you.

Examine the *motor system* systematically every time.

Inspect first for wasting (both proximally and distally) and fasciculations. Don't forget to include the shoulder girdle in your inspection (p 304).

Ask the patient to hold both his hands out with the arms extended and close his eyes. Look for drifting of one or both arms. There are only three causes for this drift:

1. upper motor neurone weakness (usually downwards owing to muscle weakness)
2. cerebellar lesion (usually upwards owing to hypotonia)
3. posterior column loss (any direction owing to joint position sense loss).

Also note any tremor and pseudoathetosis as a result of proprioceptive loss.

Feel the muscle bulk next, both proximally and distally, and note any muscle tenderness. In the presence of wasting and weakness, fasciculation indicates lower motor neurone degeneration.

Test tone at the wrists and elbows by moving the joints at varying velocities.

Assess power next.

Shoulder
- Abduction (C5, C6): tell the patient to abduct his arms with the elbows flexed and not to let you push them down.
- Adduction (C6–C8): tell him to adduct his arms with the elbows flexed and not to let you separate them.

Elbow
- Flexion (C5, C6): tell him to bend his elbow and pull, so as not to let you straighten it.
- Extension (C7, C8): tell him to bend his elbow and push, so as not to let you bend it.

Wrist
- Flexion (C6, C7): tell him to bend his wrist and not to let you straighten it.
- Extension (C7, C8): tell him to straighten his wrist and not to let you bend it.

Fingers
- Extension (C7, C8): tell him to straighten his fingers and not to let you push them down.
- Flexion (C7, C8): tell him to squeeze two of your fingers.
- Abduction (C8, T1): tell him to spread out his fingers and not to let you push them together.

Grade the power (p 306).

Next test for an ulnar lesion (loss of finger abduction and adduction) and a median nerve lesion (loss of thumb abduction) (pp 310, 311).

Examine the reflexes:
- biceps (C5, C6)—biceps muscle
- triceps (C7, C8)—triceps muscle
- supinator (C5, C6)—brachioradialis muscle (elbow flexion)
- inverted supinator jerk—when tapping the lower end of the radius, elbow extension and finger flexion are the only response; associated with an absent biceps and exaggerated triceps jerk, this indicates an intraspinal lesion compressing the spinal cord and nerve roots at C5, C6 (p 313)
- finger (C8).

Assess coordination with finger–nose testing and look for dysdiadochokinesis and rebound (p 319).

Motor weakness can be caused by an upper motor neurone lesion, lower motor neurone lesion, neuromuscular junction disorder or myopathy.

If there is evidence of a lower motor neurone lesion, consider anterior horn cell, nerve root and brachial plexus lesions, peripheral nerve lesions, or a motor peripheral neuropathy.

Examine the *sensory system* after motor testing because this can be time-consuming.

First test the spinothalamic pathway (pain and temperature).

Use a new blunt pin. One candidate accidentally pricked his own finger during the examination with a sharp pin. By the time he stopped bleeding his short case time was up. In case you believe this might be a good ploy, the candidate failed.

First demonstrate to the patient the sharpness of the pin on the anterior chest wall or forehead. Then ask him to close his eyes and tell you if the sensation is sharp or dull. Start proximally and test each dermatome. As you are assessing, try to fit any sensory loss into dermatomal (cord or nerve root lesion) (Fig 8.20), peripheral nerve, peripheral neuropathy (glove) or hemisensory (cortical or cord) distribution. Also remember that 'cape' sensory loss (neck, shoulders and arms) suggests syringomyelia, while 'shield' sensory loss (front of the chest) may occur with syphilis. It is not usually necessary to test temperature perception in the examination.

Next test the posterior column pathway (vibration and proprioception).

Use a 128-Hertz tuning fork to assess vibration sense. Place this when vibrating on the ulnar head at the wrist when the patient has his eyes closed and ask whether he can feel it. If so, ask him to tell you when the vibration ceases and then stop the

Figure 8.20 Dermatomes of the upper limb and trunk.

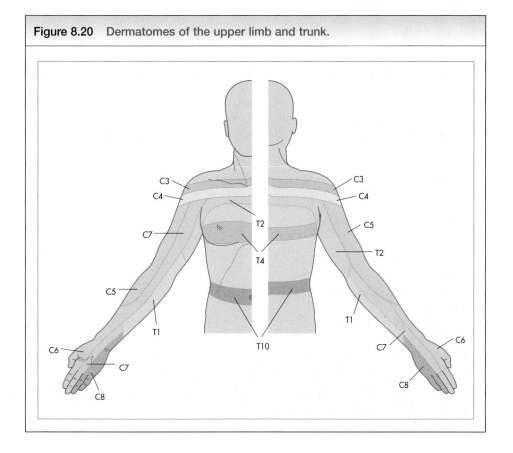

vibration. If the patient has deficient sensation, test at the elbow, then the shoulder. Test both arms.

Examine proprioception first with the DIP joint of the index finger. When the patient has his eyes open, grasp his distal phalanx from the sides and move it up and down to demonstrate, then ask him to close his eyes and repeat the manoeuvres. Normally, movement through even a few degrees is detectable, and he can tell whether it is up or down. If there is an abnormality, proceed to test the wrist and elbows similarly.

Test light touch with cotton wool. Touch the skin lightly in each dermatome.

Feel for thickened nerves—ulnar at the elbow, median at the wrist, and radial at the wrist—and feel the axillae if there is evidence of a plexus lesion. Don't forget to mention any scars that may be present. Finally examine the neck movements if relevant, and look for surgical scars in the front and back of the neck and in the axillae.

To confirm a diagnosis, it may be necessary to examine further afield. Ask the examiners whether you can do this. For example, if there is evidence of motor neurone disease, assess the lower limbs as well as the tongue. If there is evidence of a C5, C6 root lesion, assess the lower limbs for an upper motor neurone lesion and the neck for cervical spondylosis.

Shoulder girdle examination

Examine this man's shoulder girdle.

Methods

This is likely to be a muscular dystrophy or a root lesion.

Proceed by inspecting each muscle, palpating its bulk and testing function as follows.

From the back:

1. trapezius (XI, C3, C4)—ask the patient to elevate the shoulders against resistance and look for winging of the upper scapula
2. serratus anterior (C5–C7)—ask him to push his hands against the wall and look for winging of the lower scapula
3. rhomboids (C4, C5)—ask him to pull both shoulder blades together with his hands on his hips
4. supraspinatus (C5, C6)—ask him to abduct his arms against resistance, and begin with the patient's arms less than 15° from the sides
5. infraspinatus (C5, C6)—ask him to rotate the upper arms externally against resistance with his arms at his side
6. teres major (C5–C7)—ask him to rotate the upper arms internally against resistance
7. latissimus dorsi (C7, C8)—ask the patient to cough and palpate on both sides.

From the front:

1. pectoralis major, clavicular head (C5–C8)—ask the patient to lift the upper arms above the horizontal and push them forward
2. pectoralis major, sternocostal part (C6–T1) and pectoralis minor (C7)—ask him to adduct the upper arms against resistance
3. deltoid (C5, C6) (and circumflex nerve)—ask him to abduct the arms against resistance, but begin with the patient's arms more than 15° from the sides.

Lower limbs

Examine this man's lower limbs neurologically.

Method (Fig 8.21)

Figure 8.21 Lower limb neurological examination.

Lying

1. GENERAL INSPECTION
   Diagnostic facies (Table 8.29)
   Scars, skin
   Urinary catheter

2. GAIT

3. MOTOR SYSTEM
   Inspect
     Wasting
     Fasciculation
     Tremor
   Palpate
     Muscle bulk
     Muscle tenderness
   Tone
     Knee—and test for clonus
     Ankle—and test for clonus
   Power
     Hip
     Knee
     Ankle
     Foot
   Reflexes
     Knee

Ankle
Plantar
Coordination
   Heel–shin test
   Toe–finger test
   Foot tapping test

4. SENSORY SYSTEM
   Pain
   Vibration
   Proprioception
     Light touch

5. SADDLE REGION SENSATION

6. ANAL REFLEX

7. BACK
   Deformity
   Scars
   Tenderness
   Bruits

8. OTHER
   Upper limbs
   Cranial nerve
   Urine analysis, etc.

Test the gait first. Ask the examiners whether this is possible—sometimes they will not let you examine the gait.

Note the general appearance. Especially look for upper limb girdle wasting and the presence of a urinary catheter.

Have the patient lie in bed with the legs entirely exposed. Place a towel over the groin.

Look for muscle wasting and fasciculation. Note any tremor. Feel the muscle bulk of the quadriceps and run your hand up each shin, feeling for wasting of the anterior tibial muscles.

Test tone at the knees and ankles. Test clonus at this time. Push the patella sharply downwards. Sustained rhythmical contractions indicate an upper motor neurone lesion. Also test the ankle by sharply dorsiflexing the foot with the knee bent and the thigh externally rotated.

Assess power next.

Hip
- Flexion (L2, L3): ask the patient to lift up his straight leg and not let you push it down (having placed your hand above his knee).
- Extension (L5, S1, S2): ask him to keep his leg down and not let you pull it up.
- Abduction (L4, L5, S1): ask him to abduct his legs and not let you push them together.

- Adduction (L2, L3, L4): ask him to keep his legs adducted and not let you pull them apart.

Knee
- Flexion (L5, S1): ask him to bend his knee and not let you straighten it.
- Extension (L3, L4): with the knee slightly bent, ask him to straighten the knee and not let you bend it.

Ankle
- Plantarflexion (S1): ask him to push his foot down and not let you pull it up.
- Dorsiflexion (L4, L5): ask him to bring his foot up and not let you push it down.
- Eversion (L5, S1): ask him to evert the foot against resistance; loss of this may also indicate a common peroneal (lateral popliteal) nerve palsy (p 312).
- Inversion (L5): ask him to invert his *plantarflexed* foot against resistance.

Elicit the reflexes:
- knee (L3, L4)—quadriceps muscle
- ankle (S1, S2)—calf muscle
- plantar response (S1).

Test coordination with the heel–shin test, toe–finger test and tapping of the feet (p 319).

Examine the sensory system as for the upper limbs (p 301): pin prick, then vibration and proprioception, and then light touch (Fig 8.22).

If there is a peripheral sensory loss, attempt to establish a sensory level on the abdomen.

Examine the saddle region sensation (S3–5). Test the anal reflex (S2–4); if intact, there is brief contraction of the external sphincter of the anus to scratching the perianal skin.

Go to the back. Look for deformity, scars and neurofibromata. Palpate for tenderness over the vertebral bodies and auscultate for bruits. Test straight leg raising.

It may be relevant to ask whether you can proceed to the upper limbs and cranial nerves (pp 283, 301).

Notes on the neurological examination of the limbs
Grading muscle power (Medical Research Council)

0. Complete paralysis.
1. Flicker of contraction.
2. Movement with *no* gravity.
3. Movement with gravity only (any resistance stops movement).
4. Movement with gravity plus some resistance.
5. Normal power.

This grading is weighted towards severe weakness (grades 0–3 are all severe). A more sensible scale would be the following.

1. Complete paralysis.
2. Severe weakness.
3. Moderate weakness.
4. Mild weakness.
5. Normal.

Signs of a lower motor neurone lesion

1. Weakness.
2. Wasting.

Figure 8.22 Dermatomes of the lower limb.

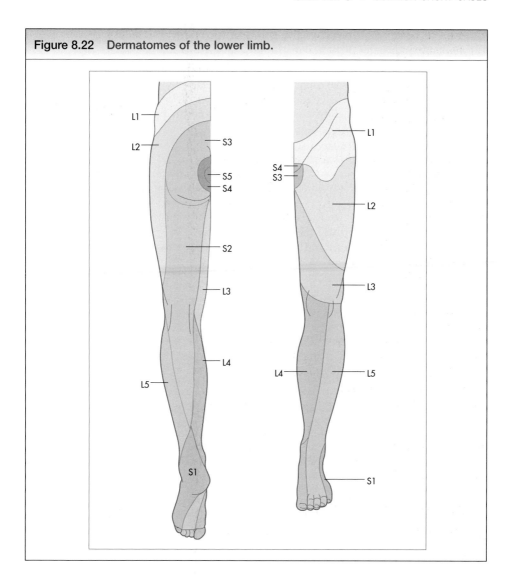

3. Hypotonicity.
4. Decreased or absent reflexes.
5. Fasciculation (prominent in anterior horn cell diseases unless far advanced).

Signs of an upper motor neurone lesion

1. Weakness in an 'upper motor neurone pattern'. All muscle groups are weak but this may be more marked in upper limb abductor and extensor muscles—shoulder abduction, elbow and wrist extensors—and lower limb flexor muscles—hip flexion, knee flexion, ankle dorsiflexion.
2. Spasticity.
3. Clonus.
4. Increased reflexes and extensor plantar response.

An approach to peripheral neuropathy

This may be sensory (glove and stocking), motor or both.

Causes of peripheral neuropathy (mnemonic 'DAM IT BICH')

But remember: diabetes 30%, hereditary 30%, idiopathic 30%, all others 10%.

1. Drugs and toxins—isoniazid, vincristine, phenytoin, nitrofurantoin, cisplatinum, amiodarone, large doses of vitamin B_6, heavy metals.
2. Alcohol (with or without vitamin B_1 deficiency); amyloid.
3. Metabolic—diabetes mellitus, uraemia, hypothyroidism, porphyria.
4. Immune-mediated—Guillain-Barré syndrome.
5. Tumour—lung carcinoma.
6. Vitamin B_{12}, B_1, B_5 or B_6 deficiency.
7. Idiopathic.
8. Connective tissue diseases or vasculitis—SLE, polyarteritis nodosa.
9. Hereditary.

Causes of a predominantly motor neuropathy

1. Guillain-Barré syndrome and chronic inflammatory demyelinating polyradiculoneuropathy (CIDP).
2. Hereditary motor and sensory neuropathy (Charcot-Marie-Tooth disease)
3. Acute intermittent porphyria.
4. Lead poisoning.
5. Diabetes mellitus.
6. Multifocal motor neuropathy.

Note: Motor neurone disease and neuromuscular junction disorders must always be considered in the differential diagnosis.

Causes of a predominantly sensory neuropathy (sensory neuronopathy)

This is unusual and results in sensory ataxia and pseudoathetosis. Causes include the following:

1. carcinoma (e.g. lung, ovary, breast)
2. paraproteinaemia
3. vitamin B_6 intoxication
4. Sjögren's syndrome
5. diabetes mellitus
6. syphilis
7. vitamin B_{12} deficiency (occasionally)
8. idiopathic.

Causes of a painful peripheral neuropathy

1. Diabetes mellitus.
2. Alcohol.
3. Vitamin B_{12} or B_1 deficiency.
4. Carcinoma.
5. Porphyria.
6. Arsenic or thallium poisoning.
7. Heredity (most are not painful).

Note: Burning soles of the feet can be caused by a painful peripheral neuropathy, tarsal tunnel syndrome or an S1 lesion.

Mononeuritis multiplex

Mononeuritis multiplex refers to separate involvement of more than one peripheral or rarely cranial nerve (e.g. a common peroneal nerve palsy plus an axillary nerve palsy).

Common causes of mononeuritis multiplex

Acute (usually vascular):

1. diabetes mellitus
2. polyarteritis nodosa or connective tissue diseases—SLE, rheumatoid arthritis.

Chronic:

1. multiple compressive neuropathies, especially with joint-deforming arthritis
2. sarcoidosis
3. acromegaly
4. leprosy
5. Lyme disease
6. carcinoma (rare)
7. idiopathic.

Causes of thickened nerves

1. Hereditary motor and sensory neuropathy.
2. Acromegaly.
3. Chronic inflammatory demyelinating polyradiculoneuropathy.
4. Amyloid.
5. Leprosy.
6. Others—sarcoid, neurofibromatosis.

Fasciculation

Fasciculation is *not* always motor neurone disease.

Causes of fasciculation

1. Benign idiopathic fasciculation (by far the most common).
2. Motor neurone disease.
3. Motor root compression.
4. Malignant neuropathy.
5. Any motor neuropathy (less commonly).

Note: Myokymia resembles benign coarse fasciculation of the same muscle group (e.g. eyelids). Electromyographic myokymia can occur in multiple sclerosis, brain stem neoplasm, Bell's palsy, radiculopathy or radiation plexopathy, or chronic nerve compression.

Hereditary motor and sensory neuropathy (HMSN)

Charcot-Marie-Tooth disease: usually autosomal dominant.

Clinical features

1. Pes cavus (short, high-arched feet with hammer toes).
2. Distal muscle atrophy owing to peripheral nerve degeneration. Not usually extending above the elbows or above the middle one-third of the thighs.
3. Absent reflexes.
4. Slight to no sensory loss in the limbs.
5. Thickened nerves.
6. Optic atrophy; Argyll Robertson pupils (rare).

An approach to brachial plexus lesions

Complete lesion

1. Lower motor neurone signs affect the whole arm.
2. Sensory loss (whole limb).

3. Horner's syndrome (an important clue but only if the lesion is proximal in the lower plexus.

Note: This is often painful. Remember always to feel for axillary lymphadenopathy at the end of your examination.

Upper trunk (Erb Duchenne) (C5, C6) lesion
1. Loss of shoulder movement and elbow flexion—hand is held in the 'waiter's tip' position.
2. Sensory loss is present over the lateral aspect of the arm and forearm and over the thumb.

Lower trunk (Klumpke) (C8, T1) lesion
1. True claw hand with paralysis of all the intrinsic muscles.
2. Sensory loss along the ulnar side of the hand and forearm.
3. Horner's syndrome.

Cervical rib syndrome
1. Weakness and wasting of the small muscles of the hand (true claw hand).
2. Sensory loss over the medial aspect of the hand and forearm.
3. Unequal radial pulses and blood pressures.
4. Subclavian bruit and loss of the pulse on arm manoeuvring (this sign is often also present in normal persons).
5. Palpable cervical rib in the neck (uncommon).

Important peripheral nerves

Radial nerve (C5–C8) lesions

Clinical features
1. Wrist and finger drop (wrist flexion normal).
2. Triceps loss (elbow extension loss) if lesion is above the spiral groove.
3. Sensory loss over the anatomical snuff box.
4. Finger abduction *appears* to be weak because of the difficulty of spreading the fingers when they cannot be straightened.

Median nerve (C6–T1) lesions
This nerve supplies all muscles on the front of the forearm except flexor carpi ulnaris and half of flexor digitorum profundus. It also supplies the following short muscles of the hand (LOAF):

L lateral two lumbricals
O opponens pollicis
A abductor pollicis brevis
F flexor pollicis brevis (this sometimes has ulnar innervation).

Clinical features
1. Loss of abductor pollicis brevis with a lesion at or above the wrist. Pen touching test: with the hand flat, ask the patient to abduct the thumb vertically to touch the examiner's pen.
2. Loss of flexor digitorum sublimis with a lesion in or above the cubital fossa. Ochsner's clasping test: ask the patient to clasp the hands firmly together—the index finger on the affected side fails to flex.
3. Sensory loss over the thumb, index, middle and lateral half of the ring finger (palmar aspect only).

Note: Causes of carpal tunnel syndrome:

1. idiopathic
2. arthropathy—rheumatoid arthritis
3. endocrine disease—myxoedema, acromegaly
4. pregnancy
5. trauma and overuse.

Ulnar nerve (C8–T1) lesions

Clinical features
1. Wasting of the intrinsic muscles of the hand (except LOAF muscles).
2. Weak finger abduction and adduction (loss of interosseous muscles).
3. Ulnar claw-like hand. (*Note*: A higher lesion causes less deformity, as an above-the-elbow lesion also causes loss of flexor digitorum profundus.)
4. Froment's sign: ask the patient to grasp a piece of paper between the thumb and lateral aspect of the forefinger with each hand—the affected thumb will flex (loss of thumb adductor).
5. Sensory loss over the little and medial half of ring finger (both palmar and dorsal aspects).

Wasting of the small muscles of the hand
Examine as for the upper limbs and make sure you feel the pulses and examine the neck, unless the cause is very obvious (e.g. rheumatoid arthritis).

Causes
1. Nerve lesions:
   (a) median and ulnar nerve lesions
   (b) brachial plexus lesions
   (c) peripheral motor neuropathy (in the examination, don't forget hereditary motor and sensory neuropathy).
2. Anterior horn cell disease:
   (a) motor neurone disease
   (b) polio
   (c) spinal muscular atrophies (e.g. Kugelberg–Welander disease).
3. Myopathy:
   (a) dystrophia myotonica—forearms more affected than the hands
   (b) distal myopathy.
4. Spinal cord lesions:
   (a) syringomyelia
   (b) cervical spondylosis with compression of C8 segment
   (c) other (e.g. tumour).
5. Trophic disorders:
   (a) arthropathies (disuse)
   (b) ischaemia, including vasculitis
   (c) shoulder–hand syndrome.

Note: When distinguishing an ulnar nerve lesion from a C8 root/lower trunk brachial plexus lesion, remember that the sensory loss of a C8 lesion extends proximal to the wrist, and the thenar muscles are involved with a C8 root or lower trunk brachial plexus lesion. Distinguishing a C8 root from a lower trunk brachial plexus lesion is difficult clinically, but the presence of Horner's syndrome or an axillary mass suggests that the brachial plexus is affected.

Femoral nerve (L2, L3, L4) lesions

Clinical features
1. Weakness of knee extension (quadriceps paralysis).
2. Slight hip flexion weakness.
3. Preserved adductor strength.
4. Loss of knee jerk.
5. Sensory loss involving the inner aspect of the thigh and leg.

Sciatic nerve (L4, L5, S1, S2) lesions

Clinical features
1. Weakness of knee flexion (hamstrings involved).
2. Loss of power of all muscles below the knee causing a foot drop, so the patient may be able to walk but cannot stand on his toes or heels.
3. Knee jerk intact.
4. Loss of ankle jerk and plantar response.
5. Sensory loss along the posterior thigh and total loss below the knee.

Common peroneal (lateral popliteal) nerve (L4, L5, S1) lesions

Clinical features
1. Foot drop and *loss of foot eversion only*.
2. Sensory loss (minimal) over the dorsum of the foot.

Note: The reflexes are normal.

When distinguishing a common peroneal and L5 root lesion, the L5 lesion causes mild weakness of knee flexion, loss of foot inversion as well as eversion, with a sensory loss involving the L5 distribution sparing the little toe and sole.

Lateral cutaneous nerve of the thigh lesion
Meralgia paraesthetica is caused by compression of this nerve, which may result in sensory loss and/or hyperaesthesia over the lateral aspect of the thigh, but no motor loss.

Causes of foot drop
1. Common peroneal nerve palsy.
2. Sciatic nerve palsy.
3. Lumbosacral plexus lesion.
4. L4, L5 root lesion.
5. Peripheral motor neuropathy.
6. Distal myopathy.
7. Motor neurone disease.
8. Precentral gyrus lesion.
9. Spinal cord lesion.

Note: Remember, if there is a foot drop, test the ankle jerk carefully. As a very rough rule of thumb, if it is absent, an S1 lesion should be suspected; if it is normal, a common peroneal palsy should be considered; if it is increased, an upper motor neurone lesion is likely.

Notes on spinal cord lesions

Assessment of the paraplegic patient

1. Is there also a sensory level? Patterns of sensory loss depend on the level and type of lesion.

Consider:
(a)   cord compression, which causes a loss of all modalities bilaterally below the level involved (*Note*: Extrinsic compression may spare the perineum), and radicular pain and lower motor neurone weakness are present at the level of spinal compression
(b)   transverse myelitis
(c)   anterior spinal artery occlusion (posterior column function is spared)
(d)   intrinsic cord lesion
(e)   multiple sclerosis.
2.   Back examination:
For example, deformity, tenderness or bruits may provide clues about the underlying disease process.
3.   Arm involvement?
Consider:
(a)   cervical spondylosis
(b)   syringomyelia
(c)   motor neurone disease
(d)   multiple sclerosis.
4.   Cranial nerve lesions?
Consider:
(a)   motor neurone disease
(b)   multiple sclerosis.
5.   Peripheral neuropathy?
Consider:
(a)   vitamin B_{12} deficiency
(b)   Friedreich's ataxia
(c)   carcinoma
(d)   hereditary spastic paraplegia
(e)   syphilis.
6.   Cerebral lesions?

Note: Intracranial lesions (e.g. parasagittal meningioma) cause paraplegia in *extension* only, while spinal cord lesions cause paraplegia in *flexion* or *extension* (i.e. flexor reflexes are released with spinal lesions).

Important motor and reflex changes of spinal cord and conus compression

Lower motor neurone signs occur at the level of the root lesion and upper motor neurone signs occur below the lesion.

Upper cervical
• Upper motor neurone signs in the upper and lower limbs. Paralysis of the diaphragm occurs with a lesion above C4.

C5
• Lower motor neurone weakness and wasting of the rhomboids, deltoids, biceps and brachioradialis.
• Upper motor neurone signs affect the rest of the upper and all the lower limbs.
• The biceps jerk is lost.
• The supinator jerk is 'inverted'.

C8
• Lower motor neurone weakness and wasting of the intrinsic muscles of the hand.
• Upper motor neurone signs in the lower limbs.

Midthoracic
- Intercostal paralysis (cannot be detected clinically).
- Loss of upper abdominal reflexes at T7 and T8.
- Upper motor neurone signs in the lower limbs.

T10–T11
- Loss of the lower abdominal reflexes and upward displacement of the umbilicus on contraction (Beevor's sign).
- Upper motor neurone signs in the lower limbs.

L1
- Cremasteric reflexes lost (normal abdominal reflexes).
- Upper motor neurone signs in the lower limbs.

L4
- Lower motor neurone weakness and wasting of the quadriceps. Knee jerks lost.

L5 and S1
- Lower motor neurone weakness of knee flexion and hip extension (S1) and abduction (L5) plus calf and foot muscles.
- Knee jerks present.
- No ankle jerks or plantar response.
- Anal reflex present.

S3–S4
- No anal reflex.
- Saddle sensory loss.
- Normal lower limbs.

Note: Look for a urinary catheter.

Important syndromes

Subacute combined degeneration of the cord (vitamin B$_{12}$ deficiency)

Clinical features
1. Symmetrical posterior column loss (vibration and position sense), causing an ataxic gait.
2. Symmetrical upper motor neurone signs in the lower limbs with absent ankle reflexes. Knee reflexes may be absent or, more often, exaggerated.
3. Peripheral sensory neuropathy (less common and mild).
4. Optic atrophy (occasionally).
5. Dementia (occasionally).

The combination of upper motor neurone signs causing an extensor plantar response plus peripheral neuropathy causing loss of knee and ankle jerks is a distinctive pattern.
    Causes of an extensor plantar response plus absent ankle jerks include:

1. subacute combined degeneration of the cord (vitamin B$_{12}$ deficiency)
2. conus medullaris lesion
3. combination of an upper motor neurone lesion with cauda equina compression or peripheral neuropathy
4. syphilis (tabo-paresis)
5. Friedreich's ataxia
6. diabetes mellitus (uncommon)
7. adrenoleucodystrophy or metachromatic leucodystrophy.

Brown-Séquard syndrome (hemisection of the spinal cord)

Clinical features

Motor changes:

1. upper motor neurone signs below the hemisection on the *same* side as the lesion
2. lower motor neurone signs at the level of the hemisection on the *same* side.

Sensory changes:

1. pain and temperature loss on the *opposite* side of the lesion (*Note*: The upper level of sensory loss is usually a few segments below the level of the lesion.)
2. vibration and proprioception loss occurs on the *same* side
3. light touch is often normal
4. there may be a band of sensory loss on the same side at the level of the lesion (afferent nerve fibres).

Common causes:

1. multiple sclerosis
2. angioma
3. glioma
4. trauma
5. myelitis
6. postradiation myelopathy.

Causes of dissociated sensory loss (usually indicates spinal cord disease but may occur with peripheral neuropathy)

Spinothalamic (pain and temperature) loss only
1. Syringomyelia ('cape' distribution).
2. Brown-Séquard syndrome (contralateral leg).
3. Anterior spinal artery thrombosis.
4. Lateral medullary syndrome (contralateral to the other signs).
5. Peripheral neuropathy (e.g. diabetes mellitus, amyloid, Fabry's disease).

Dorsal column (vibration and proprioception) loss only
1. Subacute combined degeneration.
2. Brown-Séquard syndrome (ipsilateral leg).
3. Spinocerebellar degeneration (e.g. Friedreich's ataxia).
4. Multiple sclerosis.
5. Tabes dorsalis.
6. Sensory neuropathy or ganglionopathy (e.g. carcinoma).
7. Peripheral neuropathy from diabetes mellitus or hypothyroidism.

Syringomyelia (a central cavity in the spinal cord)

Clinical triad
1. Loss of pain and temperature over the neck, shoulders and arms ('cape' distribution).
2. Amyotrophy (weakness, atrophy and areflexia) of the arms.
3. Upper motor neurone signs in the lower limbs.

Note: There may also be thoracic scoliosis owing to asymmetrical weakness of paravertebral muscles.

An approach to myopathy

Causes of proximal muscle weakness

1. Myopathic (see below).
2. Neuromuscular junction disorder—myasthenia gravis.
3. Neurogenic—Kugelberg-Welander disease (proximal muscle wasting and fasciculation as a result of anterior horn cell damage—autosomal recessive), motor neurone disease, polyradiculopathy.

Causes of myopathy

1. Hereditary muscular dystrophy (qv).
2. Congenital myopathies (rare).
3. Acquired (mnemonic PACE, PODS):
   (a) polymyositis or dermatomyositis
   (b) alcohol
   (c) carcinoma
   (d) endocrine (e.g. hypothyroidism, hyperthyroidism, Cushing's syndrome, acromegaly, hypopituitarism)
   (e) periodic paralysis (hyperkalaemic or hypokalaemic or normokalaemic)
   (f) osteomalacia
   (g) drugs (e.g. clofibrate, chloroquine, steroids)
   (h) sarcoidosis.

Note: Causes of proximal myopathy and a peripheral neuropathy include:

1. paraneoplastic syndrome
2. alcohol
3. connective tissue disease.

Muscular dystrophies

1. Duchenne's (pseudohypertrophic) (sex-linked recessive disorder):
   (a) affects only males (or females with Turner's syndrome)
   (b) the calves and deltoids are hypertrophied early and weak later
   (c) early proximal weakness
   (d) tendon reflexes are preserved in proportion to muscle strength
   (e) severe progressive kyphoscoliosis
   (f) heart disease (dilated cardiomyopathy)
   (g) creatine kinase level markedly elevated
   (h) patients die in the second decade, usually from heart disease.
2. Becker (sex-linked recessive disorder). Same features as Duchenne's but less severe, has a later onset and is less rapidly progressive.
3. Limb girdle (autosomal recessive):
   (a) shoulder or pelvic girdle affected (onset third decade)
   (b) face and heart usually spared.
4. Facioscapulohumeral (autosomal dominant):
   (a) facial and pectoral girdle weakness with hypertrophy of the deltoids (normal pelvic muscles early).
5. Distal dystrophies:
   (a) autosomal dominant disease, which is rare and causes distal muscle atrophy and weakness
   (b) dystrophia myotonica (autosomal dominant).

Tests for myopathy

1. Creatine kinase (highest in Duchenne's).
2. Electromyogram (EMG).

3. Electrocardiogram (particularly Duchenne's and dystrophia myotonica).
4. Muscle biopsy.

Dystrophia myotonica

This man has noticed some arm weakness. Please examine him.

Method

Stand back and you fortunately notice the features of myotonic dystrophy. Proceed as follows.

Observe the face for frontal baldness (the patient may be wearing a wig), dull triangular facies ('hatchet' face), temporalis, masseter and sternomastoid atrophy, and partial ptosis. Note thick spectacles, as these patients develop cataracts, and fine subcapsular deposits, which are virtually diagnostic.

Look at the neck for sternomastoid atrophy, then test neck flexion (neck flexion is weak, while extension is normal).

Go to the upper limbs. Shake hands (for grip myotonia) and test percussion myotonia. Tapping over the thenar eminence causes contraction then slow relaxation of abductor pollicis brevis (Table 8.44).

Table 8.44   **Causes of myotonia**

1. Dystrophia myotonica
2. Myotonia congenita (myotonia of the tongue and thenar eminence, the recessive form being more severe)
3. Paramyotonia congenita (episodic myotonia after cold exposure)

Note: Drugs (e.g. clofibrate) can also cause myotonic discharges on EMG, but do not cause clinical myotonia.

Examine the arm now for signs of wasting and weakness, especially of the forearm muscles. Sensory changes from the associated peripheral neuropathy are usually very mild.

Go to the chest and inspect for gynaecomastia.

Next palpate the testes for atrophy.

Examine the lower limbs if there is time. Always ask to test the urine for sugar (diabetes mellitus is more common in this disease) and ask to examine the cardiovascular system for cardiomyopathy. Finally test mental status (mild mental retardation is usual).

Note: Remember the classic EMG finding in dystrophia myotonica of a 'dive bomber' effect with needle movement in the muscle at rest.

Gait

Please examine this man's gait.

Method (Fig 8.23)

Make sure the patient's legs are clearly visible. Ask him to 'hop out' of bed (look carefully while he is doing so for focal disease), watch him walk normally for a few metres, and then ask him to turn around quickly and walk back towards you.

Figure 8.23   Gait examination.

Standing (legs fully exposed)

1. **GENERAL INSPECTION**
   Deformity
   Diagnostic facies (Table 8.29)
   Upper limb lesions
   Focal neurological disease (e.g.
     wasting)
   Fasciculation
   Abnormal movements

2. **ASK THE PATIENT TO:**
   Walk normally and turn around
     quickly (abnormal gait)

Heel–toe walking (cerebellar
  disease)
Walk on toes (S1)
Walk on heels (L4 or L5)
Squat (proximal myopathy)
Romberg's sign—feet together with:
   Eyes closed (posterior columns)
   Eyes open (cerebellar disease)

3. **EXAMINE LOWER LIMBS**

Next ask him to walk heel-to-toe to exclude a midline cerebellar lesion.

Ask him then to walk on his toes (an S1 lesion will make this difficult) and then on his heels (a lesion causing foot drop will make this difficult).

Test for proximal myopathy by asking the patient to squat and then stand up or sit in a chair and then stand.

Look for Romberg's sign (posterior column loss causes inability to stand steadily when the feet are together with the eyes closed, while cerebellar disease causes difficulty when the eyes are open too). Go on to examine the lower limbs depending on your findings.

The typical gaits to recognise are listed in Table 8.45.

Table 8.45   Typical gaits

1. Hemiparetic—the foot is plantarflexed and the leg swung in a lateral arc
2. Paraparetic (scissor gait)
3. Extrapyramidal (e.g. Parkinson's disease)
   (a) hesitation in starting
   (b) shuffling
   (c) freezing
   (d) festination (the patient hurries forward, trying to catch up with his centre of gravity)
   (e) propulsion (pull him towards you gently—he will be unable to stop), retropulsion
4. Cerebellar (a drunken gait that is wide-based or reeling on a narrow base; the patient staggers towards the affected side)
5. Apraxic (prefrontal lobe) (feet appear glued to the floor when erect, but move more easily when the patient is supine)
6. Posterior column lesion (clumsy slapping down of the feet on a broad base)
7. Distal weakness (high-stepping gait)
8. Proximal weakness (waddling gait)

Cerebellum

This man has noticed a problem with his coordination. Please examine him.

Method

This patient is likely to have a cerebellar problem (Table 8.46). The only other likely possibilities are posterior column loss or extrapyramidal disease. Proceed as follows for assessment of cerebellar disease.

Look first for nystagmus, usually jerky horizontal nystagmus with an increased amplitude on looking towards the side of the lesion.

Assess speech next. Ask the patient to say 'British Constitution' or 'West Register Street'. Cerebellar speech is jerky, explosive and loud, with irregular separation of syllables.

Go to the upper limbs. Ask the patient to extend his arms and look for arm drift and static tremor as a result of hypotonia of the agonist muscles. Test tone. Hypotonia is caused by loss of a facilitatory influence on the spinal motor neurones in acute unilateral cerebellar disease.

Table 8.46 Causes of cerebellar disease

Unilateral
1. Space-occupying lesion (tumour, abscess, granuloma)
2. Ischaemia (vertebrobasilar disease)
3. Paraneoplastic syndrome
4. Multiple sclerosis
5. Trauma

Bilateral
1. Drugs (e.g. phenytoin)
2. Friedreich's ataxia
3. Hypothyroidism
4. Paraneoplastic syndrome
5. Multiple sclerosis
6. Trauma ('punch drunk')
7. Arnold-Chiari malformation
8. Alcohol
9. Large space-occupying lesion, cerebrovascular disease, rare metabolic diseases

Midline
1. Paraneoplastic syndrome
2. Midline tumour

Rostral vermis lesion (only lower limbs affected)
1. Alcohol (commonest cause of a cerebellar lesion)

Next perform the finger–nose test—the patient touches his nose, then rotates his finger and touches your finger. Note any intention tremor (erratic movements increasing as the target is approached owing to loss of cerebellar connections with the brain stem) and past pointing (the patient overshooting the target).

Test rapid alternating movements; the patient taps alternately the palm and back of one hand on his other hand or thigh. Inability to perform this movement smoothly is called dysdiadochokinesis.

Test rebound—ask the patient to lift his arms quickly from the sides and then stop. Hypotonia causes the patient to be unable to stop his arms.

Always demonstrate each movement for the patient's benefit, asking him to copy you.

Go on to examine the legs. Again test tone here. Then perform the heel–shin test, looking for accuracy of fine movement when the patient slides his heel down the shin slowly on each side for several cycles. Next ask him to lift his big toe up to touch your finger, looking for intention tremor. Ask the patient then to tap each foot rapidly on a firm surface.

Look for truncal ataxia by asking the patient to fold his arms and sit up. While he is sitting, ask him to put his legs over the side of the bed, and test for pendular knee jerks.

Test gait (the patient will stagger towards the affected side).

If there is time, look for possible causes of the problem. If there is an obvious unilateral lesion, auscultate over the cerebellum, then proceed to the cranial nerves and look for evidence of a cerebellopontine angle tumour (fifth, seventh, eighth nerves affected) (pp 294–5) and the lateral medullary syndrome. Always look in the fundi for papilloedema. Next examine for peripheral evidence of malignant disease and vascular disease (carotid bruits).

If there is a midline lesion only (i.e. truncal ataxia or abnormal heel–toe walking or abnormal speech), consider either a midline tumour or a paraneoplastic syndrome. If there is bilateral disease, look for signs of multiple sclerosis (p 205), Friedreich's ataxia (pes cavus being the most helpful initial clue) (Tables 8.47 and 8.48) and hypothyroidism (rare). Alcoholic cerebellar degeneration (which affects the anterior lobe of the cerebellar vermis) classically spares the arms.

If there are, in addition, upper motor neurone signs, consider the causes in Table 8.49.

Table 8.47 Clinical features of Friedreich's ataxia (autosomal recessive)

Usually a young person with:
1. cerebellar signs (bilateral), including nystagmus
2. posterior column loss in the limbs
3. upper motor neurone signs in the limbs (although ankle reflexes are absent)
4. peripheral neuropathy
5. optic atrophy
6. pes cavus, cocking of the toes and kyphoscoliosis
7. cardiomyopathy (ECG abnormalities occur in more than 50% of cases)
8. diabetes mellitus

Table 8.48 Causes of pes cavus

1. Friedreich's ataxia or other spinocerebellar degenerations
2. Hereditary motor and sensory neuropathy (HMSN)
3. Neuropathies in childhood
4. Idiopathic

Table 8.49	Causes of spastic and ataxic paraparesis (upper motor neurone and cerebellar signs combined)

In adolescence
- Spinocerebellar degeneration (e.g. Marie's spastic ataxia)

In young adults
- Multiple sclerosis
- Syphilitic meningomyelitis
- Spinocerebellar degeneration
- Arnold-Chiari malformation or other lesions at the craniospinal junction

In later life
- Multiple sclerosis
- Syringomyelia
- Infarction (in upper pons or internal capsule bilaterally—'ataxic hemiparesis')
- Lesion at the craniospinal junction (e.g. meningioma)
- Spinocerebellar degeneration

Don't forget, common unrelated diseases (e.g. cervical spondylosis and cerebellar degeneration from alcohol) may occur together by chance.

Parkinson's disease

This man has Parkinson's disease. Please assess him.

Method

Look at him first. Note the obvious lack of facial expression ('mask-like') and paucity of movement.

Ask him to walk, turn quickly, and stop and restart. Particularly note difficulty starting, shuffling, freezing and festination. It is probably a little dangerous to look for propulsion or retropropulsion (see Table 8.45).

Ask the patient to return to bed and look for a resting tremor with the arms relaxed (Table 8.50). The characteristic movement is described as pill rolling and may be unilateral early on. On finger–nose testing, a resting tremor diminishes, but an action tremor may appear. Test wrist tone, feeling for cogwheel or lead pipe rigidity. Reinforce this by asking him to turn his head from side to side. Test for abnormal rapid alternating movements. Look also for involuntary movements produced by medication use.

Go to the face. Note tremor, absence of blinking, dribbling of saliva and lack of expression. Test the glabellar tap; the sign is positive when the patient continues to blink after the middle finger taps several times over the glabella from behind—it is important that your finger is out of his line of vision. Test speech then, which is typically monotonous, soft, poorly articulated and faint. Look at the ocular movements for supranuclear gaze palsies. Feel for a greasy or sweaty brow (owing to autonomic dysfunction).

Ask the patient to write (looking for micrographia), and test the frontal lobe reflexes and higher centres (looking for evidence of dementia).

Table 8.50   A classification of tremor

1. Parkinsonian—resting tremor
2. Action tremor—present throughout movement but resolves at rest:
   (a) thyrotoxicosis
   (b) anxiety
   (c) drugs
   (d) familial
   (e) idiopathic (most common)
3. Intention tremor (cerebellar disease)—increases towards the target
4. Cerebellar outflow tract tremor ('red nucleus')—abduction–adduction movements of upper limbs with flexion–extension of wrists (usually associated with intention tremor, e.g. in multiple sclerosis or brain injury)

Note: Flapping (asterixis) is not strictly a tremor but a sudden brief loss of tone in hepatic failure, cardiac failure, respiratory failure or renal failure.

Causes of parkinsonism

1. Idiopathic (Parkinson's disease).
2. Drugs (e.g. phenothiazines, methyldopa).
3. Postencephalitis.
4. Other—toxins (carbon monoxide, manganese), Wilson's disease, Steele-Richardson syndrome, Shy-Drager syndrome, syphilis, tumour.

Note: Atherosclerosis is controversial as a cause of parkinsonism.

Chorea

Examine this man's arms.

Method

Happily you notice an extrapyramidal choreiform movement disorder. Choreiform movements are non-repetitive, abrupt, involuntary, more distal jerky movements, which the patient often attempts to disguise by completing the involuntary movement with a voluntary one. This is caused by a lesion of the corpus striatum. *Hemiballismus* is unilateral and usually involves rotary movements of proximal joints. It is caused by a subthalamic nucleus lesion on the opposite side. *Athetosis* involves slow, sinuous distal writhing movements at rest. It is caused by a lesion of the outer segment of the putamen.

If the patient has chorea, proceed as follows.

First shake the patient's hand, for a lack of sustained grip ('milkmaid grip'). Ask the patient to hold his hands out and look for a choreic posture (finger and thumb hyperextension and wrist flexion as a result of hypotonia). Note any signs of vasculitis. Go to the face and look at the eyes for exophthalmos, Kayser-Fleischer rings and conjunctival injection (ataxia-telangiectasia). Ask the patient to poke his tongue out and note a serpentine tongue (moving in and out). Notice any rash (e.g. SLE).

If the patient is young, examine the heart for signs of rheumatic fever.

Test the knee jerks (pendular) and the higher centres (for Huntington's disease). The causes are summarised in Table 8.51.

Table 8.51   **Causes of chorea**

1. Huntington's disease (autosomal dominant)
2. Sydenham's chorea (rheumatic fever)
3. Senility
4. Wilson's disease
5. Drugs (e.g. phenothiazines, the contraceptive pill, phenytoin, L-dopa)
6. Vasculitis or connective tissue disease (e.g. SLE)
7. Thyrotoxicosis (very rare)
8. Polycythaemia or other causes of hyperviscosity (very rare)
9. Viral encephalitis (very rare)

Imaging for physician trainees

Associate Professor Ross O'Neil, Radiologist, The Canberra Hospital, ACT

The diagnosis of disease is often easy, often difficult, and often impossible.

Peter Mere Latham, 1878

During the discussion stage of the long case and after the presentation of the short-case examination findings, candidates will often be asked to say what investigations might be appropriate. Plain X-rays, computed tomography (CT) scans and magnetic resonance imaging (MRI) scans are often indicated, especially for patients with cardiac, respiratory, neurological or rheumatological problems. These films may well be available for the candidate to comment upon. It is important to be able to justify the requested investigation and explain its advantages over other tests. This means that candidates must know why an MRI, for example, is more appropriate imaging for a patient with multiple sclerosis than a CT scan. The examiners may want to know what type of scan or MRI should be ordered (e.g. when a high-resolution CT scan is more appropriate than a spiral CT or when contrast should be used). They may expect the candidate to know some technical information (e.g. the difference between a T1- and T2-weighted MRI scan). Finally, candidates must be able to comment sensibly when given the scan requested.

In this chapter some important X-rays and scans are shown and discussed. An approach to appropriate assessment of the images is outlined.

The chest radiograph

The chest X-ray is often the first investigation for respiratory and cardiac problems. Although it is relatively simple to perform and to order, it is a difficult investigation to interpret well. The usual films are posteroanterior (PA) and lateral radiographs. Antero-posterior (AP) films are only performed on immobile and very ill patients. AP films are usually marked *mobile* or *AP*. AP films are more difficult to assess and the heart size and lung fields are more difficult to interpret. AP films are unlikely to appear in the examinations but failing to notice that a film is marked *mobile* will lead to trouble. It is also wise to take a moment to look at the date and patient's name on the film.

The chest X-ray in heart disease

One needs to be aware of the normal anatomy visualised on a chest X-ray (Fig 9.1). The *heart size* should be less than half the transverse diameter of the chest on the PA film (Figs 9.1 and 9.2a). The heart size cannot be accurately assessed on an AP film or if there is chest wall deformity, such as pectus excavatum.

Specific cardiac chamber enlargement can often be appreciated on plain X-rays. Left ventricular dilatation is typically seen with left heart failure (Fig 9.2). Left atrial

Figure 9.1   Normal chest X-ray.

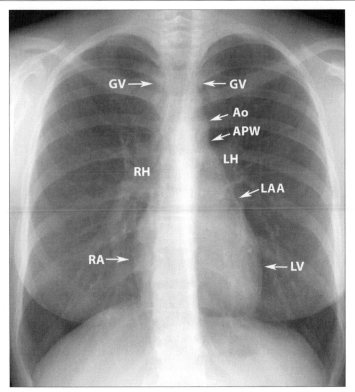

The right heart border (from superior to inferior) is composed of the great vessels (GV), the ascending aorta (especially when unfolded), the right hilum (RH), and the right atrium (RA). The left heart border (from superior to inferior) is composed of the great vessels (GV), the aortic arch (Ao), the aorto-pulmonary window (APW), the left hilum (LH), the left atrial appendage (LAA) and the left ventricle (LV). It should be noted that the aorto-pulmonary window is concave and the left atrial appendage is usually concave but may be flat on a normal chest X-ray.

enlargement resulting from mitral valve disease is a common finding (Fig 9.3). Right ventricular hypertrophy may be seen with congenital heart disease, particularly tetralogy of Fallot (Fig 9.4), pulmonary stenosis and Eisenmenger reaction (the severe pulmonary hypertension and shunt reversal that can complicate congenital heart disease) associated with chronic left-to-right shunts (Fig 9.5).

Valvular calcification may accompany rheumatic heart disease. The position of the calcification can be a useful indicator of the involved valve (Fig 9.6). The aorta should be specifically assessed for size, position, appearance and situs (position) (Fig 9.7). The ribs should also be reviewed (Fig 9.7).

The chest X-ray and lung disease

The *hila* should be assessed for size (Fig 9.9) and position (Fig 9.10). The hilar structures are among the most difficult areas to assess on the chest X-ray. Even experienced radiologists may be unwilling to commit themselves in the face of subtle changes. If there is no obvious abnormality, candidates should probably follow this example and

Figure 9.2   Chest X-ray features of left ventricular failure (AP film).

a

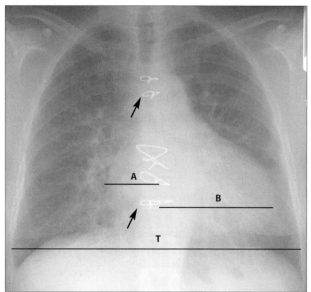

b

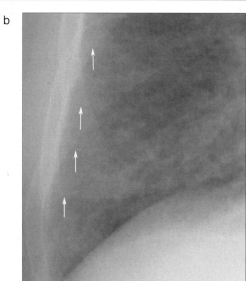

(a)   The cardiothoracic ratio $\left(\dfrac{A + B}{T}\right)$ is greater than the normal 50%. The thoracic measurement (T) is the maximum internal transverse diameter of the rib cage. The cardiac diameter is the addition of the two widths A and B. Other features include:
- large left ventricle (apex downwards and outwards) (*Note*: A large right ventricle causes the apex to pass upwards and outwards.)
- sternotomy wires from previous coronary artery bypass grafting (CABG) (arrows)
- upper lobe blood diversion (upper lobe vessels more prominent than lower lobe vessels).

(b)   Interstitial pulmonary oedema with septal (Kerley B) lines (arrows).

Figure 9.3   Mitral valve disease with left atrial enlargement (p 232).

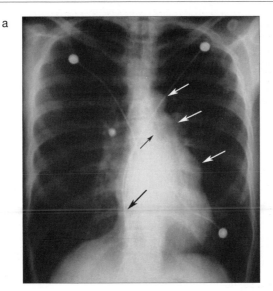

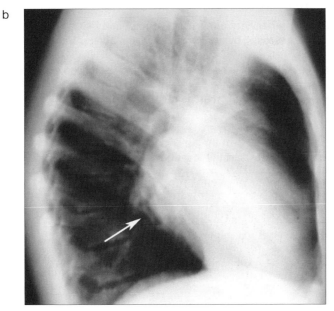

(a)   PA film. There are three prominences of the left heart border (white arrows): the aorta, the pulmonary outflow tract and the left atrial appendage. Prominence of the left atrial appendage is a useful and reliable sign. The right side of the left atrial border (LAB) (large black arrow) is also visible. This is an unreliable sign of left atrial enlargement. The left main bronchus (LMB) (small black arrow) does not appear elevated. This is also an inconsistent sign. Increase in the left atrial diameter (the distance from LMB to LAB) is a good sign but distances vary depending on the patient's age, sex and size.

(b)   Focal prominence of the left atrium on the lateral film (arrow).

Figure 9.4 Atrial septal defect (ASD) with Eisenmenger reaction (p 245)—typical chest X-ray findings.

a

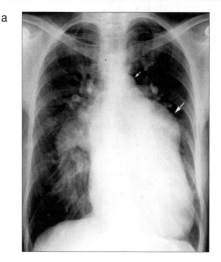

b

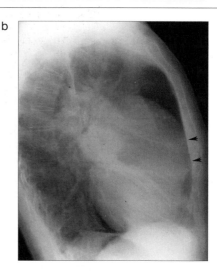

(a) Findings on the PA film:
- large heart
- dilated main pulmonary artery (large arrow) and its central branches (vessel size can be assessed by comparison with the adjacent bronchi, which should be of similar calibre)
- aortic knuckle is small (small arrow), reflecting decreased aortic flow in ASD
- the Eisenmenger reaction shows as an abrupt narrowing of the peripheral vessels—in ordinary ASD there is pulmonary plethora.

(b) Findings on the lateral film:
- right ventricular enlargement (arrows)—the right ventricle should only lie against the lower third of the anterior chest wall between the antero-inferior costophrenic recess and the manubriosternal junction.

Figure 9.5 Tetralogy of Fallot (p 246): AP film.

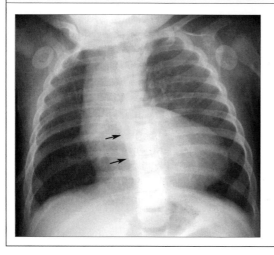

- Boot-shaped heart (*coeur en sabot*) as a result of right ventricular enlargement (apex is directed upwards and outwards).
- Paucity of lung vessels.
- The aortic knuckle is not visualised but the descending aorta (arrows) is clearly right-sided (present in 25%).
- This patient is a child but the same signs are found in adults. In this case, the thymus overlies the enlarged aorta, which cannot be seen.

Figure 9.6 Calcification of the mitral annulus: (a) PA film. (b) lateral film.

a

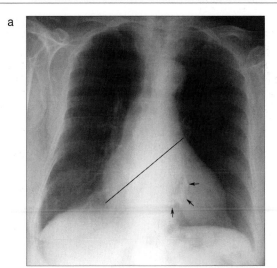

b

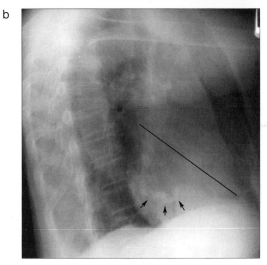

- The mitral annulus is calcified (arrows).
- Valvular calcification has a smaller diameter than calcification of the annulus.
- Valvular calcification is always associated with valvular disease.
- Annulus calcification may be an incidental finding or occasionally associated with valvular regurgitation. It is more common in the elderly, in women, diabetes and in renal failure.

Position of the valves
The mitral valve lies below, behind, and slightly to the left of the aortic valve.

To distinguish the valves if calcification is present, draw imaginary lines. The PA view line passes from the right cardiophrenic angle to the inferior aspect of the left hilum. The lateral view line passes from the antero-inferior angle through to the midpoint of the hilum. The aortic valve lies above these lines and the mitral valve below.

> **Figure 9.7**   Coarctation of the aorta.
>
>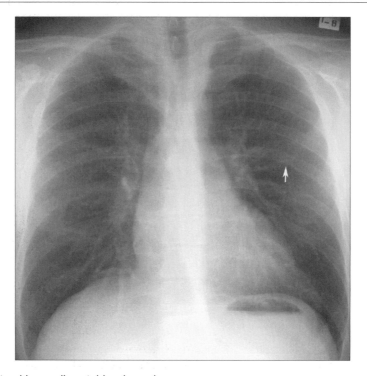
>
> - Bilateral lower rib notching (arrow).
> - Aortic knuckle is obscured. (Other knuckle abnormalities that may be seen are high knuckle, low knuckle and double knuckle.)
> - This patient has not yet developed left ventricular failure.
>
> *Differential diagnosis of inferior rib notching*
> Inferior rib notching is usually associated with abnormalities of the neurovascular groove (typically enlargement of the intercostal artery, vein or nerve).
> - Vascular (caused by shunting of blood):
>   Coarctation of the aorta
>   Blalock-Taussig procedure (unilateral) for tetralogy of Fallot (p 246)
>   Venous obstruction (superior or inferior vena cava, innominate or subclavian)
>   Arteriovenous fistula of chest wall
>   Pulmonary stenosis
>   Pulmonary atresia
>   Tetralogy of Fallot
> - Neurogenic: nerve sheath tumour, especially in neurofibromatosis, which also causes upper rib notching and 'ribbon ribs' (Fig 9.8)
> - Metabolic: hyperparathyroidism (also causes upper rib notching)
> - Normal variant

say 'there is no obvious hilar abnormality' and move on to a possibly more rewarding part of the film.

Assess the *lung fields* more generally. It is important to look behind the heart and at the apices (Fig 9.11).

Figure 9.8   Neurofibromatosis.

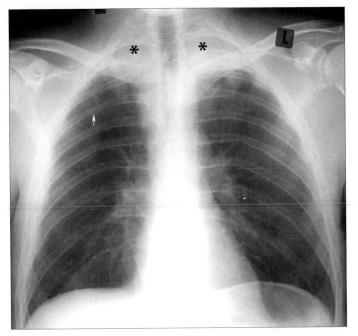

There is bilateral rib notching. Rib modelling deformity ('ribbon ribs') is also present (arrow). There are bilateral apical soft tissue masses as a result of plexiform neurofibroma (asterisks).

Homogeneous opacity is typically caused by collapse, consolidation or effusion (Table 9.1). One could imagine shading this with a crayon. Air bronchograms are seen within an area of consolidation (Fig 9.12). There are numerous causes of the 'consolidative' pattern (Table 9.1).

Interstitial lung disease manifests on the chest X-ray as increased linear (reticular) (Fig 9.13a), nodular (Fig 9.13b) or mixed (reticulonodular) markings (Fig 9.13c). One could imagine drawing these lines with a sharp pencil. Septal (Kerley B) lines are a useful diagnostic feature (Table 9.1).

Desperate candidates may suggest that there is a 'subtle interstitial infiltrate'. Be reluctant to make this observation. Although interstitial infiltrates can be subtle, other more obvious abnormalities must be excluded before this suggestion is made. If this diagnosis seems the only possibility, ask for a high-resolution CT scan to clarify matters.

The silhouette sign

This is one of the most important signs in chest radiology. An edge is visible on a chest X-ray film when there is an interface between two structures of different density (typically soft tissue and air). The silhouette sign occurs when the normal interface is lost because of disease. For example, when the left lower lobe collapses, there is no air in that part of the lung and it is no longer possible to see the medial aspect of the left hemidiaphragm. Similarly, the right heart border is lost when there is middle lobe disease and the left heart border disappears when there is collapse or consolidation of the lingula (Fig 9.14).

Figure 9.9 Sarcoidosis (p 97), showing bilateral hilar adenopathy (arrows).

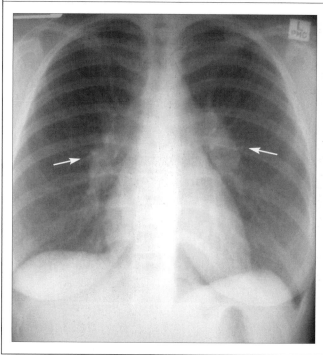

Differential diagnosis of bilateral hilar lymphadenopathy
1. Sarcoidosis
2. Lymphoma, lymphatic leukaemia
3. Metastases
4. Glandular fever

Figure 9.10 Tuberculosis (p 103).

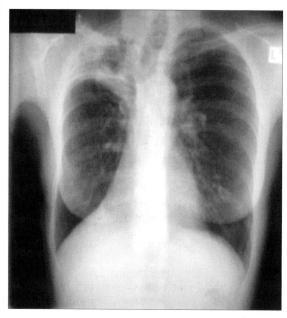

There is scarring of the upper lobes, more marked on the right. Note that both hila are elevated and there is upward bowing of the horizontal fissure and deviation of the trachea to the right, indicating upper lobe volume loss. There is consolidation and cavitation, suggesting active disease (Table 9.1).

Figure 9.11 Pancoast tumour with rib destruction.

a

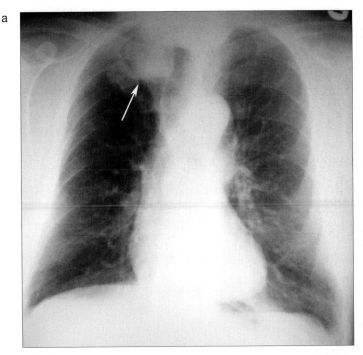

b

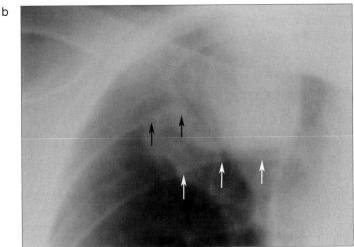

It is easy to overlook both the mass and the rib destruction if this area is not looked at specifically. Note that the rib below the mass can be seen clearly to extend medially (white arrows). The rib at the level of the mass (black arrows) is eroded and cannot be visualised through the mass.

The lack of a silhouette sign is also a useful abnormality. For example, a mass lesion that is projecting through the aortic arch cannot lie posteriorly if the normal aortic knuckle is seen through the mass (Fig 9.15).

Figure 9.12   Right upper lobe consolidation.

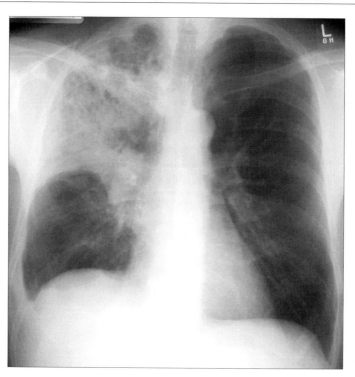

- Dense shadow in right upper zone.
- Air bronchograms are seen as lucent dark lines within the opacity.

Computed tomography (CT)

In computed tomography, a highly focused X-ray beam and a powerful computer are used to form transverse (axial) images of the body. These images represent density maps. Comparative density is measured as Hounsfield units (HU), and water is arbitrarily assigned a value of zero. On this scale, soft tissues measure +30 to +70 HU, fat measures −30 to −100 HU, air measures −1000 HU and dense bone measures +1000 HU. These can be directly measured on any image and, in some cases, this tissue characterisation will enable a specific diagnosis to be made.

Most often, however, tissues are appreciated as a visual difference. The denser an object, the whiter it appears on the image, and the less dense an object, the darker it appears. As the eye can only distinguish 16 shades of grey between white and black, it is necessary therefore to manipulate the window level (WL) and window width (WW) to allow optimal interpretation of pathology. This is like varying the brightness (WL) and contrast (WW) on a monitor.

Black	Grey	White
	WL (midpoint)	

$\leftarrow$————————————————WW————————————————$\rightarrow$

Different windows are used in different parts of the body.

Table 9.1   Differential diagnosis of radiological appearances in the chest X-ray film

Homogeneous opacity
Consolidation—alveoli full of something—look for air bronchogram (see Fig 9.12)
Pus—pneumonia
Blood—infarct, trauma
Cells—bronchoalveolar cell carcinoma, lymphoma
Water—pulmonary oedema
Protein—alveolar proteinosis
Collapse—look for volume loss (elevation of diaphragm and mediastinal shift to affected side)
Effusion—look for increased volume (shift of mediastinum to unaffected side)
Collapse and effusion—seen with lung carcinoma or chronic effusion with underlying passive collapse—look for opaque hemithorax with no mediastinal shift

Diffuse opacities
These are usually interstitial and classified as reticular (linear), nodular (or often both—reticulonodular)

Nodular
• Tuberculosis (see Fig 9.16)
• Metastatic carcinoma
• Sarcoidosis (Figs 9.9, 9.13b)
• Pneumoconiosis
• Lymphoma
• Viral pneumonia
• Vasculitis (e.g. polyarteritis)

Reticular (linear opacities)
• Fibrosis—idiopathic pulmonary fibrosis (IPF)—usually usual interstitial pneumonia (UIP) (see Fig 9.13a)
   —secondary to connective tissue disorder or non-specific interstitial pneumonitis (NSIP)
   —asbestosis—look for other features of asbestos exposure, such as pleural plaques
   —drugs
• Sarcoidosis (see Figs 9.9, 9.13b)
• Pulmonary oedema
• Lymphangitis carcinomatosis

Causes of septal (Kerley B) lines
Common
• Pulmonary oedema
• Lymphangitis carcinomatosis

Uncommon
• Sarcoidosis
• Lymphoma

Nodular calcification
Tuberculosis (see Fig 9.16)
Pneumoconiosis

Table 9.1	Differential diagnosis of radiological appearances in the chest X-ray film (cont.)	
Post-chickenpox pneumonia (usually in cigarette smokers) Ectopic calcification in renal failure, hyperparathyroidism Histoplasmosis and coccidioidomycosis (common in parts of the United States but not in Australia)		
Coin lesion *Common* Tumour (primary or metastatic—look closely for any rib lesion) Granuloma (e.g. tuberculosis, fungus) (see Fig 9.16) Hamartoma *Uncommon* Arteriovenous fistula Rheumatoid nodule Lung abscess Hydatid cyst		
Cavitated lesion Neoplastic	Squamous cell—primary or metastasis Lymphoma	
Infectious	Lung abscess Tuberculosis (see Fig 9.16) Fungi (e.g. coccidioidomycosis)	
Granulomatous	Wegener's granulomatosis (see Fig 9.17) Rheumatoid arthritis Histiocytosis Sarcoidosis	
Abnormal lung	Cystic bronchiectasis Infected bulla Bronchogenic cyst Sequestration	
Pulmonary infarct Traumatic lung cyst		

CT and chest disease

In the chest, dual windows are commonly used. The 'lung windows' have a WL of −600 HU and a WW of 1600 HU. Anything less dense than −1400 HU (−600 − 800) will appear black and anything denser than 200 HU (−600 + 800) will appear white. The 'mediastinal windows' have a WL of 50 HU and a WW of 400 HU. Anything less dense than −150 HU (50 − 200) will appear black and anything denser than 250 HU (50 + 200) will appear white (Fig 9.18).

CT scanning exposes a patient to more ionising radiation than does a plain radiograph but provides better spatial and density resolution. Although most patients with chest conditions have a chest X-ray as the first investigation, CT will provide much more diagnostic information. As well as the use of different window settings, varying the thickness of scan slices and the use of intravenous contrast can provide additional information. The data can also be manipulated after acquisition. The technique used

Figure 9.13   Interstitial lung disease.

a

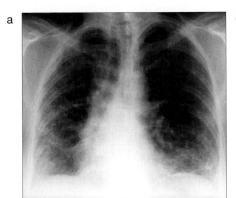

(a) Scleroderma (p 174):
- There is a marked increase in basal reticular markings, with considerable volume loss. When the volume loss is this pronounced, consider fibrosing alveolitis (UIP—usual or classical interstitial pneumonia) and scleroderma as likely diagnoses.

b

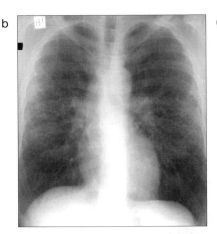

(b) Sarcoidosis (p 97):
- There are multiple small nodules in the mid and upper zones.

c

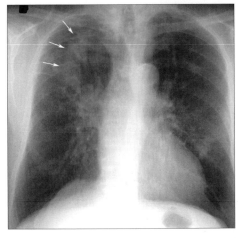

(c) Silicosis:
- There are increased reticular and nodular markings in the mid and upper zones.
- In the right upper lobe, progressive massive fibrosis (arrows) has commenced, giving the typical 'angel wing' configuration.

Figure 9.14   Lingula and middle lobe collapse in an asthmatic patient.

a 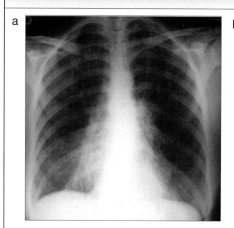 b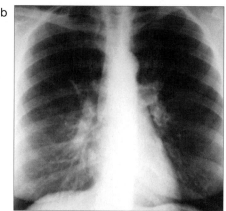

(a)   There is loss of both right and left heart borders and an associated increase in density.
(b)   A progress film shows a return to the normal appearance.

Figure 9.15   Lymphoma.

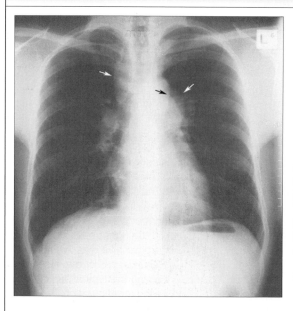

- Widening of the superior mediastinum to both sides (white arrows), suggesting an anterior location. Clear visualisation of the aorta (black arrow) through the mass indicates that the mass is not posterior. There is also enlargement of the right hilum.

Differential diagnosis (the five Ts) of superior (anterior) mediastinal mass
1. Thyroid (retrosternal goitre)
2. Thymoma
3. Teratoma
4. 'Terrible' lymphoma or carcinoma
5. Tortuous vessels, aortic aneurysm

If the mass was posterior, the differential diagnosis would be different:
1. Neurogenic tumour
2. Other tumours, including lymphoma, myeloma, metastases
3. Dilated oesophagus, hiatus hernia (more inferiorly)
4. Aortic aneurysm
5. Lateral thoracic meningocele, particularly in neurofibromatosis
6. Extramedullary haematopoiesis
7. Varices
8. Foregut cyst

Figure 9.16   Miliary tuberculosis.

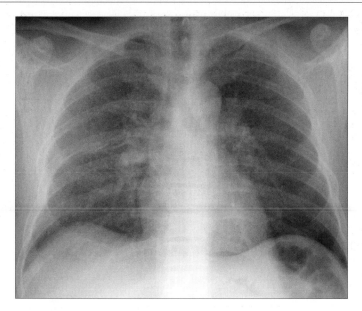

- There are multiple fine discrete nodules of soft tissue density uniformly distributed throughout both lung fields owing to haematological dissemination.
- This condition does not cause miliary calcification.

Figure 9.17   Wegener's granulomatosis.

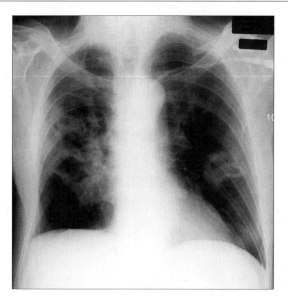

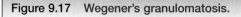

- There are multiple nodules, many of which are cavitated.
- The patient has a central dialysis catheter for associated renal disease.

Figure 9.18 Bronchogenic carcinoma: (a) mediastinal window: (b) lung window.

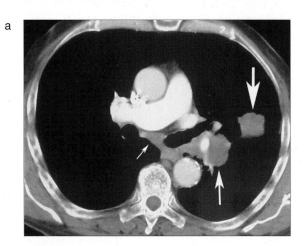

a

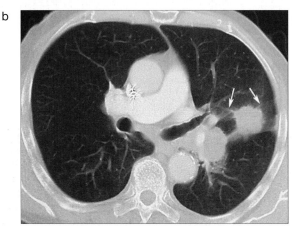

b

(a) The mass is seen as a soft tissue density (large arrow) on the mediastinal window. There are enlarged hilar (medium arrow) and subcarinal (small arrow) nodes.
(b) The irregular margins and radiating strands (arrows) seen on the lung window are features that suggest malignancy. These are not visible in (a).

most often involves improving spatial resolution and perception by edge enhancement. This technique is most useful for lung and bone images.

For chest images there are two commonly used basic CT techniques. The first, and more common, is helical scanning. This involves continuous acquisition of images from the whole chest, using slice thicknesses that vary from 1 mm to 10 mm. This is usually performed with intravenous contrast so that vessels containing moving blood can be distinguished from adjacent masses or pulmonary emboli. This technique is most useful for assessing conditions such as lung collapse, consolidation, masses and emboli. Contrast must be used with caution in patients with an allergic history (including asthma), heart disease, myeloma or renal impairment. It is contraindicated in cases of suspected phaeochromocytoma as it may precipitate a hypertensive crisis.

The second technique is called high-resolution CT (HRCT). This involves a series of slices with thickness of 0.5 mm to 1.0 mm performed at intervals of about 10 mm. This gives the best visualisation of the lung parenchyma. HRCT is therefore useful for the assessment of bronchiectasis (Fig 9.19) (p 77) and diffuse lung disease, such as interstitial fibrosis.

Although it is called high-resolution CT, this type of scan should not be requested in the expectation that it is always superior to ordinary (helical) CT. HRCT does not visualise 90% of the lungs and must not be requested with false expectations.

Interstitial lung disease often causes one of two patterns of disease. The first pattern involves thickening of the peripheral interstitial structures. This typically occurs in fibrosing alveolitis (Fig 9.20) and interstitial disease related to connective tissue disorders and asbestosis.

The second common pattern of disease involves thickening of the bronchovascular (central) interstitium. Sarcoidosis is a common cause of this pattern of disease (Fig 9.21).

A third pattern of disease is less common but produces almost diagnostic images. This is cystic lung disease. A group of rare interstitial lung diseases, Langerhan's cell histiocytosis (LCH—histiocytosis X) and lymphangioleiomyomatosis (LAM) or tuberous sclerosis (very similar to LAM but can occur in males) manifest on HRCT as cystic disease. All look similar at first glance to bronchiectasis or emphysema. Bronchiectasis can usually be diagnosed on serial slices showing dilated airways. Focal areas of emphysema have no visible walls associated with areas of lung destruction.

Figure 9.19 Bronchiectasis (p 77).

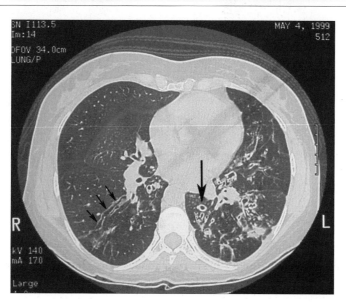

HRCT demonstrates dilated airways, which are seen as rings on axial images. The size of a normal airway should be comparable to that of the adjacent vessel. Significant bronchial dilatation gives the *signet ring* sign of bronchiectasis (large arrow). Bronchi running in the plane of the scan can be seen as non-tapering tubular structures (small arrows).

Figure 9.20   Fibrosing alveolitis.

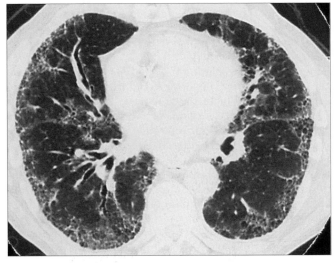

HRCT demonstrates peripheral interstitial thickening that is progressing towards 'honeycombing'.

Figure 9.21   Sarcoidosis (p 97).

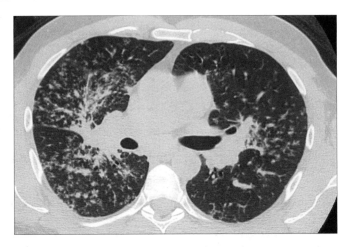

HRCT shows marked thickening of the bronchovascular bundles. Multiple small nodules are also a feature of the disease.

Langerhan's cell histiocytosis and lymphangioleiomyomatosis have cysts surrounded by walls. On HRCT, lymphangioleiomyomatosis shows numerous well-defined, thin-walled cysts. In Langerhan's cell histiocytosis (Fig 9.22), the cysts are unusual in shape and the walls are more irregular. Nodules may be present.

Asbestos exposure causes multiple lung and pleural abnormalities. The character-istic abnormality that suggests asbestos exposure is the pleural plaque. This may be of

Figure 9.22   Histiocytosis.

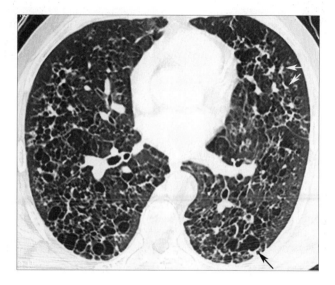

HRCT showing multiple cystic spaces with walls. Some of the cysts are of a bizarre shape and have irregular walls (black arrow). Nodules are also present (white arrows).

soft tissue density or calcified. These patients have an increased risk of bronchogenic carcinoma. Asbestosis produces a pattern of disease similar to that of fibrosing alveolitis (see Fig 9.20). Mesothelioma usually shows a nodular pleural thickening. It may be associated with pleural effusion (Fig 9.23).

CT and abdominal disease

The window most often used in the abdomen is similar to the 'mediastinal windows' used in the chest. That is, a WL of 50 HU and a WW of 400 HU, where anything less dense than −150 HU (50 − 200) will appear black and anything denser than 250 HU (50 + 200) will appear white (Fig 9.24). The skeleton is best appreciated on 'bone windows' with a WL of 800 HU and a WW of 2000 HU (Fig 9.25).

Abdominal CT scans are usually performed after the patient has been given oral and intravenous contrast. In some cases, for example, scans for renal calculi or thalassaemia (Fig 9.25), contrast is not necessary.

Oral contrast is usually given in the form of a 750-mL drink of fluid containing barium or iodine to provide radiodensity. The effect of this is to increase bowel density, especially small bowel density, and to enable it to be distinguished from soft tissue masses. One of the problems of this technique is that it can be difficult to be sure that an apparent soft tissue mass is not unopacified small bowel. This can happen even when bowel preparation has been very careful (Fig 9.26).

Intravenous contrast can be used to differentiate masses from vessels (Fig 9.27).

The timing of scans after intravenous contrast injection can be varied to optimise visualisation of different organs. The earliest contrast scan is the 'arterial' or 'hepatic arterial phase' scan. The scan is usually performed 30–40 seconds after the injection of contrast into a cubital fossa vein. These scans are best for demonstrating lesions that enhance during the 'arterial phase', such as abdominal aortic aneurysms and

Figure 9.23 Mesothelioma.

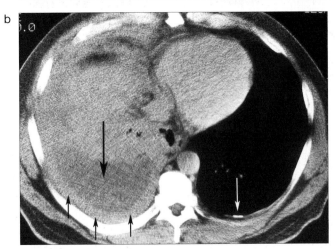

a

b

(a) There is extensive pleural thickening at the level of the aortic arch. Nodularity, thickness of greater than 1 cm, involvement of the mediastinal pleura (arrows) and lung encasement are all features that suggest malignancy. Metastatic adenocarcinoma can produce a similar appearance.

(b) At the lung bases, the tumour (small black arrows) can be differentiated from an associated pleural effusion that is of water density (large black arrow). There is a calcified pleural plaque (white arrow), indicating previous asbestos exposure.

hypervascular islet cell tumours of the pancreas. Liver lesions that have an hepatic arterial supply will appear more dense than the surrounding normal liver parenchyma. These include hepatocellular carcinoma and hypervascular metastases from melanoma and pancreatic islet cell tumours.

The commonest contrast abdominal scan is a 'portal' venous phase' scan. This is usually performed 70 seconds after an injection of contrast into a cubital fossa vein. As its name implies, the intention is to opacify the portal venous system with contrast.

Figure 9.24   Tuberous sclerosis.

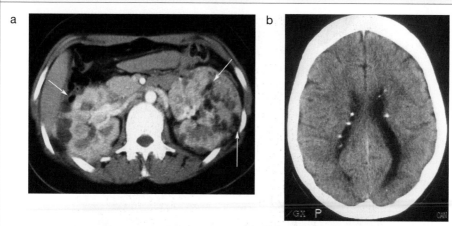

a   b

(a) Contrast-enhanced helical scan of the abdomen. There are multiple masses in each kidney. Some have density measurements of fat (–80 HU), indicating that they are multiple angiomyolipomata. The fat density can be appreciated visually by comparing the renal masses with the subcutaneous and intraperitoneal fat and by appreciating that the density is less than half that of the cerebrospinal fluid (CSF, equals water) within the thecal sac.

(b) The same patient's CT brain scan showing multiple calcified (+300 HU) periventricular tubers.

Figure 9.25   Thalassaemia (p 132).

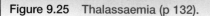

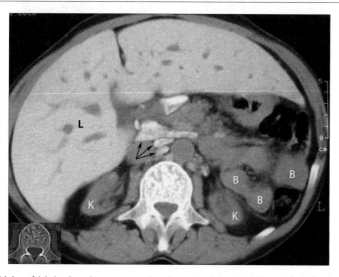

The liver (L) is of high density, suggesting haemosiderosis. A splenectomy has been performed and unopacified bowel (B) fills the splenic bed. There are small end-stage renal failure kidneys (K). High-density retroperitoneal nodes (arrows) are also a feature of the disease. The vertebral bone texture is abnormal. This is best appreciated on the 'bone' windows (insert).

Figure 9.26   Normal bowel scan.

a

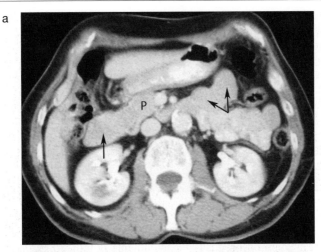

b

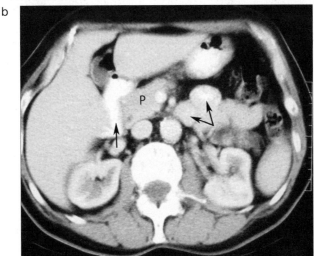

(a) The proximal small bowel (arrows) is not well opacified with contrast. It is difficult to differentiate it from the adjacent head of pancreas (P) and it is not easy to exclude lymphadenopathy in these scans.

(b) After further oral contrast, the normal appearances can be appreciated.

Liver abnormalities that are seen on these scans will appear as lower density lesions within the enhancing liver parenchyma.

The 'triple phase scan' for liver lesions includes a scan without intravenous contrast followed by 'hepatic arterial' and 'portal venous' scans (Fig 9.28).

The other commonly used contrast scan is the delayed scan. This can be performed at a number of different times but is typically taken about 5 minutes after contrast injection. These scans are most often used to assess renal contrast excretion. The collecting systems, ureters and bladder are very dense in these scans in normal people (Fig 9.29).

Figure 9.27   Lymphoma (p 146).

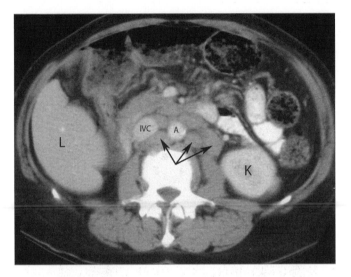

Multiple enlarged lymph nodes (arrows) are readily differentiated from adjacent bowel that contains oral contrast and the aorta (A) and inferior vena cava (IVC), which are opacified by intravenous contrast. The density of the liver (L) and kidney (K) are also increased by intravenous contrast.

Magnetic resonance imaging of the brain and spine

MRI is the modality of choice for most neurological disease. MRI is able to show disease processes more clearly because it provides better anatomical definition and more subtle analysis of signal alteration. MRI does not involve the use of ionising radiation. The main contraindications to its use include the presence of implanted pacemakers, metallic foreign bodies (e.g. old penetrating eye injuries with fragments of metal) and implanted metallic devices. Most prosthetic heart valves, aneurysm clips and joint prostheses implanted over the last 10 years are made of non-magnetic metals and are safe. Scans should not be performed in patients within a month of the implantation of an arterial stent.

Images are produced by examining the properties of nuclei in a strong magnetic field after stimulation by a radiofrequency pulse. In clinical practice, the hydrogen nucleus is almost always used for this purpose. The parameters that are most commonly measured and displayed are T1 and T2. In a T1-weighted scan, water (equals cerebrospinal fluid [CSF]) shows as black (or dark grey) and in a T2-weighted scan, water (CSF) shows as white.

Most diseases of the brain and spinal cord show up as an alteration in both anatomy and signal. Some show predominantly as an anatomical disturbance. These are mainly the developmental disorders and the degenerative diseases. T1-weighted scans are good for demonstrating disturbances in anatomy. Syringomyelia (p 315) is well demonstrated by these scans (Fig 9.30).

Contrast may also be useful. Scans performed after intravenous contrast are normally T1-weighted. A good example of this is MRI of a pituitary adenoma (Fig 9.31).

Most diseases of the brain and spine involve tissue oedema. Water-weighted scans are therefore most sensitive for this. The scans most commonly used for this purpose

Figure 9.28 Hepatocellular carcinoma.

a

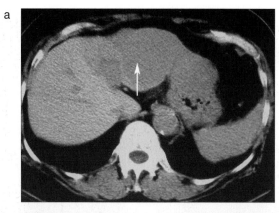

b

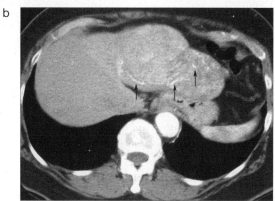

c

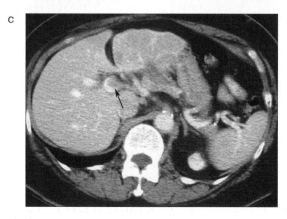

(a) The initial plain scan shows the tumour as a large, low-density lesion (arrow) replacing the left lobe of the liver.

(b) The hepatic arterial scan demonstrates an irregular enhancement pattern with supply by abnormal hepatic arterial branches (arrows).

(c) The late arterial scan, taken a little more inferiorly, again shows the tumour as a low-density lesion within the liver parenchyma. Tumour extension into the portal vein is seen as a filling defect within the early enhancing vein (arrow).

| Figure 9.29 | Retroperitoneal fibrosis secondary to an inflammatory abdominal aortic aneurysm. |

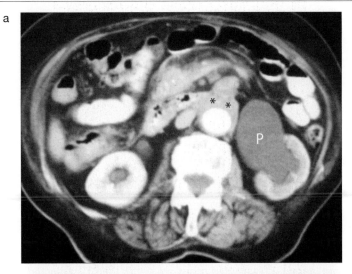

a

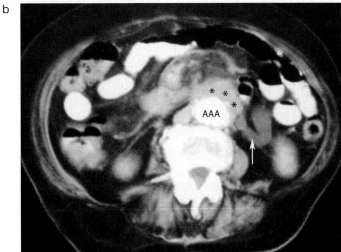

b

(a) There is an abnormal cuff of tissue (asterisks) anterior to the aorta. Both pel-vicalyceal systems are dilated. The changes are much more marked on the left, where the cortex is also less dense because of markedly reduced contrast excretion. The urine in the renal pelvises (P) remained of low density in the 5-minute scan (not shown), indicating a marked delay in contrast excretion.

(b) More inferiorly, the tortuous left ureter (arrow) is pulled medially by the fibrotic tissue (asterisks) anterior to the abdominal aortic aneurysm (AAA).

are T2-weighted (Fig 9.32) and FLAIR (fluid attenuated inversion recovery) (Fig 9.33). FLAIR scans are designed to show free water as dark. Because oedema (water in soft tissues) has different signal characteristics to free water, it will be seen as white on a background where almost everything else is dark. This sequence (like T2-weighted) is good for diseases that cause signal alteration but will make the

---

Figure 9.30   Syringomyelia decompressed by surgery (p 315).

a

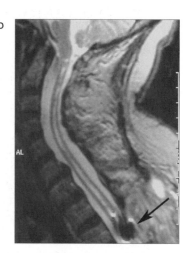

b

(a) T1-weighted scan shows an elongated cavity of water (CSF) intensity within the spinal cord (arrow). T1-weighted scans are better than T2-weighted scans when cord oedema may be confused with syringomyelia.

(b) Corresponding T2-weighted scan. There is metallic artefact from previous surgery (arrow).

Figure 9.31   Pituitary tumour.

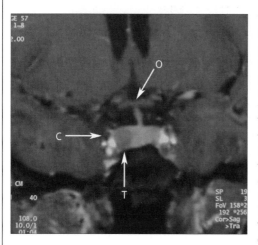

The pituitary tumour (T) shows as a filling defect within the enhancing pituitary gland. The enhancing structures of the cavernous sinus are seen lateral to the gland. The carotid artery (C) is seen as a signal void within the cavernous sinus. The pituitary stalk extends superiorly from the pituitary gland towards the horizontal optic chiasm (O). This tumour measures 7 mm in maximum diameter and is therefore a microadenoma. A macroadenoma has a similar appearance but is larger than 10 mm. Macroadenomas may extend into the adjacent cavernous sinuses, encase the carotid arteries or impinge on the undersurface of the optic chiasm.

Figure 9.32   Multiple sclerosis (p 205).

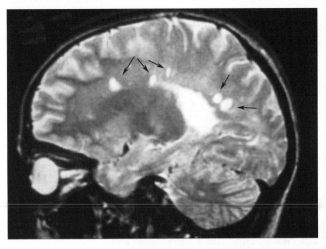

Multiple sclerosis is seen as multiple areas of high signal on T2-weighted scans (arrows). These most commonly lie in the cerebral white matter, particularly in periventricular locations. Foci of demyelination (arrows) are often linear or flame-shaped and oriented at right angles to the ventricular system. Lesions within the corpus callosum are usually caused by demyelination rather than ischaemia.

---

changes even more obvious. The FLAIR scans are a good place to start if you have multiple sheets of film.

The spine is usually well imaged with a combination of sagittal and axial T1- and T2-weighted scans (Fig 9.34).

Imaging and the rheumatology case

From an imaging point of view, arthropathies can be divided into three groups:

1. inflammatory (synovial)
2. chondropathic
3. depositional.

These different disease processes cause characteristic radiological changes. All are associated with erosions of some type. The changes that need to be looked for specifically (and commented upon) include:

1. the site of the erosion
2. the symmetry of the disease
3. bone density
4. periosteal reaction
5. malalignment
6. presence of osteophytes/syndesmophytes.

Inflammatory (synovial) arthropathies

In these patients, the inflammation involves the synovium and the first erosions occur at the joint margins where the synovium inserts into the bare bone adjacent to the hyaline

Figure 9.33 Infarction: (a) FLAIR scan; (b) T2-weighted scan.

a

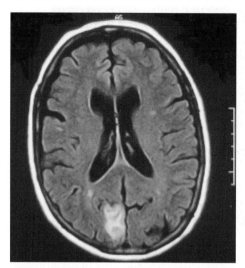

This occipital infarct is more apparent on the (a) FLAIR scan than on the corresponding (b) T2-weighted scan. Small foci of high signal (white) are caused by deep white matter ischaemia. Infarcts typically show straight margins and are often rectangular or triangular in shape.

b

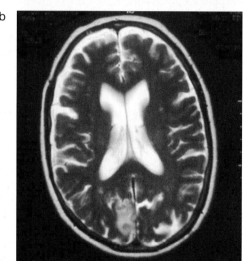

cartilage. These are sometimes called *marginal erosions*. It is very important to know where the synovium (and adjacent joint capsule) insert so that these can be differentiated from the extra-articular erosions that occur with depositional disease (Fig 9.35).

Rheumatoid arthritis is the most common synovial arthropathy seen in examinations and in clinics. It typically involves the metacarpophalangeal (MCP), metatarsophalangeal (MTP) and proximal interphalangeal (PIP) joints of the hands and feet but any joint can be involved. It is a symmetrical arthritis (i.e. involvement in one hand is similar to that in the other). With time, periarticular osteoporosis progresses to generalised osteoporosis; erosions become more extensive and involve all of the joint surface and the joint becomes subluxed or dislocated. There are usually no osteophytes, no periosteal reaction nor ankylosis (Fig 9.36).

Figure 9.34 Disc protrusion.

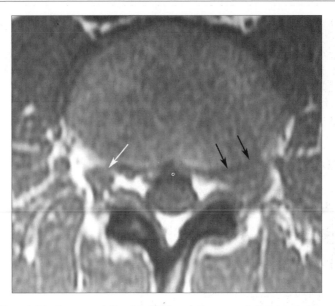

The axial T1-weighted scan at the L3–L4 level shows a left lateral disc protrusion (black arrows) impinging on the L3 nerve root in the neuroforamen. The normal right L3 nerve root is seen (white arrow). Note that a more medial protrusion (a paracentral or posterolateral protrusion) would impinge on the L4 nerve root in the lateral recess.

The seronegative synovial arthropathies (p 280), including psoriatic arthritis, enteropathic arthropathy, ankylosing spondylitis, Reiter's disease and juvenile chronic arthritis, give a different pattern of disease. The erosions are still marginal but involvement is asymmetrical. Large joints and the spine are more typically involved. In the hands and feet, the distal interphalangeal (DIP) joints are most commonly affected. Osteoporosis is not a prominent feature. Periosteal reaction may be present (Fig 9.37) and ankylosis (bony fusion of joints) may be seen in chronic disease (Fig 9.38).

Spinal involvement is more common with the seronegative arthropathies. Sacroiliitis may be seen in most arthropathies. Bilateral symmetrical sacroiliitis occurs in ankylosing spondylitis (p 283), enteropathic arthropathy and hyperparathyroidism. Bilateral asymmetrical sacroiliitis is seen in Reiter's disease, occasionally in severe rheumatoid arthritis and gout. Psoriasis may produce symmetrical or asymmetrical arthritis (Fig 9.39).

Ankylosing spondylitis will often progress to complete fusion of the sacroiliac joints. Bridging syndesmophytes in the spine will result in varying degrees of spinal fusion (Fig 9.40).

Rheumatoid arthritis does not usually cause ankylosis in the spine (or elsewhere). An important spinal abnormality caused by rheumatoid arthritis is atlanto–axial instability, which is a result of disease involving the odontoid peg and adjacent ligaments. Lateral views of the cervical spine in flexion and extension will demonstrate this complication (Fig 9.41).

Figure 9.35   Acute rheumatoid arthritis (p 159).

a

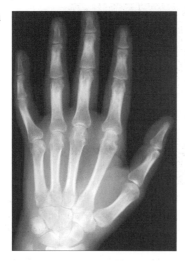

b

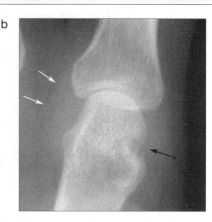

(a)   There is generalised periarticular osteoporosis (marked reduction in bone density adjacent to the joints). This pattern is typical of acute inflammatory arthroses and particularly of rheumatoid arthritis.

(b)   The magnified view of the second metacarpophalangeal joint shows capsular distension (white arrows) owing to synovial thickening and a joint effusion. There is an erosion (black arrow) at the joint margin. This is a typical site for an inflammatory arthrosis.

Figure 9.36   Chronic rheumatoid arthritis.

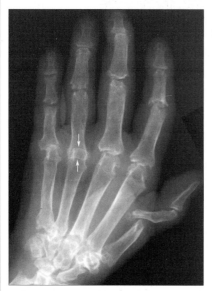

There is generalised osteoporosis. Note on this film the thinness of the cortices of the shafts and the relative prominence of the soft tissues. These are characteristic changes of osteoporosis. Extensive erosive changes involve all the joints in this X-ray. There is dislocation of the first MCP joint. The fourth MCP joint is also dislocated with overlap of the articular surfaces (arrows) on the AP film. The fifth MCP joint is subluxated.

Figure 9.37   Reiter's disease.

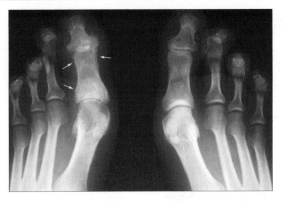

There is asymmetrical disease involving the left great toe. The right foot appears normal. Erosive changes are seen in the DIP joint. Irregular periosteal reaction is seen along the shaft of the proximal phalanx (arrows). The bone density is normal. These are all features of a seronegative synovial arthropathy.

Figure 9.38   Psoriatic arthropathy.

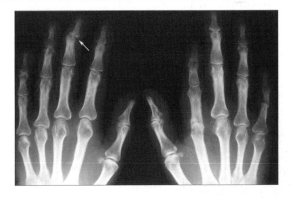

The bone density is normal. Erosive change is seen in the left third DIP joint, which is subluxated (arrow). There is ankylosis of the second MCP, PIP and DIP joints of the right hand, in keeping with chronic disease. Again, these are all features of a seronegative arthritis.

Chondropathic arthropathies

These arthropathies result from abnormalities of the articular cartilage. As a result, erosions tend to be subchondral rather than marginal. Subchondral sclerosis may be present and osteophytes may form on the joint margins. The bone density is normal. Periosteal reaction and ankylosis are not typical features.

The cartilage abnormality may be 'degenerative' in conditions such as osteoarthritis (Figs 9.42, 9.43), or occur as a result of damage in neuropathic joints or haemophilia (Fig 9.44). In these conditions involvement is more marked in the load-bearing joints.

Figure 9.39   Psoriasis with bilateral asymmetrical sacroiliitis.

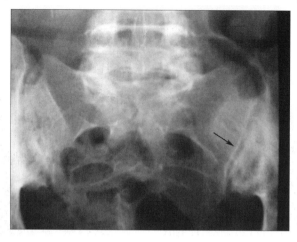

Extensive erosive change is seen in the sacroiliac (SI) joints. The joint margins are poorly defined and there is adjacent lysis and sclerosis (increased bone density). The ilium is more involved than the sacrum. (This is the usual pattern of the disease.) The right SI joint is more affected than the left. A more normal section of the left SI joint shows as a dark band with thin white margins (arrow).

Figure 9.40   Chronic ankylosing spondylitis (p 283).

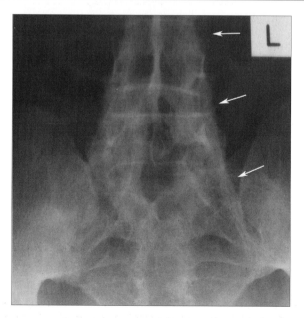

There is bony fusion of the sacroiliac joints. Syndesmophytes are fusing the L4, L5 and S1 vertebrae (arrows).

Figure 9.41   Rheumatoid arthritis with atlanto-axial instability.

a   b

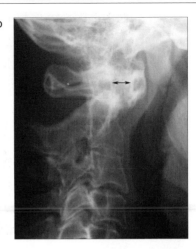

(a) Lateral film in neutral position. The distance from the anterior aspect of the peg to the atlas appears slightly widened beyond the normal upper limit of 2 mm.
(b) Lateral film in extension. There is clear widening of the atlanto-axial space to 7 mm (arrow).

Figure 9.42   Osteoarthritis of the right hip.

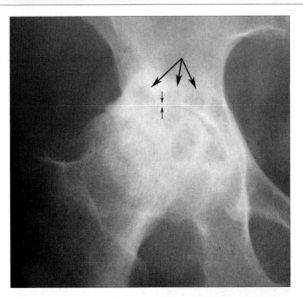

There is marked joint space narrowing (small arrows) indicating loss of cartilage. Subchondral sclerosis is present. The 'erosions' (large arrows) lie beneath the cartilage, not in marginal locations. These are often called *synovial cysts*, *subchondral cysts* or *geodes*. There are osteophytes on the joint margins, most obvious superolaterally.

Figure 9.43 Osteoarthritis.

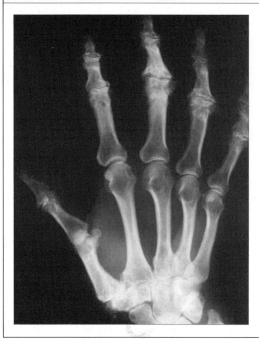

Joint space narrowing, subchondral sclerosis and marginal osteophytes are seen in the first metacarpo-phalangeal (MCP) joint and in many of the interphalangeal (IP) joints. There are subchondral erosive changes, most obvious in the third PIP joint, typical of 'erosive osteoarthritis'. The marginal osteophytes on the IP joints correspond to Heberden's and Bouchard's nodes.

Figure 9.44 Haemophilia.

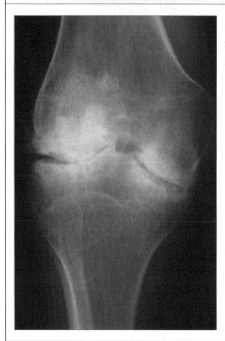

There is diffuse joint space narrowing and subchondral sclerosis. Small osteophytes are seen at the joint margins. There are numerous small subchondral cysts. The changes are essentially those of osteoarthritis, although an underlying cause should be suspected in this 23-year-old man. Haemophilia most often affects the large hinge joints (knee, ankle and elbow).

In the hands, the DIP joints and the first carpometacarpal (CMC) joints are most often involved.

The chondropathic arthropathies may also be caused by metabolic conditions that result in deposition of calcium in hyaline cartilage (chondrocalcinosis). These conditions include calcium pyrophosphate deposition disease (CPPD), hyperparathyroidism, Wilson's disease, acromegaly (p 272), haemochromatosis (p 128) and alkaptonuria. The changes are similar to those seen in the degenerative conditions but the sites are different. For example, in degenerative osteoarthritis, the most commonly affected joint surface in the knee is the medial compartment (the primary weight-bearing surface). In CPPD, one may see advanced arthropathy of the patellofemoral joint with little change in the medial or lateral compartments (Fig 9.45). Although chondrocalcinosis may be a feature of gouty arthritis, this condition is considered separately as a depositional arthropathy.

Figure 9.45   Calcium pyrophosphate deposition disease (CPPD).

a

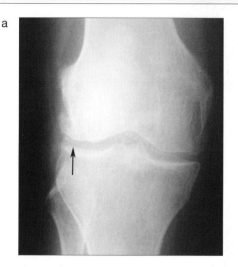

b

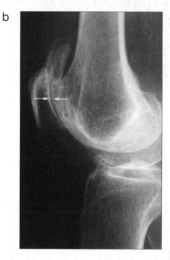

(a) AP view. The medial and lateral compartment joint spaces are preserved. There is chondrocalcinosis in both compartments but it is most obvious laterally (arrow).

(b) Lateral view. The patellofemoral joint space is diffusely narrowed (arrows) and prominent osteophytes project from the upper pole of the patella.

Depositional arthropathies

The hallmark of the depositional arthropathies is the soft tissue mass that may not always be visible on plain films. Erosions occur in association with these deposits. The erosions may therefore be articular or extra-articular in location. The presence of extra-articular erosions is very suggestive of a depositional arthropathy. The bone density is normal. Ankylosis and periosteal reaction are not features. Gout is a typical example (Fig 9.46).

Amyloid and reticulo-histiocytosis (a rare destructive polyarthritis, often involving the DIP joints and associated with cutaneous nodules) are also causes of depositional

Figure 9.46   Gout.

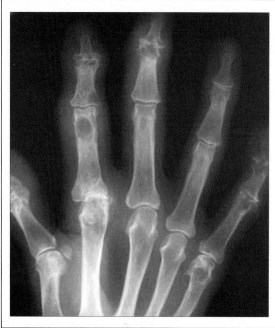

There is a soft tissue mass adjacent to the second PIP joint. There are multiple well-defined (*punched out*) erosions. Many are associated with joints. There is also, however, a clear extrasynovial erosion in the shaft of the second metacarpal. The bone density is normal.

arthropathy. Note that rheumatoid arthritis can cause soft tissue nodules but the location of erosions and the presence of osteoporosis makes this easy to distinguish from depositional arthropathy.

Further reading

You will find it very good practice always to verify your references, sir.

Martin Ruth (1755–1854)

Candidates for any medical examination must read widely. This particularly applies to the postgraduate candidate who wishes to pass both the written and oral tests. It is very important to spend plenty of time on your weak areas, where you have had the least clinical experience.

We have listed below some of the texts that may be useful to candidates. The sections are divided into two parts where applicable. Concise textbooks refer to books that are particularly useful to undergraduates but do have some relevant material for postgraduate students of internal medicine. Specialist textbooks refer to texts that are of particular relevance to postgraduates, although undergraduates may also find them useful. For further suggestions, see the recommendations from the American College of Physicians entitled 'A Library for Internists' published every 3 years in the *Annals of Internal Medicine*. Although it is unlikely that even the hardest-working candidates will read all these books, we believe reference to some of them will be invaluable.

General texts

Concise textbook

Tierney LM et al (eds) 2005 Current medical diagnosis and treatment. Lange, Norwalk.

Specialist textbooks

American College of Physicians 2005 Medical knowledge self assessment program. ACP, Philadelphia. Online. Available: http://www.acponline.org.

Goldman L et al (eds) 2004 Cecil textbook of medicine, 22nd edn. Saunders, Philadelphia.

Kasper DL et al (eds) 2005 Harrison's principles of internal medicine, 16th edn. McGraw-Hill, New York.

Talley NJ, Frankum B, Currow D 2000 Internal medicine: the essential facts, 2nd edn. MacLennan & Petty, Sydney.

Wiener CM et al (eds) 2005 Harrison's principles of internal medicine. Self-assessment and board review. Pretest self-assessment and review. McGraw-Hill, New York.

Aids to physical examination
Concise textbooks

Afzal Mir M 2003 Atlas of clinical diagnosis, 2nd edn. Saunders, Edinburgh.
McDonald FS et al (eds) 2004 Mayo Clinic images in internal medicine: self-assessment for board exam review. CRC Press, Boca Raton.
McGee S 2001 Evidence based physical diagnosis. Saunders, Philadelphia.
Springhouse (ed.) 2002 Auscultation skills: breath and heart sounds (book with 2 audio CD-ROMs). Lippincott, Williams & Wilkins, Baltimore.
Talley NJ, O'Connor S 2006 Clinical examination: a systematic guide to physical diagnosis, 5th edn. Elsevier, Sydney.
Zatouroff M 1996 Physical signs in general medicine, 2nd edn. Wolfe, London. (*Note*: Useful colour guide.)

Subspecialty texts
Cardiology

Specialist textbook
Braunwald E et al (ed.) 2004 Heart disease: a textbook of cardiovascular medicine, 7th edn. WB Saunders, Philadelphia.

Respiratory

Concise textbook
Fishman A, Elias J 2002 Fishman's manual of pulmonary diseases and disorders, 3rd edn. McGraw-Hill, San Juan.

Specialist textbook
Fraser RS et al 2005 Synopsis of diseases of the chest. Elsevier/Saunders, Sydney.

Gastroenterology and liver disease

Concise textbook
Talley NJ, Martin CJ (eds) 2006 Clinical gastroenterology: a practical problem-based approach, 2nd edn. Saunders, Sydney.

Specialist textbooks
Feldman M et al 2005 Sleisenger & Fordtran's gastrointestinal disease, 8th edn. Saunders, Philadelphia.
Friedman SL et al (eds) 2002. Current diagnosis and treatment in gastroenterology, 2nd edn. Lange, Norwalk.

Haematology

Concise textbook
Hoffbrand V, Moss P, Pettit JE 2001 Essential haematology, 4th edn. Blackwell, Oxford.

Specialist textbook
Jandl J 2003 Blood: a textbook of hematology, 3rd edn. Little Brown, Boston.

Rheumatology and immunology

Concise textbooks
Goldsby RA et al 2002 Immunology, 5th edn. WH Freeman, New York.
Imboden JB et al (eds) 2004 Current rheumatology diagnosis and treatment. Lange, Norwalk.

Specialist textbooks

Hochberg MC et al 2003 Rheumatology, 3rd edn. Mosby, St Louis.

Hunter GG 2003 Atlas of rheumatology. Lippincott, Williams & Wilkins, Baltimore.

Klippel JH 2001 Primer on the rheumatic diseases, 12th edn. Arthritis Foundation, Atlanta, GA.

Neurology

Concise textbooks

Fuller G 2004 Neurological examination made easy, 3rd edn. Churchill Livingstone, Edinburgh.

Greenberg DA et al 2002 Clinical neurology, 5th edn. Lange, Los Altos, CA.

Weiner HL, Levitt LP 2004 Neurology for the house officer, 5th edn. Williams & Wilkins, Baltimore. (*Note*: A practical approach to neurology is succinctly outlined, making this a valuable book.)

Specialist textbooks

Donaghy M 2001 Brain's diseases of the nervous system, 11th edn. Oxford University Press, Oxford.

Medical Research Council 1997 Memorandum no. 45. Aids to examination of the peripheral nervous system. Her Majesty's Stationery Office, London. (*Note*: Very clear photographs and illustrations make this an invaluable reference book.)

Patten J 1996 Neurological differential diagnoses—an illustrated approach, 2nd edn. Harold Starke, London. (*Note*: Refer to this book for the clear, useful illustrations.)

Rowland LP (ed.) 2000 Merritt's textbook of clinical neurology, 10th edn. Williams & Wilkins, Baltimore.

Renal disease

Specialist textbook

Johnson R et al 2003 Comprehensive clinical nephrology, 2nd edn. Mosby, St Louis.

Endocrinology

Concise textbook

Larsen PR et al 2002 William's textbook of endocrinology, 10th edn. Saunders, Philadelphia.

Specialist textbook

DeGroot LJ (ed.) 2001 Endocrinology, 4th edn. Saunders, Philadelphia.

Dermatology

Concise textbook

Wolff K et al (eds) 2005 Fitzpatrick's color atlas and synopsis of clinical dermatology. McGraw-Hill, New York.

Pharmacology

Concise textbook

Katzung BG 2003 Basic and clinical pharmacology, 8th edn. Lange, Norwalk.

Specialist textbook

Hardman JG et al (eds) 2001 Goodman and Gilman's pharmacological basis of therapeutics, 10th edn. McGraw-Hill, New York. (*Note*: Still the leading text.)

Radiology

Concise textbook

Hughes J 2000 Radiology for the MRCP. Churchill Livingstone, Edinburgh.

Infectious diseases

Specialist textbook

Mandell GL et al (eds) 2004 Principles and practice of infectious diseases, 6th edn. Churchill Livingstone, New York.

Journals

All postgraduate candidates must read the journals because textbooks are always somewhat out of date by the time they are published.

The following journals are specifically recommended by the Royal Australasian College of Physicians:

1. *Lancet*
2. *New England Journal of Medicine*
3. *British Medical Journal*
4. *Annals of Internal Medicine*
5. *Internal Medicine Journal*
6. *American Journal of Medicine*

Note: The excellent review articles and editorials should be studied. *The Medical Journal of Australia* is also worth a look. The consensus statements on management produced by the specialist societies are also most useful. Topics often crop up from these articles, particularly those published in the 3 years or so prior to the setting of the multiple-choice questions.

Index

non-Hodgkin's lymphoma 146–7, 148, 149, 150–2, 158
nystagmus 206, 213, 284, 286, 287, 293, 319, 320

O
oedema 248–9
one-and-a-half syndrome 287, 293
optic atrophy 185, 266, 268, 270, 273, 284, 287, 309, 314
optic neuropathy 291
Osler's nodes 41, 227, 228
osteoporosis (and osteomalacia) 177–82
ostium primum 242, 244
ostium secundum 242–4

P
Paget's disease of the bone 179, 180, 184–7, 272, 273, 283
panhypopituitarism 267–9
papillitis 206, 290
papilloedema 98, 185, 247, 264, 270, 273, 287
Parinaud's syndrome 288, 293
Parkinson's disease 318, 321–2
patent ductus arteriosus 229, 230, 231, 233, 244
Pemberton's sign 250, 252, 265, 266
peptic ulceration 108–10
peripheral neuropathy 307–9
Phalen's wrist flexion test 267, 272, 280
pleural effusion 80, 252, 253, 258
pneumothorax 81, 83, 101, 102, 253
pituitary tumour 268, 270, 289, 350
POEMS syndrome 155
polyarteritis nodosa (PAN) 89, 90, 170, 171, 172
polycystic kidneys 142, 143, 197, 202, 258, 260
polycythaemia 80, 84, 141–5, 245, 246, 247
polycythaemia rubra vera 125, 141, 142, 143–4, 247, 262
portal hypertension 125, 126–7
pregnancy and diabetes 196
primary biliary cirrhosis 99, 122, 123, 124, 132, 178, 257, 259
prophylaxis 85, 141, 151, 157
  antibiotic 41, 46, 77, 237
  for endocarditis 45–6
  for rheumatic fever 41, 45–6
pseudogout 182, 183, 199, 261, 272, 273, 280
ptosis 251, 258, 283, 284, 286, 287, 291, 317
pulmonary fibrosis 88–91
pulmonary hypertension 91–6
pulmonary stenosis 52, 227, 228, 231, 233, 241, 325, 330
pyrexia of unknown origin (PUO) 45, 215–18

R
radiotherapy 149–50
Raynaud's phenomenon 159, 166, 168, 169, 172, 174–5, 176
reflux nephropathy 197, 199
renal masses 143, 246, 260, 345
renal system 196–205
renal transplantation 41, 196, 204–5
respiratory examination 87, 106, 249–54, 288
respiratory system 77–108, 183, 217, 249–54
revascularisation 38–41
rheumatoid arthritis 159–64, 353–4
rheumatology 159–77, 351, 362–3
Riedel's thyroiditis 268
Rinné's test 285, 295
Romberg's sign 318
Roth's spots 41, 217, 230

S
sarcoidosis 90–1, 97–100
scleroderma *see* systemic sclerosis
seroconversion illness 218, 219
shoulder girdle examination 301, 302, 304
Shy-Drager syndrome 88, 322
sickle cell anaemia 133–4
Sjögren's syndrome 159, 161, 162, 164, 173, 206, 308
sleep apnoea 86–8
smoking 47, 59, 79, 83, 86
speech 298–9, 300–1
spinal cord lesions 312–17
splenomegaly 262
splinter haemorrhages 228, 227
Steele-Richardson-Olszewski syndrome 293
superior vena caval obstruction 80, 228, 249, 265
supranuclear palsy 293
syringomyelia 287, 288, 303, 311, 313, 315
systemic lupus erythematosus (SLE) 45, 132, 159, 164–70, 206, 215
systemic sclerosis 52, 79, 80, 157, 167, 168, 173, 174–7
systemic vasculitis 170–3
systolic click–murmur syndrome *see* mitral valve prolapse (systolic click–murmur syndrome)

T
tetralogy of Fallot 245, 246, 325, 328, 330
thrombophilia 138–41
thyroid gland 249, 265–7, 272, 273
thyrotoxicosis 76, 251, 266, 267
training requirements 1–4
transient ischaemic attacks and 'funny turns' 142, 212–15
transoesophageal echocardiography 41, 42, 43, 92, 214
tricuspid regurgitation 240–1
Trousseau's sign 265, 266